Nursing for Continence

SECOND EDITION

Editor
Christine Norton
MA, RGN

Clinical Nurse Specialist (Continence),
St Mark's Hospital, Harrow, Middlesex, UK

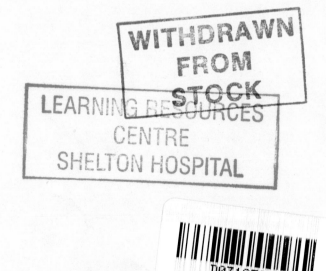

BEACONSFIELD PUBLISHERS LTD

First published in 1996
Reprinted 1998

This edited work © Christine S. Norton 1996
Individual chapters © as credited 1996

British Library Cataloguing in Publication Data
Nursing for Continence. - 2 Rev.ed
  I. Norton, Christine
  610.7369

ISBN 0–906584–42–6

Illustrations by Barbara Hyams and Jenny Valentine.
Phototypeset by Gem Graphics, Trenance, Mawgan Porth, Cornwall in 10 on 12 point Times.
Printed and bound by Biddles Ltd, Guildford and King's Lynn, UK.

Preface

Continence is a human skill basic to living in a complex social environment. Helping people to achieve continence or manage incontinence is a core nursing skill, which all nurses will need at some point, and which many will use on a daily basis. I use the word 'skill' deliberately – this is not just a matter of common sense and TLC. There is today a growing body of research evidence and specialist consensus on which to base clinical practice, and this is an area of care where the use of skilled nursing can have a tremendous impact on each individual patient. The knowledgeable and skilled nurse has many tools with which to promote continence.

This book is written primarily for trained nurses working in clinical settings with patients who are, or who are at risk of becoming, incontinent. This includes district nurses, health visitors, midwives, practice nurses, specialists in elderly care, disability, psychiatry and learning disability, as well as those working in nursing homes or acute care – indeed almost any acute or community setting that can be imagined. It should also be of interest to nurse teachers at the basic and post-basic level, to nurse learners wishing to pursue the topic in greater detail, and to nurse managers wishing to support their clinical colleagues in improving this aspect of care. Continence advisers may find it a useful starting point in acquiring the more in-depth knowledge needed by a clinical nurse specialist. It should also be of interest to other professionals working with incontinent people – hospital and community doctors, physiotherapists, occupational therapists, social workers and pharmacists.

Much has changed since the publication of the first edition of *Nursing for Continence* a decade ago. Continence services have developed throughout the UK, and are an established and valued part of the National Health Service. The Department of Health has identified continence as a priority area, and much investment has gone into research and service development. Major initiatives in public awareness have meant that more and more people seek help for continence problems.

This second edition builds on the success of the first, keeping essentially the same format and style, aiming to be an accessible and practical book rather than an academic literature review. The content is

iii

research-based, where research evidence is available (which remains far from always the case); where no valid research evidence exists, the opinions of expert practitioners are used. This has been achieved by recruiting the UK's leading nurse specialists to revise and update individual chapters from the first edition.

We have not attempted to make this book exhaustively comprehensive. We concentrate on describing nursing interventions in some detail, and while the contribution of other team members is mentioned, the interested reader will need to follow up the references and further reading at the end of each chapter and the books listed in Appendix 4 for more detail.

For simplicity we generally refer to the nurse as 'she' and the patient as 'he' (except when describing specifically female problems). Where continence products are mentioned we have generally described a principle, rather than naming a brand, except where a product is unique or tends to be difficult to locate.

Thanks are due to many people. First and foremost to the chapter editors, who were given the difficult task of using a style not their own, and who have been more than patient in awaiting the finished result. To Lesley Irvine and Val Bayliss, who provided a constructive analysis of the first edition in the early planning stages of the second; to Angela Shepherd, Ros Waldron and Dawn Wilson, who reviewed drafts of the manuscript; to Jo Laycock, who contributed her pelvic floor expertise; to Barbara Hyams and to Jenny Valentine for their beautiful and sympathetic illustrations; to Barbara Haydon for secretarial support; and as always to John Churchill, for being such an imaginative and supportive publisher. It has been a great pleasure and privilege to work with so many enthusiastic and committed people in producing this book which will, I hope, inform and inspire all those who read it to genuinely 'nurse for continence'.

Christine Norton

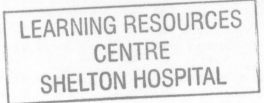

Contents

Contents

Contents

Contents

Contents

Chapter 1

Introduction to Incontinence

Christine Norton, MA, RGN

Clinical Nurse Specialist (Continence),
St Mark's Hospital, Harrow, Middlesex

Incontinence is an unpleasant and distressing symptom. Those affected often feel embarrassed, ashamed and alone. Many incontinent people hide their problem from society, from their family and friends, from health professionals, even from themselves. From the playground to the continuing care facility, incontinence attracts ridicule and blame, the incontinent person is often ostracised and avoided. Health care professionals may see only a small part of the misery and distress that accompany incontinence.

Many health care professionals lack in-depth knowledge about the causes and management of incontinence and passively accept the symptom in people who come into their care. Incontinence is often regarded as an inevitable condition, rather than as a symptom of an underlying disorder. It has been largely ignored as a research topic until recently, and there are still insufficient clinics or resources to help incontinent people. Reluctant to seek assistance, many incontinent people attempt to cope alone or with the help of long-suffering relatives.

There have been many positive advances in recent years. Both the public and professionals are talking more about the subject. It is now being discussed in the media, articles in women's magazines and in occasional television and radio programmes. Retail pharmacists may display incontinence products rather than hiding them under the counter. Most areas of the UK have at least one continence adviser in post. Study days, seminars and courses are becoming widespread. Incontinence is coming to be seen as a 'respectable' symptom, and in spite of a feeling of shame, more people are seeking help. It is evident that in many instances incontinence will respond to appropriate treatment and can often be cured completely. Hundreds of research papers from all parts of the world are submitted to the International Continence Society's annual conference, with evidence of an ever-increasing range of successful treatment options. Where cure is not attained, good management can enable the incontinent person to live a 'normal' life. To be incontinent should not mean inevitable and irreversible discomfort and embarrassment.

At one time incontinence was seen largely as a nursing problem, with nurses providing 'custodial' care to keep the patient as clean and comfortable as possible and to prevent the development of pressure sores. Nurses can now approach incontinence with a much more positive attitude than in the days when the only equipment available was a mop and an underpad, and 'regular toileting' was the only regime thought suitable. There is now a wide range of nursing interventions and equipment available, although not yet universally known or used. While there is still a long way to go, nurses are now in a position to see incontinence as a nursing challenge rather than as a problem to be tolerated. They are also often ideally placed to empower their patients to seek appropriate help from other health or social care professionals.

Nurses are not alone in acknowledging that incontinence is a symptom requiring investigation and treatment. Many other professions are developing their own specialist skills for helping. This book aims to highlight the role of the nurse within the context of a multidisciplinary team approach to incontinence.

WHAT IS INCONTINENCE?

All nurses deal with incontinence at some time in their career, and recognise only too well the wet bed, the puddle on the floor, and the tell-tale odour. Some nurses deal with incontinence many times each day. Yet how many could offer a clear definition of the term? 'Continence' is not an absolute concept. We all have to pass urine and faeces. Incontinence is not to do with the fact of excretion, but with its location and timing. Continence very much depends on society's rules for acceptable excretory behaviour. Those who cannot or will not abide by these rules are thereby defined as 'incontinent'. This will obviously vary between cultures and over time.

At the simplest level, continence is passing urine and faeces only in a socially accepted place, and incontinence is doing so in the 'wrong' place. The rules are often quite arbitrary. The person who parks his car in a lay-by at night and relieves himself behind a tree is not normally classed as incontinent, because this is an accepted practice. To do the same in broad daylight in a crowded street behind a lamppost invites at best public censure, at worst arrest and criminal proceedings. If urine or faeces are passed in the wrong place, whether into clothing, in bed or onto the ground, or into the wrong receptacle, this will usually be called 'incontinence'.

Some definitions note the fact that incontinence is 'involuntary' – the individual cannot help it. The distinction between voluntary and involuntary excretion in the wrong place is largely academic and the results are similar. The International Continence Society takes the definition a step further and defines urinary incontinence as 'involuntary loss of urine which is objectively demonstrable and a social or hygienic problem' (Anderson et al., 1988). This emphasises that the results of the event should be considered. Incontinence is the state where passing urine in the 'wrong' place has become a problem (whether to the individual or those around him). This may vary between people and circumstances.

What amounts to a problem for one person may be ignored by another. No absolute values can be given for the volume or frequency of loss that will constitute 'incontinence' for any individual (although a consistent definition is necessary for research purposes and should always be stated explicitly for a research study).

The general public's interpretation of the term 'incontinence' is often different from the medically accepted usage, if indeed the term is understood at all. Many people would only use the term to describe total lack of control. Often it is used pejoratively to reflect on the character or self-control of the incontinent person – misunderstandings between professional and patient can easily arise because of this. The individual who denies he is incontinent may admit to 'wetting', 'soiling' or 'leaking'.

It is important to recognise that incontinence is a symptom, not a diagnosis. It gives an indication that something has impaired the individual's ability to comply with societal norms, but of itself does not constitute an explanation, nor give a clear indication of what the cause is, or what can be done about it. Later chapters of this book explore in detail the causes, assessment and treatment of urinary and faecal incontinence.

Incontinence can have widespread ramifications for the individual, for family and friends, and for society. Some cope reasonably well with little apparent disruption of lifestyle. Others experience anxiety, embarrassment, sexual difficulties, impaired social and mental well-being and are unwilling to undertake a wide range of activities (Norton, 1982; Wyman,1987; Norton et al., 1988). The degree of problems experienced does not necessarily correlate with the actual volume of incontinence. Hunskaar and Vinsnes (1991) have found that while incontinence has an adverse effect upon quality of life, the extent depends on the type of incontinence and age. For those who cope less well it can become the dominant factor in their life. For a few it can tip the balance between living independently and needing residential care. Those close to an incontinent person, whether relatives, friends or professional carers, are usually also affected. On occasion the relationship may be reduced to an endless round of washing and changing, which can become an intolerable burden.

The costs of incontinence to the country as a whole are vast. The health and social services spend huge amounts on the problem. Incontinence products alone were estimated to cost the National Health Service £56 million in 1991 (CEST, 1991), and this takes no account of services (such as home help, laundry, residential care), prolonged hospital stay, and possibly the most neglected item – nursing time and morale. In both hospital and community far too many nurses spend much of their time and energy dealing with the results rather than actively treating incontinence. Estimates in the United States have suggested that urinary incontinence may account for up to 2% of the health care budget (Hu, 1990).

WHO IS INCONTINENT?

It is commonly supposed that incontinence is a problem exclusive to older people. A common image is of a confused, dependent, elderly woman, usually in long-stay care. People with physical or mental disabilities, and possibly a child who wets the bed, may also come to mind. It is only recently that the public and professionals have started to realise that incontinence can affect almost anyone. Far from being a problem confined to elderly or disabled people, it is common at all ages. Prevalence does increase with age and disability, but the majority of incontinent people are neither elderly nor disabled. Most live at home and lead otherwise 'normal' lives, with incontinence being their major or only health care problem.

Evidence about who suffers from incontinence remains patchy and inconclusive. Table 1.1 shows the results obtained from a large-scale prevalence study based on over 18,000 replies to a postal questionnaire conducted in several locations and in both community and institutional settings in the UK (Thomas et al., 1980). The definition of 'regular' incontinence was 'involuntary excretion or leakage of urine

Table 1.1   Prevalence of 'Regular' Urinary Incontinence

SEX	AGE 15–64 years	65 years +
Male	1.6%	6.9%
Female	8.5%	11.6%

('Regular' = twice or more per month) (Thomas et al., 1980)

in inappropriate places or at inappropriate times twice or more a month, regardless of the quantity of urine lost'. The table shows that in those under 65 years of age, urinary incontinence was far more common in women, but that this difference tended to equalise in the older age-groups. In addition, nearly twice as many people reported 'occasional' urinary incontinence occurring less than twice per month.

Overall, Thomas found that 72.4% of women and 89.2% of men said they were *never* incontinent of urine, i.e. one in four women and one in ten men had some incontinence. For around 5% of the total population this was 'regular'.

In the same study, a figure was obtained for 'recognised' incontinence by asking the health, social, and voluntary services in the same areas to identify people they knew to be incontinent. Table 1.2 shows the results. By comparing this with Table 1.1 it is obvious that only a tiny proportion of those with incontinence were presenting for professional help. Of those people with recognised incontinence, one half of the total were resident in long-stay institutions, so the vast majority of incontinent people outside long-stay care were unknown to the health and social services. In total, 10% of people with urinary incontinence were in touch with statutory services.

Of the total number of people in the questionnaire reporting incontinence, 22% were judged to have a moderate or severe problem, involving extra laundry or expenses, use of pads, some restriction of

Table 1.2   Prevalence of 'Recognised' Urinary Incontinence

SEX	AGE 15–64 years	65 years +
Male	0.1%	1.3%
Female	0.2%	2.5%

('Recognised' = known to be incontinent by health, social, or voluntary services) (Thomas et al., 1980)

activities, and possibly requiring help from others. Of those with a moderate or severe problem, less than one-third were receiving help from health or social services for incontinence.

Extrapolations from these results suggest that between two and three million people in the UK may be incontinent of urine at least twice a month. Care should be taken not to assume that all these people see their incontinence as a problem. Over three quarters of this total had only minimal or slight incontinence, which may or may not be seen as a problem depending on the characteristics of each individual.

Although this study is now quite old, it remains the most comprehensive survey in the UK. Other studies have found different results. For example Wolin (1969), by asking young nurses who had never had a baby if they had *ever* experienced involuntary leakage, found that 51% had at some time in their life. Jolleys (1988) found that 41% of women have some incontinence, although for 70% of them it is damp pants only. One quarter delay seeking help for more than five years after symptoms have become troublesome (Norton et al., 1988). Mohide (1992) and Williams et al. (1995) have provided reviews of prevalence studies. They highlight the difficulty of attempting to compare studies using different definitions of incontinence.

Brocklehurst (1993), in a survey of 4007 adults over 30 years old, living in their own homes, found that 14% of women and 6.6% of men admit to having had 'bladder problems' such as leaking or damp pants at some time, and for 7.5% of women and 2.8% of men this was within the previous two months. Over half (61%) had had the problem for over four years. Over half had seen their doctor about the bladder problem (as compared to the 10% found by Thomas a decade earlier, which may indicate a substantial change in reaction to incontinence). In addition, the results emphasise the danger of assuming that everybody who leaks urine sees it as a problem. Only sixty per cent said that they were concerned or worried about their incontinence and 34% that it affected their lifestyle considerably.

Figures for childhood incontinence are given in chapter 5. Nocturnal enuresis (bedwetting) affects one to two adults in every hundred over 15 years old (Pierce, 1980; Rutter, 1973).

Faecal incontinence is less common than urinary incontinence. About one adult in two hundred living in the community suffers regular faecal incontinence. Table 1.3 gives a detailed breakdown (Thomas et al., 1984). It tends to be a significantly under-reported symptom which many elderly or disabled people and those with ano-rectal and colonic disorders accept and disguise, because of shame

Table 1.3   The Prevalence of Faecal and Double Incontinence

SEX	AGE 15–64 years	65 years +
Men	0.42%	1.09%
Women	0.17%	1.33%
Total % Adults	0.43%	

Definition: Two or more episodes in the past month.

(Thomas et al., 1984.)

and embarrassment without seeking medical help (Leigh and Turnberg, 1982). Most people with faecal incontinence receive no professional help (Table 1.4). As with urinary incontinence, there are also problems of definition. Should minor staining of underwear be classified as faecal incontinence? Inability to control flatus can be as embarrassing as actual leakage of faeces.

Table 1.4   The Prevalence of 'Recognised' Faecal and Double Incontinence

SEX	AGE 15–64 years	65 years +
Men	0.05%	0.49%
Women	0.04%	0.88%
Total % Adults	0.19%	

Note: Over two-thirds of people with recognised faecal incontinence were resident in institutions.

(Thomas et al., 1984.)

The prevalence of incontinence among people in institutional care should be easier to discover than in the general population, yet reports vary so widely that it is difficult to generalise. Studies have used very different (and often unquoted) definitions of incontinence. In hospitals, probably 80% of the total number of incontinent people are in acute or general wards, with only 20% of the overall total being in long-stay or continuing care wards (Egan et al., 1983). However, in long-stay wards the *proportion* of patients who are incontinent is much higher than on acute wards. Between 32% and 55% of people in long-stay care are incontinent of urine or catheterised (Mohide, 1992).

Some studies have suggested that only 10% of long-stay patients who are mentally infirm are totally continent (McLaren, 1981). In residential homes one third of residents are reported to be incontinent of urine (Tobin and Brocklehurst, 1986).

It must be noted that these overall percentages disguise huge variations locally. Although useful for planning services, they do little to predict how many incontinent people there are in an individual home or hospital. In some there is very little incontinence; in others virtually everyone is incontinent. The reasons for these variations are many and complex.

Is all this incontinence unavoidable or inevitable? Probably not. Many types of incontinence are curable. For example, research suggests that, if accurate diagnosis is made prior to treatment, continence is attainable for up to 80–90% of selected women with stress incontinence, and 70–80% with urge incontinence. It is likely that many more people could benefit than are at present receiving treatment. The potential of preventive measures is still largely unexplored.

ATTITUDES AND INCONTINENCE

Attitudes towards incontinence continue to present a major problem. As nurses we can usefully begin by examining our own attitudes. Passive acceptance of incontinence, as an inevitable part of working in certain situations or with certain patient groups, is common. With increased knowledge and awareness this is gradually changing towards a more positive problem-solving approach for each individual. As we move towards individualised patient-centred nursing, incontinence can be identified as a symptom in a patient who has a unique combination of problems, needs and potentials.

Incontinence may arouse a negative response in a nurse, as in anyone else. Few people enjoy dealing with other people's excreta, or even with their own. Yet nurses are expected, right from the beginning of their training, to ignore their own automatic reactions. Emptying bedpans and cleaning incontinent people must be one of the most unpleasant aspects of nursing, and is what members of the public usually mean when they say that they could never be a nurse, or that nurses are wonderful for putting up with the things they have to do for people. Nurses are not encouraged to discuss or express their emotions about this aspect of their work. A nurse must expect and accept incontinence as part of the job, and get on and deal with it. Feelings of distaste are considered unworthy and best ignored – 'you will soon get used to it'. It is this very 'getting used to it' that leads to a tendency to deal with incontinence as quickly as possible, usually in a manner which detaches the individual nurse from the personal reality of the situation. Incontinence is cleared away and forgotten so that the nurse may move on to a more pleasant aspect of care – until the next time. This, combined with the patient's embarrassment, can lead to a situation of 'mutual pretence' (Schwartz, 1977) between nurse and patient that nothing abnormal has occurred. Neither nurse nor patient talks about the incontinence, even while it is actually being cleared up. The nurse wishes to spare the patient's feelings, and the patient is ashamed and assumes it cannot be helped. It is seldom openly and frankly discussed. Alternatively, the nurse may take a patronising attitude, reassuring the patient that it does not matter and that it happens all the time: 'Don't worry, we have plenty more sheets in the cupboard'. Neither pretence nor bland platitudes help to identify the cause of the incontinence and there are many missed opportunities.

Nurses need to be able to discuss their own feelings more openly, without fear of censure. Nurses may feel embarrassed, both for themselves and for the patient. There may be guilt, since incontinence is sometimes interpreted as a sign of 'bad' nursing care. Anger with a patient is particularly difficult to admit. Anger may result from the extra, unpleasant work created by incontinence, or because the patient is felt to be lazy, or wetting on purpose to gain attention or annoy the staff. Many of these feelings – revulsion, guilt, embarrassment, and anger – are understandable. They should be admitted and examined openly, rather than repressed as unworthy of a professional nurse, if the nurse is to be able to view the patient's incontinence objectively and plan a rational care regime. Constructive assessment begins with awareness of our own attitudes to the problem.

Cheater (1991) has found that while nurses have a predominantly therapeutic, rehabilitative attitude towards incontinence, a number of misconceptions remain. For example, 21% of nurses who answered her questionnaire felt that their primary role in caring for incontinent people was supplying aids. Eleven per cent thought incontinence was an inevitable part of ageing and 16% that it was due to laziness.

O'Brien et al. (1991) found in a controlled trial that a non-specialist nurse can cure or improve over two thirds (68%) of adults with a standard assessment and treatment package. There can be little doubt that nursing interventions are effective in helping the majority of incontinent people.

Nurses have a tradition of coping, whatever the situation, of putting up with problems however great or unpleasant, and making the best of them. For the sake of incontinent patients, as well as for nurses themselves, it is time to look at how the situation could be altered. The nursing profession has a responsibility to patients and their families to use the best available expertise in providing care, both for the promotion of continence and the management of incontinence, and in fostering a positive approach amongst carers.

REFERENCES AND FURTHER READING

Andersen, J., Abrams, P., Blaivas, J. G., Stanton, S. L., 1988. The standardisation of terminology of lower urinary tract function. *Scandinavian Journal of Urology and Nephrology*, Supplement, 114: 5–19.

Brocklehurst, J. C., 1993. Urinary incontinence in the community, analysis of a MORI poll. *British Medical Journal* 306: 832–4.

CEST, 1991. Advanced Medical Textiles. Centre for Exploitation of Science and Technology, London.

Cheater, F., 1991. Attitudes towards urinary incontinence. *Nursing Standard*, 5, 26: 23–7.

Egan, M., Plymat, K., Thomas, T. M., Meade, T., 1983. Incontinence in patients in two district general hospitals. *Nursing Times*, 79, 5: 22–4.

Hu, T. W., 1990. Impact of urinary incontinence on health care costs. *Journal of the American Geriatrics Society*, 38, 3: 292–5.

Hunskaar, S., Vinsnes, A., 1991. The quality of life in women with urinary incontinence as measured by the sickness impact profile. *Journal of the American Geriatrics Society*, 39: 378-82.

Jolleys, J. V., 1988. Reported prevalence of urinary incontinence in women in a general practice. *British Medical Journal*, 296: 1300–2.

Leigh, R. J., Turnberg, L. A., 1982. Faecal incontinence; the unvoiced symptom. *Lancet*, 1: 1349–51.

McLaren, S. M., McPherson, F. M., Sinclair, F., Ballinger, B. R., 1981. Prevalence and severity of incontinence among hospitalised female psychogeriatric patients. *Health Bulletin*, 39, 3: 157–61.

Masterton, G., Holloway, E. M., Timbury, G. C., 1980. The prevalence of incontinence in local authority homes for the elderly. *Health Bulletin*, 38, 2: 62–4.

Mohide, E.A., 1992. The prevalence of urinary incontinence. In: Roe, B. (ed), *Clinical Nursing Practice*. Prentice Hall, Hemel Hempstead.

Norton, C., 1982. The effects of urinary incontinence in women. *International Rehabilitation Medicine*, 4: 9–14.

Norton, P. A., MacDonald, L. D., Stanton, S. L., 1988. Distress and delay associated with urinary incontinence, frequency, and urgency in women. *British Medical Journal*, 297: 1187–9.

O'Brien, J., Austin, M., Sethi, P., O'Boyle, P., 1991. Urinary incontinence: prevalence, need for treatment, and effectiveness of intervention by a nurse. *British Medical Journal*, 303:1308–12.

Pierce, C. M., 1980. Enuresis. In: Kaplan, H. I., Friedman, A. M., Sadock, B. J. (eds), *Comprehensive Textbook of Psychiatry* (3rd edn). Williams and Wilkins, Baltimore.

Rutter, M., Yule, W., Graham, P., 1973. Enuresis and behavioural deviance: some epidemiological considerations. In: Kolvin, I., MacKeith, R. C., Meadow, S. R. (eds), *Bladder Control and Enuresis*. William Heinemann Medical Books, London.

Schwartz, D. R., 1977. Personal point of view, a report of 17 elderly patients with a persistent problem of urinary incontinence. *Health Bulletin*, 35, 4: 197–204.

Thomas, T. M., Plymat, K. R., Blannin, J., Meade, T. W., 1980. Prevalence of urinary incontinence. *British Medical Journal*, 281: 1243–5.

Thomas, T. M., Egan, M., Walgrove, A., Meade, T. W., 1984. The prevalence of faecal and double incontinence. *Community Medicine*, 6: 216–20.

Tobin, G. W., Brocklehurst, J. C., 1986. The management of urinary incontinence in local authority residential homes for the elderly. *Age and Ageing*, 15: 292–8.

Williams, K., Roe, B., Sindhu, F., 1995. An evaluation of nursing developments in continence care. National Institute for Nursing (Report 10), Oxford.

Wolin, L. H., 1969. Stress incontinence in young healthy nulliparous female subjects. *Journal of Urology*, 101: 545–9.

Wyman, J., Harkins, S., Choi, S., Taylor, J., Fantl, J., 1987. Psychosocial impact of urinary incontinence in women. *Obstetrics and Gynaecology*, 70: 378–80.

Chapter 2

The Development of Urinary Continence, and Causes of Incontinence

Mandy Wells, RGN, SCM, DipN, FETC

Clinical Services Manager/Lead Nurse, Continence and Stoma Services, St Pancras Hospital, London

None of us is born continent. Continence is a skill acquired, at a variable age, and retained often only with difficulty. This chapter aims to provide a framework for understanding, in a simplified form, the mechanism of continence and the most common causes of urinary incontinence. Subsequent chapters explain in greater depth many of the types of incontinence introduced here.

Any nurse who wishes to help incontinent patients needs a thorough knowledge of the normal functioning of the bladder and the ways in which it may become disordered. This will make it possible to assess the causes of an individual's incontinence (see Chapter 3) and to set appropriate and realistic goals during care planning.

THE BABY'S BLADDER

The bladder of the newborn baby is controlled by a sacral reflex arc (Figure 2.1). As the bladder fills with urine (which drains from the kidneys via the ureters), stretch and pain receptors in the bladder wall send sensory impulses via afferent fibres to the sacral bladder centre in the spinal cord (located in sacral segments S_2, S_3, and S_4). When these impulses become strong and persistent enough a spinal reflex arc is completed, and motor impulses (via efferent fibres) cause a bladder contraction, coordinated with relaxation of the urethral sphincter. The bladder empties completely. The whole filling and emptying cycle is then repeated. Babies are therefore not continuously wet, but empty the bladder in episodes throughout the 24-hour period. At this stage the baby's immature central nervous system cannot consciously appreciate or voluntarily control this cycle.

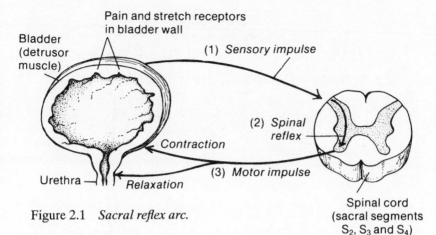

Figure 2.1   *Sacral reflex arc.*

Spinal cord
(sacral segments
S_2, S_3 and S_4)

Acquisition of Continence

Continence is acquired by the interaction of two processes – socialisation of the infant, and maturation of the central nervous system. Potty-training is dealt with in Chapter 5. Suffice it to say here that without society's expectation of continence, and without broadly accepted definitions of correct behaviour, the whole concept of 'incontinence' would be meaningless.

As the central nervous system matures with age, the baby is increasingly aware of its various bodily functions, including bladder emptying. Between 1 and 2 years of age the infant gradually becomes aware of bladder sensations, when the bladder is full and when it is emptying. However, it is not generally until the child approaches 2 years that there can be any influence over micturition. With practice, voluntary control becomes possible, just as control of limb movements becomes more purposeful. Reasonable control is usually mastered in the third year of life and by the age of 4 years the child can usually void voluntarily on command, even if the bladder is not full. By 5 or 6 years of age most children can delay micturition when the bladder is full and hold on until they get to a toilet.

Figure 2.2 (overleaf) shows that the sensory messages from the bladder are relayed, via several intermediate centres such as the pons, to the cerebral cortex, where the voluntary micturition control centre is situated in the frontal lobe. As maturation progresses, the infant is able to interpret these signals as indicating a full bladder; and, with practice, to initiate inhibitory motor impulses to block the completion of the sacral reflex arc, and thus prevent micturition.

13

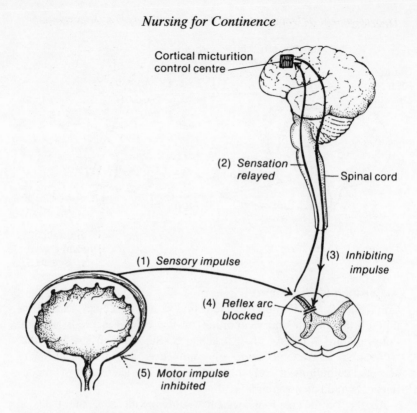

Figure 2.2 *Inhibition of the sacral reflex arc.*

Continence involves an active inhibition of nerve impulses, not merely the passive absence of micturition. Eventually the child learns to delay micturition reliably until the appropriate time and place are reached. Then cerebral inhibition is removed, the pelvic floor is relaxed, the sacral reflex arc is completed, and the bladder contracts and empties (Figure 2.3). Micturition is coordinated by very complex neurological links between the bladder, spinal cord and pontine micturition centre in the brain stem. These ensure that bladder contraction is simultaneous with, and coordinated with, sphincter relaxation (in other words, is 'synergic'), and that voiding is sustained until the bladder is completely empty.

With time, this control no longer involves continuous conscious effort between the first sensation of bladder filling and micturition. In most circumstances continence becomes subconscious and automatic.

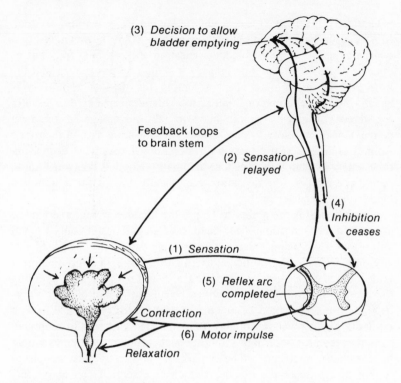

(3) *Decision to allow bladder emptying*

Feedback loops to brain stem

(2) *Sensation relayed*

(4) *Inhibition ceases*

(1) *Sensation*

(5) *Reflex arc completed*

Contraction

(6) *Motor impulse*

Relaxation

Figure 2.3   *Micturition.*

THE 'NORMAL' ADULT BLADDER

Bladder control and function is taken for granted by most people from an early age, and few adults pay it any attention. Indeed, few people are able to give an accurate account of how often they pass urine, until something goes wrong with voluntary control.

The boundaries of 'normality' are quite wide, and possibly 'normal' should be defined as the absence of any problem for each individual. Most people empty the bladder between three and six times in twenty-four hours. Some people do so more or less often than this and would still class themselves as normal. Most people seldom have to get up at night as the body has a diurnal rhythm of antidiuretic hormone production that ensures that less urine is produced at night. A few people always have to get up once. Urgency (having to rush to the toilet) should be rare, and only experienced if bladder sensations have been ignored for too long or if fluid intake has been excessive.

15

Generally the bladder has a very effective early warning system. Most people have a margin of one to two hours between the first conscious appreciation of bladder sensation and reaching the limit of bladder capacity. During this interval it should be possible to find the time and an appropriate place to empty the bladder. Sensation is usually first felt at about one-half of total bladder capacity. It is usually registered consciously as the need to take advantage of the next convenient opportunity to pass urine. The sensation should then fade from consciousness. It returns with increasing intensity, at decreasing time intervals, until the bladder is finally emptied. Between these periodic reminders the sensation can usually be forgotten until the bladder is very nearly full.

A useful skill is the ability to empty the bladder at will, even in the absence of any sensation of the need to do so and despite only a small volume of urine being present. Most people can empty the bladder at any time. This enables 'anticipatory micturition', for example before a long journey or a meeting, or during a meal break, thereby avoiding the need to interrupt future activities because of a full bladder. Ordinary civilised life would be much more difficult if we all had to wait until the bladder was absolutely full and then rush off to empty it. Cinemas, lectures, meetings and other such structured activities would be constantly interrupted. The remarkable ability of most people to inhibit and activate the bladder (which is essentially an autonomic organ and so, in theory, outside voluntary control), enables organised modern life to proceed uninterrupted by 'calls of nature'.

Most adult bladders have a capacity of between 400ml and 600ml, although many people micturate before this volume is reached. Incontinence should not occur at any time, even if micturition has been delayed and urgency is severe, including during strenuous exercise and while asleep.

CAUSES OF URINARY INCONTINENCE

There are many reasons why some people never acquire the control described above, or why it may break down at some point in life, and any classification of the causes is necessarily arbitrary. However, some scheme for considering the causes is needed, and in this book they are divided into three broad categories: physiological bladder dysfunction; factors directly influencing bladder function; and factors affecting the individual's ability to cope with bladder function.

Table 2.1 summarises the major types of incontinence and the most common associated symptoms. It should be remembered that these categories are intimately interrelated and that they often overlap.

Table 2.1   Common Causes of Urinary Incontinence

CAUSE	USUAL SYMPTOMS
Physiological Bladder Dysfunction	
Unstable detrusor	Frequency, urgency, urge incontinence
Genuine stress incontinence	Incontinence upon physical exertion
Outflow obstruction	Dribbling overflow incontinence, nocturia, frequency, urgency
Underactive bladder	Dribbling overflow incontinence, recurrent UTI, feeling of incomplete emptying, frequency
Factors Influencing Bladder Function	
Urinary tract infection	Frequency, dysuria, urgency and urge incontinence
Faecal impaction	Voiding difficulty with overflow incontinence or stress incontinence
Drug therapy	Various
Endocrine disorder	Various
Miscellaneous bladder pathology	Various
Factors Affecting Ability to Cope with Bladder	
Immobility	Urge incontinence or 'voluntary' wetting
Environment	Various
Mental function	Behavioural incontinence
Emotions	Urge incontinence or apathetic incontinence
Inadequate Patient Care	'Institutional' incontinence

Physiological Bladder Dysfunction

The causes of incontinence which fall into this category involve an abnormality in actual bladder function. The bladder, at its most basic, only has two functions: to hold urine until the correct time for micturition, and then to expel it completely. The first two causes described below involve a failure to hold urine reliably during bladder filling; the second two involve a failure to expel it completely and leave no residue after micturition.

Most, but not all, people who are incontinent have some underlying degree of bladder dysfunction. For many it is the only cause of their incontinence. For others it is a necessary, but not sufficient, predisposing reason. Alone, it does not explain entirely why they are wet, and many people are actually precipitated into incontinence by the coincidence of another problem from one of the other categories described below. A few incontinent people do not have any abnormality of bladder functioning and are wet solely for reasons discussed on pages 28–31.

Four basic types of bladder dysfunction may be distinguished. These are: the unstable detrusor; genuine stress incontinence; outflow obstruction; and an underactive bladder. The terms used here follow the recommendations of the standardisation committee of the International Continence Society (Andersen et al., 1988).

The Unstable Detrusor

The detrusor is the muscle of the bladder wall. The unstable detrusor (which may also be referred to as detrusor instability, bladder instability, detrusor hyperreflexia or the unstable bladder) is a condition characterised by involuntary bladder contractions or pressure rises during bladder filling. These contractions may be spontaneous or may occur only when the bladder is provoked (e.g. by a cough). It is often associated with neurological disease (when it is termed detrusor hyperreflexia), or with bladder outlet obstruction, but can also be idiopathic in origin (i.e. has no identifiable cause). In the unstable detrusor the normal inhibiting impulses are not sent from the cortical bladder centre to prevent completion of the sacral reflex arc, and the bladder begins to contract before micturition is voluntarily initiated (Figure 2.4). This will usually cause symptoms of frequency, urgency, urge incontinence, and possibly nocturia or nocturnal enuresis.

The unstable bladder may be caused by an upper motor neurone lesion affecting the cortical micturition centre (e.g. a cerebrovascular accident). Often sensation is left intact – the person appreciates the

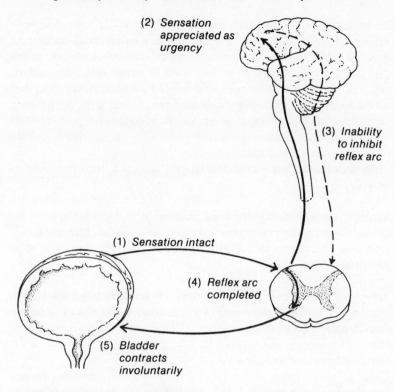

Figure 2.4   *Detrusor instability.*

need to pass urine, but cannot delay this until the lavatory is reached. Sometimes urgency is total, precipitant micturition occurs simultaneously with sensation of bladder fullness. At other times it may be less severe, with a diminished warning time between sensation and capacity, but may still result in incontinence if the lavatory is not reached in time. It is possible that general age-changes in the brain cause most very elderly people to have some degree of bladder instability (see Chapter 11).

Many people with an unstable bladder have no obvious neurological lesion to explain their inability to inhibit bladder contractions. This includes most lifelong nocturnal enuretics (bedwetters) and other people without overt neuropathy. The condition often presents in the second, third or fourth decade of life with no obvious preceding cause. It is then called 'idiopathic detrusor instability', causing exactly the same symptoms as the unstable bladder occurring secondarily to an upper motor neurone lesion. In children, detrusor instability predominantly affects boys; in young adults it is commoner in women. Some workers have postulated a psychosomatic causation, others that the bladder control centre in the brain is congenitally malformed. Learning theorists have suggested it might be caused by a failure ever to learn effective subconscious bladder control. Minimal neurological or neurochemical imbalances have also been suggested. None of these explanations has been conclusively proven, so the condition, for the present, remains 'idiopathic'.

An unstable detrusor may coexist with genuine stress incontinence in women.

Sensory urgency is urgency (and possibly urge incontinence) in the absence of unstable detrusor contractions – the bladder is hypersensitive. This can be secondary to a urinary tract infection, or have no identifiable cause.

Reflex incontinence is urine loss due to detrusor hyperreflexia (or involuntary urethral relaxation) in a neuropathic absence of sensation (e.g. in paraplegia).

Genuine Stress Incontinence

Genuine stress incontinence (also termed urethral sphincter incompetence) is caused by a failure to hold urine during bladder filling, in the absence of a detrusor contraction, as a result of an incompetent urethral sphincter mechanism. Leakage occurs because the intravesical (bladder) pressure exceeds the maximum urethral pressure. If the closure mechanism of the bladder outlet fails to hold urine under all circumstances, incontinence will occur. This is most usually manifest during physical exertion or physiological stress (the term does not refer to emotional 'stress'). It may occur in either sex, but is commoner in women because of a shorter urethra and the physical trauma of childbirth (see Chapter 6). Men may experience stress incontinence following traumatic or surgical damage to the sphincter (see Chapter 7). The mechanism of genuine stress incontinence is described in detail in Chapter 6.

Outflow Obstruction

Obstruction of the outflow of urine during voiding can lead to a variety of symptoms, including frequency, nocturia, straining to void, poor urinary stream, post-micturition dribbling, and urgency with urge

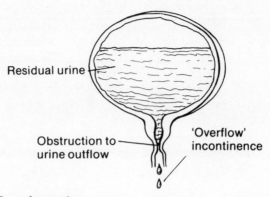

Residual urine

Obstruction to urine outflow

'Overflow' incontinence

Figure 2.5 *Outflow obstruction.*

incontinence. In severe cases the bladder is never completely emptied and a volume of residual urine builds up. Overflow incontinence may result (Figure 2.5).

This is most commonly associated with prostatic enlargement due to benign hyperplasia, malignancy or inflammation in men (see Chapter 7). It may also occur in either sex because of urethral stenosis or stricture (possibly following instrumentation or infection of the urethra). Alternatively, a neurological lesion may prevent coordinated relaxation of the urethra during voiding, resulting in obstruction to the outflow of urine ('detrusor-sphincter dyssynergia'). Instead of relaxing synergically when the detrusor contracts, the urethra is in spasm and acts as an obstruction to the passage of urine (see Chapter 8). *Dysfunctional voiding* is the term given to overactivity of the urethral sphincter in the absence of neuropathy.

The detrusor muscle of an obstructed bladder may become very powerful and hypertrophied, in an attempt to overcome the high outflow resistance. In some instances secondary detrusor instability may develop. If the obstruction is long-standing the bladder may eventually 'decompensate', give up the unequal struggle to empty, and become underactive or even acontractile.

Underactive Bladder
The underactive bladder is one which does not produce an effective voiding contraction. Emptying can be attempted by abdominal effort or manual expression, but a large residual volume builds up. Sensation may or may not be present. Frequency will be common if sensation is

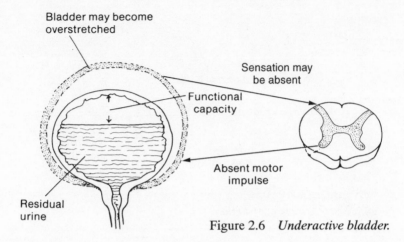

Bladder may become overstretched

Sensation may be absent

Functional capacity

Absent motor impulse

Residual urine

Figure 2.6   *Underactive bladder.*

present, as only a small proportion of bladder volume is utilised (Figure 2.6). Sensation is often diminished and the residual urine volume may reach considerable amounts (500–2000ml). Overflow incontinence will often occur. Genuine stress incontinence often coexists with an underactive bladder, because of simultaneous denervation (nerve damage) of the detrusor and sphincter.

Detrusor weakness can be caused by damage to the peripheral nerves of the bladder (e.g. in diabetic neuropathy), or by damage to the lower spinal cord or feedback loops to the brain stem (see Chapter 10). Where neurological lesions are present it is termed *detrusor hyporeflexia*.

Detrusor underactivity denotes an inadequate magnitude or duration of contraction to effect bladder emptying within the normal time span.

Detrusor areflexia is acontractility due to abnormality of nervous control and denotes the complete absence of a centrally coordinated contraction.

These four types of bladder dysfunction (the unstable detrusor, genuine stress incontinence, outflow obstruction and the underactive bladder) are very different in their mechanism of causing urinary incontinence. It is vital to distinguish between them because, as will be seen, the treatments are also very different. It is possible to have more than one of these problems at the same time, and for elderly people especially, multiple pathology is common. There are also other, rarer types of incontinence which are discussed in other chapters.

Factors Directly Influencing Bladder Function

Some problems directly affect and upset the normal functioning of the bladder. Any of these factors, if severe enough, could cause incontinence, even in someone with a normal bladder. More often they combine with one of the above bladder dysfunctions in leading to incontinence.

Urinary Tract Infection

The term urinary tract infection means the presence of micro-organisms in the urinary tract. Because of the ease of contamination of urine samples, especially in the female, it is usual to disregard the presence of small numbers of micro-organisms, and take 100,000 colony-forming units of bacteria per millilitre of urine as the threshold for 'significant' infection in women without symptoms (Kass et al., 1956). Further work has shown that in acutely symptomatic women a culture of 100 or more colony-forming units of a single species is a reliable threshold. In men a threshold of 1000 or more colony-forming units of a single species per millilitre is reliable, as contamination is less likely to occur (Stamm, 1988; Lipsky, 1989). It should, however, be remembered that these criteria were developed under very precise conditions. The urine sample was collected early in the morning by careful technique, stored at 4°C and received in the laboratory with minimal delay. In everyday practice these conditions are not always achieved.

An acute urinary tract infection (UTI) causes frequency, dysuria and can sometimes cause transient incontinence even in a fit, healthy young person who normally has no bladder problems. In community settings 90% are due to the bacteria *Escherichia coli*; in hospital this falls to 50%, with a much broader range of causative organisms implicated. Twenty per cent of women experience acute UTI at some time in their lives. Over 6% of women consult their general practitioner annually for symptoms of UTI (Wilkie et al., 1992).

The pain associated with urinary tract infections (dysuria) is usually a burning sensation which occurs either at the onset, during or after micturition. This can either be internal, arising within the bladder and urethra and experienced on initiation of micturition, or external, when the discomfort is felt around the labia by women.

If there is an associated underlying bladder dysfunction, such as an unstable bladder, an acute UTI is likely to aggravate the problem, for example increasing the number, frequency and intensity of uninhibited contractions. If a voiding problem is present, with a high residual urine volume, there is a predisposition to UTI.

However, it should be noted that not all dysuria is related to a UTI. The symptoms of an unstable bladder can include a dull ache experienced in the lower abdomen, which coincides with urgency. This is worsened if micturition has to be delayed. Interstitial cystitis manifests with a persistent dull ache in the lower abdomen, which increases as the bladder fills and is only partially relieved by micturition. The urethral syndrome, atrophic vaginitis and some sexually transmitted diseases can all cause dysuria.

A urinary tract infection in the absence of symptoms (dysuria and frequency) is termed 'covert bacteriuria' or 'asymptomatic bacteriuria'. Ronald and Pattullo (1991) highlight that there is no real evidence linking asymptomatic bacteriuria to the subsequent development of an acute infection, other than in special circumstances (such as in pregnancy or the presence of vesico-ureteric reflux). Covert bacteriuria is present in 5–10% of women and 0.5% of men. In most instances, asymptomatic bacteriuria should not be treated (Hooton and Stamm, 1991). Transient episodes of uncomplicated bacteriuria are common in women, particularly after sexual intercourse, but usually resolve spontaneously within 24–72 hours (Wilkie et al., 1992).

The role that chronic infection plays in causing incontinence is unproven (Brocklehurst et al., 1968; Milne et al., 1972). Elderly people especially have a very high prevalence of chronic urinary tract infection (see Chapter 11). Since many are also incontinent it is likely just by chance that a proportion will be both infected and incontinent. Twenty to fifty per cent of older women and 5–20% of older men who live in institutional care are found to have chronic infection. A causal role for chronic infection in incontinence has never been proven. It is generally accepted as relatively benign if asymptomatic.

When considering infection, tuberculosis must not be forgotten as the tubercle bacillus can invade the urinary tract. Although rare, it should be considered as a potential cause of symptoms, especially among those living in very poor conditions, those who have lived abroad or who are recent immigrants, and in people with a history of tuberculosis.

Faecal Impaction

Severe constipation with faecal impaction considerably disturbs bladder function. It may affect the bladder in several different ways.

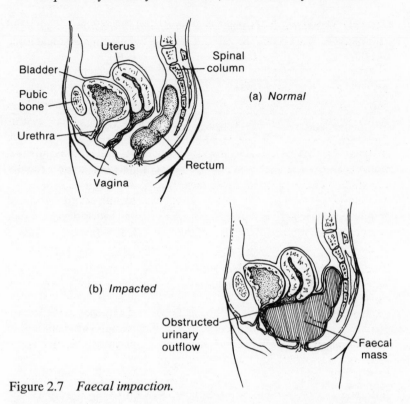

Figure 2.7   *Faecal impaction.*

Sometimes the faeces in the rectum form a physical outflow obstruction to urine (Figure 2.7) by pressing on the bladder, urethra, and local nerves, thus leading to urinary retention with overflow of urine. Direct pressure will also aggravate an unstable bladder. In other cases the impaction, by stretching the pelvic floor and inhibiting pelvic floor contractions, leads to stress incontinence.

Faecal impaction can also cause the sufferer to feel unwell, lethargic, and generally disinclined to activity. Many of the causes of faecal impaction (see Chapter 10) may also disturb urinary continence, for example a poor diet, low fluid intake, immobility, and a poor environment.

Drug Therapy

Many drugs can disturb bladder function. The most obvious category is diuretics. A large, swift diuresis will give most people frequency and urgency. If the bladder is unstable or the person is immobile it may not

Table 2.2   Drugs Affecting Bladder Function

DRUG	USE	EFFECT
Alcohol	Social	Increased urinary frequency and urgency
Anticholinesterases e.g. Neostigmine	Myasthenia gravis Irritable bowel spasm and gut spasm	Bladder sphincter muscle relaxation causing involuntary micturition Also contraction of smooth muscle and increased peristalsis
Antimuscarinic drugs (also known as anticholinergics) e.g. Benzhexol Procyclidine e.g. Hyoscine Propantheline	Parkinson's disease Drug-induced Parkinsonism	Increases bladder sphincter tone and decreases bladder contractility causing urinary retention.
Drugs with antimuscarinic side-effects:		NB: some drugs with antimuscarinic effects are used to treat urinary dysfunction (see Chapter 4).
Antihistamines e.g. Pizotifen Promethazine	Allergies – hayfever, rashes, migraine, travel sickness	
Antipsychotics e.g. Chlorpromazine Thioridazine	Schizophrenia and related psychotic illness Nausea and vomiting Agitation	
Antidepressants e.g. Amitriptyline Lofepramine Imipramine	Depression	Voiding difficulty
Calcium channel blockers e.g. Nifedipine	Angina Arrhythmias High blood pressure	Nocturia Increased frequency

Table 2.2 (continued)

DRUG	USE	EFFECT
Cytotoxics e.g. Cyclophosphamide Ifosfamide	Malignancies	Haemorrhagic cystitis
Opiate analgesics e.g. Diamorphine Morphine	Pain control (abuse)	Bladder sphincter spasm causing difficulty in micturition. Also urge incontinence
Xanthines e.g. Theophylline Caffeine	 Asthma Stimulant	Diuresis

Note: Diuretics and sedatives can cause incontinence by increasing urine output and reducing awareness of the need to micturate respectively. This is not a complete list. Please refer to the *British National Formulary* for further information.

be possible to cope with a sudden influx of urine, and urge incontinence may result. Sedation may either directly affect bladder function (e.g. diazepam may lower urethral resistance), or make the individual much less responsive to signals from the bladder and so fail to maintain continence. For example, a person with an unstable bladder may find that night sedation means a good night's sleep and a wet bed, whilst without medication he is woken several times to pass urine.

Other drugs have side-effect actions upon bladder function. Table 2.2 summarises the possible effects of some commonly prescribed drugs. Note that not all patients will experience urinary side effects from these drugs. In some instances the side effects may actually be therapeutic (e.g. a drug which makes voiding more difficult for someone with a 'normal' bladder may decrease frequency and urgency for the patient with an unstable bladder).

It is not possible in the space available to list every drug which has the potential to affect the bladder. The main point to remember is that a great many can do so, and that it is always important to ascertain which drugs are being taken by an incontinent patient. The nurse often has more contact with the patient than the prescribing physician and is therefore likely to be more aware of unwanted side effects, and can if necessary suggest a review of medication.

Endocrine Disorders

Various endocrine disorders may upset bladder function. Diabetes has already been mentioned as causing damage to peripheral nerves. It may also cause polydipsia with a consequent large volume of urine to be contained, and glycosuria may encourage urinary tract infection. Thyroid imbalances may aggravate an overactive or underactive bladder. Pituitary gland disorders can cause production of excessive urine volumes because of a deficiency of antidiuretic hormone. Oestrogen deficiency in post-menopausal women causes atrophic changes in the vagina and urethra, and may worsen both genuine stress incontinence and an unstable bladder (see Chapter 11).

Miscellaneous Bladder Pathology

Several different bladder pathologies may cause incontinence by disrupting normal functioning. A neoplasm, whether benign or malignant, or a stone in the bladder may occasionally present with incontinence as a symptom (although other symptoms such as blood in the urine are usually also present). Congenital malformations, such as a ureter which inserts directly into the urethra, and vesico-vaginal or vesico-rectal fistula may lead to total uncontrollable incontinence. These are rare causes of incontinence.

Factors Affecting Ability to Cope with the Bladder

Many people have one or more of the conditions outlined above without actually wetting themselves. People with an unstable bladder, a urinary tract infection, or who are taking diuretics often learn to prevent incontinence by visiting the lavatory at every available opportunity, never moving too far from a lavatory, or keeping a receptacle near at hand, such as a commode by the bed or a bucket under the sink, in case of being 'caught short'. They will only go shopping in a centre where they know that there are lavatories, and the first thing they do on any outing (if they will go on one) is to ascertain the quickest route to the nearest lavatory. Some isolate themselves completely and refuse to go out or mix socially.

Younger people with an unstable bladder are often not incontinent simply because they have a good urethral sphincter pressure and are agile enough to respond quickly to urgency. Many people with a tendency to stress incontinence avoid leakage by avoiding physical exertion, they stop playing sport, do not go shopping if heavy weights may have to be carried, refuse to dance, and try not to laugh when they go out. When they have a cough they are more likely to stay at home in order to avoid potential embarrassment. People with difficulties in bladder emptying may spend excessive time in the lavatory trying to strain until the bladder is empty. Many incontinent people restrict fluid intake in an attempt to prevent incontinence.

Often it takes something else, in addition to the underlying bladder problem, to 'tip the balance' and produce incontinence. This is especially true for some older and disabled people whose control is delicately balanced between continence and incontinence, a balance which can easily be tipped either way.

Any one of the following factors is in some cases sufficient reason on its own for incontinence. More often they combine with an actual bladder problem to produce incontinence.

Immobility

To be able to pass urine in the 'correct' place you have to be able to get there. Anything which impedes access is likely to induce incontinence. Immobility may be the result of the gradual worsening of a chronic condition, such as arthritis, multiple sclerosis, or Parkinson's disease, until eventually the individual is simply unable to get to the lavatory in time. Or it may be acute: an accident or illness which suddenly renders a person immobile may be the start of failure to control the bladder.

The significance of immobility is closely related to the degree of urgency experienced. If it takes longer than the person can hold on to get to the lavatory or obtain an alternative receptacle (such as a bedpan), incontinence is the inevitable result. A person with severe disabilities may become incontinent simply because he cannot get to or onto a lavatory, or because no help is at hand.

Linked closely with mobility are factors such as manual dexterity, eyesight, condition of the feet (and shoes), and suitability of clothing. (See Chapter 13 for a discussion of incontinence and physical disability.)

Environment

The physical design and layout of surroundings may or may not be ideal for maintaining continence. The situation of the lavatory, ease of access, and number of other people who share it (and might be using it) are important. In public places, including hospitals, many lavatories are considerable distances from main areas, and may be poorly marked and difficult to use if a person has any disabilities. At home, there may be stairs to negotiate or the lavatory may be outside the house. The social environment is also important. In some situations incontinence becomes the norm (especially in long-stay institutions), and the social pressure to be continent disappears. In a socially impoverished atmosphere people may lose their grip on reality and exhibit disordered behaviours, including incontinence. At home the isolated incontinent person may lose all motivation to try to maintain continence. The well-supported person with a good social network who is seen as a valid and useful member of the community (and sees himself as such) is most likely to make every effort to avoid incontinence and to seek help early if it does occur.

Mental Function

People with impaired mental capabilities, whether because of learning difficulties, confusion, or dementia, may not recognise the social need for continence or what is considered acceptable behaviour. This is seldom a sufficient reason on its own to explain incontinence. Many will also have an underlying bladder disorder (see above). The majority of people with disordered mental function are capable of continence with appropriate help and management (see Chapters 11 and 14), except possibly in cases of very advanced dementia. However, confused people are very easily disorientated, and many who can cope well in their own surroundings cannot manage in a strange environment. Flexibility of reaction may be lost, and incontinence results.

Emotions

The bladder is a sensitive emotional barometer, and many people find their bladder function disturbed when they are upset. Witness the queues for the lavatory outside an examination or interview room. The causal relationship of emotional problems to incontinence is unclear. There can be little doubt that many incontinent people appear depressed or anxious – but whether this is a cause or an outcome of incontinence is not yet known. Research has produced conflicting results as to whether some types of incontinence might be psychosomatic (Macaulay et al., 1987; Norton et al., 1990).

Incontinence may also be associated with emotional regression under stress, and in rare situations may be a symptom of protest or despair at an unacceptable life situation. Onset of incontinence may follow a traumatic life-event, such as bereavement. It may also be used as manipulative or 'attention-seeking' behaviour by a few patients. As mentioned above, some clinicians believe that idiopathic detrusor instability is psychosomatic in origin, although the evidence for this is inconclusive.

Inadequate Patient Care
Those who are dependent upon other people to some degree for their continence are 'at risk' of becoming incontinent unless those carers, whether relatives, nurses, or others, are sensitive to their needs and orientated towards the promotion of continence. If the attitude of the carer is to expect and accept that a dependent person will be incontinent, then incontinence becomes much more likely.

In some instances, carers can actually promote incontinence by making it easier to be wet than dry. An individual may find that it is much less bother for carers to come and change a pad at intervals than to struggle to get to the lavatory. If incontinence seems to be the expected norm, and if it is rewarded by attention and physical and social contact, it may soon become established behaviour.

These and many other potential 'causes' of incontinence are dealt with in greater depth in the relevant chapters of this book. Any combination of problems is possible. Young, otherwise fit, incontinent people tend to have just one single bladder dysfunction underlying their symptom. People who are older or who have disabilities tend to have complex problems, with many different factors combining to render them incontinent.

The multiplicity of possible causes emphasises the importance of seeing incontinence as a symptom, the causes of which must be investigated and diagnosed accurately if treatment is to stand a chance of success. It should never simply be accepted as an inevitable consequence of ageing, disease, or disability. Often the assumed 'cause' is only part of the story. Today it is possible to modify most of the underlying bladder dysfunctions and in many cases to remedy them completely. Most of the factors in the two categories discussed on pages 23–31 are also amenable to treatment or modification.

There is no incontinent person for whom it is pointless to enquire 'Why?'. There must always be a cause; incontinence does not just happen. If nurses can keep that question – WHY? – in the forefront of their thinking when caring for incontinent people, many who are currently suffering from this symptom will stand a good chance of regaining continence.

REFERENCES AND FURTHER READING

Andersen, J. T., Abrams, P., Blaivas, J. G., Stanton, S. L., 1988. The standardisation of terminology of lower urinary tract function. *Scandinavian Journal of Urology and Nephrology*, Supplement 114: 5–19.

Brocklehurst, J. C., Dillane, J. B., Griffiths, L., Fry, J., 1968. The prevalence and symptomatology of urinary tract infection in an aged population. *Gerontologica Clinica*, 10: 242–53.

Hooton, T. N., Stamm, W. E., 1991. Management of acute uncomplicated urinary tract infection in adults. *Medical Clinics of North America*, 75: 339–57.

Kass, E. H., 1956. Asymptomatic infections of the urinary tract. *Transactions, American Association of Physicians*, 69: 56–63.

Lipsky, B. A., 1989. Urinary tract infections in men: epidemiology, pathophysiology, diagnosis and treatment. *Annals of Internal Medicine*, 110: 138–40.

Macaulay, A. J., Stanton, S. L., Stern, R. S., Holmes, D M., 1987. Micturition and the mind: psychological factors in the aetiology and treatment of urinary disorders in women. *British Medical Journal*, 294: 540–3.

Milne, J. S., Williamson, J., Maule, M. M., Wallace, E. T., 1972. Urinary symptoms in older people. *Modern Geriatrics*, 5: 198–212.

Norton, K. R. W., Bhat, A. V., Stanton, S. L., 1990. Psychiatric aspects of urinary incontinence in women attending an outpatient urodynamic clinic. *British Medical Journal*, 301: 271–2.

Ronald, A. R., Pattullo, A. L. S., 1991. The natural history of urinary infection in adults. *Medical Clinics of North America*, 75: 299–311.

Stamm, W. E., 1988. Protocol for diagnosis of urinary tract infection – reconsidering the criterion for significant bacteriuria. *Urology*, 32: 6–12.

Wilkie, M. E., Almond, M. K., Marsh, F. P., 1992. Diagnosis and management of urinary tract infection in adults. *British Medical Journal*, 305: 1137–41.

(See Appendix 4 for books providing general reviews of the causes of incontinence.)

Chapter 3

Assessment and Investigation of Urinary Incontinence

Ann Winder, RGN

Continence Adviser,
Southmead Health Services NHS Trust, Bristol

Several different professionals may be involved in assessing and managing an incontinent patient. There can be little doubt that the team approach offers the optimum help for many patients, and the contribution of various paramedical personnel is dealt with in more detail in Chapter 4. This chapter concentrates on the nursing and medical aspects of assessment, but it should not be forgotten that under some circumstances a member of another profession may contribute part of the total picture.

Accurate assessment of the individual's incontinence is the key to successful outcome. It is not possible to tackle incontinence until you know the cause. Assessment is the first phase in the process of nursing care. However, the idea that it is a once-only activity must be discouraged and the nurse must recognise that it is an ongoing process. The assessment should include:

- collecting information from/about the patient,
- reviewing the collected information,
- identifying the patient's problems,
- identifying priorities amongst problems (Roper et al., 1990).

Most commonly, the individual presenting for help with incontinence will be assessed and investigated by a nurse or doctor. Ideally, a joint nursing and medical assessment should be made. Both professions have a valuable contribution to make in forming a comprehensive picture of why incontinence is occurring and how it is affecting the patient. However, we do not live in an ideal world and often nursing and medical assessments are made independently, with little liaison. Indeed, in many cases one or the other assessment is omitted completely.

This chapter describes a comprehensive assessment, without specifying who should do what, as this will often be a matter for local time, interest and expertise to determine. Every trained nurse should be able

33

to carry out a baseline assessment as outlined in the first part of this chapter. Assessment does not have to be done by a continence adviser, but these nurse specialists may be used for help and support when necessary. Nurses can do much of this assessment alone, but without medical support and interest the patient will not obtain the fullest diagnosis possible.

PRESENTATION

The first bridge to be crossed in assessing incontinence is to find out who has the problem. (This may sound ridiculous to a nurse working in a long-stay unit where the problem is only too obvious and pervasive.) The vast majority of incontinent people live outside institutional settings and only rarely come into contact with the health service. As already mentioned, many people hide their incontinence because of embarrassment or guilt, or accept it without question as an inevitable concomitant of age or disability. It is often assumed to be irreversible and incurable once established. If the patient is demotivated at assessment, it can be difficult to obtain his or her cooperation, for example, in completing fluid volume charts.

Many incontinent people become demoralised and withdraw from social contact. Not many people would wish to admit to a friend, neighbour, or relative that they were incontinent – it must be one of the least acceptable symptoms as a subject for conversation. Many others feel that as it is not 'serious' (i.e. not life-threatening), and therefore not worth bothering their busy and overworked general practitioner with. Some are too shy to discuss the topic with a doctor of the opposite sex.

Even when a nurse is already involved in a patient's care (whether as an inpatient or outpatient), the subject is seldom brought up. Once incontinence has been admitted, all too often the sufferer is met by a nurse or doctor who accepts it as a chronic untreatable condition. 'It is probably your age' is not an uncommon remark, or 'You'll have to learn to live with it'.

Sometimes this may be because of lack of knowledge – the nurse or doctor genuinely does not realise how much can be done to relieve incontinence or else feels inadequate or hopeless. Acceptance may be compounded by embarrassment and the inability to talk easily about such problems. If the professional is embarrassed, the patient will often pick this up and avoid further discussion. If incontinence has been mentioned during the course of a consultation or hospitalisation for another problem, and not taken up by the nurse or doctor, there is a temptation to revert to a 'safer', more acceptable topic. There are therefore many missed opportunities to start to tackle the problem.

Starting to talk about incontinence can be difficult if the sufferer has an inadequate vocabulary and does not know what terms to use. The word 'incontinent' is usually avoided or else used to denote total lack of control (see Chapter 11). Every care must be taken to establish a mutually understood terminology before the assessment is made. The patient who denies 'incontinence' may quite happily admit to an 'occasional leak'.

Assessment should ideally be carried out as early as possible after the onset of symptoms. In reality it is often not possible to collect extensive information, for example, within a few hours of admission to hospital. However, the first stage of the history format provides enough information for the nurse to start identifying the patient's needs and planning care; then it is followed as soon as possible by a more detailed second stage (McFarlane and Castledine, 1982).

HISTORY

The first essential in assessing the nature and extent of incontinence is to obtain an accurate and full history. It is vital that whoever is taking this history has a sound basic knowledge of the subject and knows what questions to ask, and why. Also, that he or she understands the significance of the answers and knows which leads should be followed up. This history is not gathered for its own sake, but as a tool to aid accurate diagnosis and to help in planning treatment and care. It also provides a baseline from which to monitor progress, and a point of reference for other workers.

Where possible, the information should be gathered in a relaxed, informal atmosphere, preferably in the patient's usual environment. Plenty of time should be allowed, as this will often be the first time the patient has discussed the problem with anyone, and a hurried consultation may result in missing the main point or the extent of the problem. Incontinent people usually take a while to feel comfortable and able to discuss their incontinence, especially with a stranger.

The patient will often be able to answer all the necessary questions. Where this is not possible for reasons of poor memory, communication difficulties, or mental impairment, other sources of information should be used, for example medical records, talking to relatives or carers, and observation of the patient interacting with the surroundings. When the patient is mentally alert, permission should be sought before talking to relatives, as he may have gone to great lengths to disguise the problem, and may not wish others to know about it.

Much of this information will be gathered routinely in a nursing process assessment and will not need to be repeated as a separate 'incontinence assessment'. Unfortunately in many nursing process assessments questions about 'elimination' are not expanded upon enough by the nurse. Everyone who is, or who is at risk of becoming, incontinent needs to have a detailed micturition and defaecation history taken, and the findings acted upon (Brocklehurst, 1990; Duffin, 1992; Bernard, 1994).

CHECKLIST

Table 3.1 (overleaf) gives an example of an assessment checklist which may be used as an aide-memoire when taking an incontinence history. It is not intended to be used inflexibly or administered as a question-naire, but merely to ensure that all relevant areas are covered and that accurate and complete records are kept in a systematic fashion. Some questions require simply a 'Yes/No' answer; others will require elaboration. Not all questions are likely to be relevant to every incontinent person. It has been found to be a useful tool for assessing both inpatients and outpatients. For some people a much more detailed history of specific aspects may be required (for instance, behavioural assessment for people with a learning difficulty, see Chapter 14, and confused people, see Chapter 11). A briefer assessment tool using Roy's model of nursing has been developed in the USA (Joseph, 1992).

The assessor should be constantly aware of the relevance and implications of each question. These are now discussed in detail.

Main Complaint

It is important to find out what the most important problem is, either from the perspective of the patient or that of the primary carer. An individual may have a great variety of different symptoms, of varying importance to him, and treatment or management should usually be directed in the first instance at solving those which are causing the greatest problem. The patient may rate the severity of symptoms very differently from a nurse or doctor, so it is vital to ask his opinion: 'What, to you, is the main problem with your bladder/waterworks?' is a useful way of wording the question. The answer may be a common symptom, for example wetting on the way to the lavatory or wetting the bed; or it may be a highly idiosyncratic problem which is altering the sufferer's lifestyle, perhaps leaking when taking a swing at a golf ball, or during sexual intercourse.

Urinary Symptoms
It is important to ascertain the patient's normal pattern of micturition or defaecation prior to their presenting problem.

Urinary symptoms are notoriously unreliable indicators of underlying bladder dysfunction. It is impossible to make a totally reliable diagnosis of which bladder problem is present on a history of symptoms alone. However, symptoms do give broad clues as to the likely diagnosis, and together with the rest of the history and a thorough examination, can predict the most likely dysfunction (such as an unstable detrusor, genuine stress incontinence, or retention with overflow incontinence). However, if surgery is contemplated, or if the presumptive diagnosis has not led to successful treatment, the bladder dysfunction needs to be confirmed by urodynamic tests (see pages 55–74). Patients who have a complex mixture of symptoms, or who have failed to respond to previous treatment, will often need urodynamic tests in the first instance.

Frequency
Frequency of passing urine by day may be indicated by recording either the number of times urine is passed between rising and retiring, or the average time interval between visits to the lavatory. Most people pass urine between three and six times per day (3- to 4-hourly). Ten or more times is usually classed as abnormally high frequency. When establishing frequency a careful note must be made of the fluid intake, and types of fluids, (large quantities of tea or coffee can result in frequency or urgency, either because of fluid volume or because the caffeine content stimulates unstable bladder contractions).

Nocturia
This means rising at night to pass urine. It is important to ascertain whether the patient is actually woken by bladder sensation, or whether he is already sleeping badly and simply getting up from boredom or to 'make sure' before getting back to sleep. Nocturia is a classic early symptom of prostatic enlargement in men. Some people always have to get up once in the night, although most rarely do so. Being

Table 3.1   Incontinence Assessment Checklist

Note: These headings will elicit the basic information needed for an assessment. The reader should construct a checklist using these headings (and any others found necessary and relevant for specific circumstances), leaving adequate space for filling in the answers and any comments.

PERSONAL DETAILS

Name: Date of Birth:
Address:
General Practitioner:
Assessed by: Date: Referred by:

MAIN COMPLAINT (as perceived by patient/carer):

URINARY SYMPTOMS
Frequency: Nocturia?: (?Woken):
Urgency: Average warning time: Urge incontinence:
Stress incontinence: Passive incontinence:
Nocturnal enuresis: Number of nights per week:

Symptoms of voiding difficulty
Hesitancy: Poor stream: Straining:
Manual expression: Post-micturition dribble:
Dysuria: Haematuria:

Incontinence
Onset – when?   Circumstances:
Is incontinence improving/static/worsening?
How often does incontinence occur?   How much is lost?
Are aids or pads used?   Type of aid:
Number per day: Source of supply:
Are aids effective?   Problems:
How wet are pads at each change?
Average cost of pads if bought privately:
Type and amount of fluid intake: Fluid restriction?

Other urinary symptoms:

MEDICAL HISTORY
Neurological problems:
Previous illnesses/operations:
Parity: Difficult deliveries?
Current medication:
Any previous treatment for incontinence?

Table 3.1   (continued)

BOWELS
Usual bowel habit: Constipation?
Laxatives or diet regulation used?
Faecal incontinence?

PHYSICAL ABILITIES
Problems with mobility: Aids used?
Needs assistance?   Who is available?
Difficulties in transfer to/onto lavatory?   Comments:
Foot problems: Manual dexterity:
Clothing suitability: Eyesight:
Observe self-toileting and comment on problems:
Problems with personal hygiene:

PSYCHOLOGICAL STATE
Attitude to incontinence:
Anxiety?   Depression?
Impaired mental abilities?

SOCIAL NETWORK
Usual activities: Are these restricted by incontinence?
Who does patient live with?   Who visits regularly?
Relationship problems because of incontinence?   Sexuality issues?
Official services received:

ENVIRONMENT
Lavatory facilities: Are urinals or commode used?
Obstacles to using lavatory: Washing/laundry facilities:
Comments on general physical and social environment:

RESULTS OF PHYSICAL EXAMINATION
Skin problems: Prolapse (women):   Atrophic changes (women):
Rectal examination: Post-micturition residual urine volume:
MSSU/urine test result: Other findings:

RESULTS FROM CHART:

SUMMARY OF PROBLEMS:

AIMS/GOALS:

PLANNED ACTION:

REFERRAL TO:

URODYNAMIC RESULTS:

REVIEW DATE:

FOLLOW-UP NOTES:

---

woken twice or more is abnormal, although it becomes commonplace in extreme old age, probably because the normal diurnal variation in urinary excretion is lost (younger people produce more urine by day than at night; older people may have an even rate of production throughout the 24 hours).

If abnormally high frequency by day or by night is reported, the patient should be asked why this is so. Mostly it is because of feeling the desire to void. Occasionally, however, it is caused by old habits (for example, following childhood advice not to hold urine for too long). The patient may feel a compulsion to use every available opportunity to empty the bladder because of an anxious or obsessional personality trait. High frequency accompanied by discomfort may indicate a urinary tract infection or atrophic urethritis (see Chapter 11). Sometimes frequency is high simply because fluid intake is excessive (especially in women who have been advised to drink a lot following bouts of cystitis), or because diuretic medication is being taken. A very low frequency of micturition might indicate a high-capacity bladder, deliberate fluid restriction, dehydration, or retention of urine.

Excessive frequency is most commonly associated with an unstable detrusor, the bladder contractions giving frequent sensations of the desire to void. It may also occur in genuine stress incontinence, because urine in an open bladder-neck makes the patient feel the need to empty the bladder. A patient with a large residual volume may pass small amounts of urine frequently because the functional capacity of the bladder (the actual volume available for filling and emptying) is considerably reduced.

Urgency
Urgency is the symptom of having to hurry to pass urine. The warning time between the first sensation of bladder filling and an urgent need to empty the bladder is curtailed. There may only be ten minutes' warning instead of an hour or so, or the need can be so urgent that normal activities have to be interrupted and a lavatory found immediately. Sometimes *precipitancy* is present, the bladder starts to empty simultaneously with first bladder sensation, with no prior warning at all. If urgency is not responded to, or if the environment is unsuitable, *urge incontinence* may result. This is the symptom of not being able to get to or onto the lavatory in time. Again, this may be partial or complete, and will often depend on how fast the sufferer can move and how far it is to the nearest lavatory.

Urgency and urge incontinence are most commonly due to an unstable detrusor. However, they can also occur with most other bladder problems.

Stress Incontinence

Stress incontinence is the symptom of leaking urine coincidentally with physical exertion or effort (not emotional stress), such as coughing, laughing or lifting. It may be mild, occurring only on strenuous exercise. In severe cases the effort of rising from a chair or walking may be sufficient to cause incontinence.

Stress incontinence is usually associated with genuine stress incontinence, i.e. a weakness or incompetence of the urethral sphincter mechanism. It may also occur in people with an unstable bladder (for example, a cough may trigger a bladder contraction) or with overflow incontinence.

Passive Incontinence

Passive incontinence is wetting at rest without any coincident activity or sensation. Typically the patient will complain of 'just finding myself wet' for no apparent reason. The underlying bladder problem is most often retention with overflow.

Nocturnal Enuresis

This is bedwetting whilst asleep. It must be distinguished from nocturia with urge incontinence, where the patient wakes but cannot get up in time. In people of all ages, from childhood to old age, nocturnal enuresis is often associated with an unstable detrusor.

Voiding Difficulty

Any symptoms of voiding difficulty should be elicited. Hesitancy is having to wait for the flow of urine to start. Most men will know if their stream has diminished in force, but many women cannot answer this unless the problem is severe and urine dribbles out very slowly. Straining, having to use abdominal effort, or manual expression (applying pressure above the pubic bone) may be necessary to empty the bladder.

Post-micturition dribbling is a small, usually passive, leak of urine 'when you think you have finished', most usually when clothing has been replaced. It may indicate trapping of urine in the bulbar urethra in men (see Chapter 7), or a urethral diverticulum in women. Some people feel that they never completely empty the bladder but are unable to pass the rest, however much they try.

All these symptoms of a voiding difficulty may be caused by either an obstructed bladder outlet or by an underactive bladder.

Dysuria
Dysuria means pain or burning while actually passing urine. This is most usually caused by a urinary tract infection or by an atrophic urethritis secondary to oestrogen deficiency.

Haematuria
Haematuria (blood in the urine) is a serious sign and immediate medical investigation should be performed, as a bladder carcinoma may be present.

Characteristics of the Incontinence
Questions must be asked about the incontinence itself. Too often it is just reported as a fact without any further elaboration. The nurse should enquire when it started, and whether there were any specific circumstances associated with the onset of symptoms. Is the condition static, or is it worsening or improving? Does it vary, and under what circumstances is it worse or better? How often does incontinence occur? The actual volume of leakage is important as it may determine the most appropriate management. This can be difficult to estimate, especially as a little urine can spread a long way. A simple indication of the scale of the problem will suffice for most assessments, e.g. 'a few drops', 'wet pants', 'a moderate amount', 'soaked'.

The only way to gauge the volume of incontinence accurately is by weighing pads before and after use. Pad tests are now commonly used to establish a guide to urine loss. The patient wears a pre-weighed pad prior to a set routine of exercises. At routine intervals the pad is re-weighed and urine loss estimated (one millilitre of urine weighs approximately one gram). The International Continence Society has defined a standard pad weighing test to be used by researchers, so that results are comparable (Andersen et al., 1988).

Individual perceptions and tolerances of incontinence vary greatly. What is a problem to one person will be classed as 'normal' by another. Some fastidious people are very disturbed by a few drops leaking once per month. Others seem unconcerned by incontinence occurring several times a day. Volume and frequency of loss are not directly related to the amount of distress caused (Norton, 1982). Current symptoms will be interpreted according to pre-morbid bladder habits and expectations.

Product Usage

Aids, pads, or appliances may be already used. If so, it should be noted how many and what type are used. Pad usage is not a reliable indicator of incontinence volume, as many people change pads routinely rather than waiting until they are soaked to capacity. Often the aid will not be the ideal one and any problems (e.g. leakage, discomfort, odour) should be noted, together with the source of the product (e.g. self-purchase, district nurse, or prescription), and any problem with supply.

Fluid Intake

Fluid restriction is used by many incontinent people in an attempt to control their problem. Concentrated urine can irritate the bladder and aggravate any tendency to urine infections, diminished bladder capacity and/or frequency. Some people find that certain types of fluid particularly upset the bladder, those containing caffeine (such as tea, coffee, cola), and alcohol being the most common offenders.

The most useful way of determining the pattern of continence and incontinence is by using a chart (see Figure 3.1, page 51).

Medical History

Note should be made of any medical history that could influence either bladder or bowel function, or the ability to cope with it. A woman's obstetric history should record the number of babies, type of delivery, any particular difficulties, or heavy babies. A history of gynaeco-logical, urological or neurological disease or surgery may be relevant, as may psychiatric problems or learning difficulties. It is advisable to ask if there have ever been any minor or major accidents to the back or pelvic area.

Current medical problems and general state of health should be noted. Any drug therapy may be relevant because so many drugs have an effect upon bladder function (see Table 2.2, pages 26–7).

Bowels

Careful enquiry is needed to determine the person's 'normal' bowel habit and any significant change which has occurred. Bowel function varies greatly (see Chapter 10) and care must be taken not to impose arbitrary criteria for disturbed function. 'Constipation' is related more to the difficulty of passing motions and their consistency than to frequency of defaecation. Faecal incontinence should be specifically asked about since it is even more embarrassing than urinary incontinence, and many people who will discuss the latter are unwilling to volunteer the fact that they also suffer soiling. Chapter 10 gives a format for a fuller history of bowel problems if preliminary assessment should indicate faecal incontinence or other bowel problems.

Physical Abilities

Mobility

Information about mobility problems will be gathered both by interview and direct observation. Mobility may be impaired directly or because movement is painful, or the patient may be unsteady and afraid to move. Any mobility aids (stick, frame, wheelchair) should be inspected for suitability and ease of use in the context of usual surroundings – for example, is the lavatory space adequate to accommodate the walking frame?

For people with physical disabilities, speed of mobility should be assessed in conjunction with the degree of urgency and the availability of help at the times it is needed. Ability to transfer safely from bed to commode or from wheelchair to lavatory will depend both on physical abilities and on the suitability of any equipment used. On occasion, mobility is restricted by something as simple as inappropriate footwear (such as sloppy slippers which are difficult to walk in), painful toenails which a visit to the chiropodist could remedy, or by unsafe loose mats.

Manual Dexterity

Linked closely to mobility is the degree of manual dexterity. It is useless being able to get to the lavatory in time if, once there, pants cannot be removed, zips undone, or skirts pulled up out of the way. It is very nearly as distressing to be incontinent in the lavatory as it is to be so on the way there. The best way to assess manual abilities is to watch the patient toilet himself. The temptation may be great to offer assistance, but this should be resisted during assessment.

Sometimes the problem is that an incontinence pad is not completely removed and urine is accidentally passed onto it while the patient is on the lavatory, or that a pad has not been correctly applied and has fallen out through loose fitting underwear. The style of clothing may make dexterity problems worse: many layers of tight clothing, or buttons and stiff zips, may be the deciding factor between continence and incontinence, especially for people with urgency. Some people have praxis disorders (for example following a stroke). Their manual abilities are disorientated in space so that they lose the ability to manipulate objects accurately. They are likely to make mistakes, like replacing a pad with the wrong side to the body, or be unable to dress and undress correctly.

Eyesight

Eyesight is also relevant. Impaired vision can limit ability to get to or onto the lavatory, or lead to the incomplete removal of clothing or to missing a hand-held urinal. This can be a particular problem for men using a bottle. Pads may also be incorrectly applied, especially by people who also have poor sensation in their hands.

Personal Hygiene

Physical disabilities may impair the ability to cope well with personal hygiene. Effective bathing or washing depends on having reasonable use of the hands and arms in particular. Even using lavatory paper may become impossible for those with arthritic shoulders or a weak grasp. Good personal hygiene is very important in preventing skin problems and odour. Even slight incontinence can cause an unpleasant odour and sore skin if hygiene is poor. Occasionally the incontinent person seems totally unconcerned about hygiene, and unaware of how far outside accepted social standards he has become. More often the converse is true, and the incontinent person becomes overly obsessed by a fear of smelling. For most people this is an unrealistic and unnecessary fear, since with reasonable care odour need not arise. Showers, although used by many elderly and disabled people because they are easier and safer than a bath, often do not solve the problem of hygiene in the genital area if the patient sits down to shower. Portable bidets are now readily available and easy to use as often as the patient wishes.

Psychological State

Physical factors alone will not give a full picture of the individual and his incontinence. The patient's *attitude* to incontinence will affect the treatment options. Most incontinent people are understandably distressed by incontinence and are more than anxious to try anything that might help. Some people seem apathetic – they are convinced it is irreversible and have learned to accept it. This has often been reinforced by professional advice. People who are apathetic or depressed may be helped by counselling or medical treatment.

Others deny the problem, even in the face of obvious evidence to the contrary. It may be denied because of shame, and the individual may blame someone or something else for a puddle (e.g. the cat, or a spilled flower vase). A few people seem to deny incontinence even to themselves. It may be so unacceptable to them to admit the problem that they are genuinely unaware of it. This reflects a grave psychological conflict between reality and the individual's self-image.

Many people who live in care only have a small hand mirror and never see themselves as a whole. Therefore their body image may be forgotten. They do not see the wet patches and therefore do not accept that there is a problem. One way to help preserve their self-image is to ensure access to long mirrors. Hopefully, if a problem of incontinence occurs, it will be admitted and help accepted earlier.

It may take a long time and much effort to gain the patient's confidence and bolster up his self-concept before he can admit the problem. A few never do and helping them becomes very difficult, as any treatment or aids are rejected as unnecessary.

Some incontinent people appear very anxious or depressed. This may even be severe enough to constitute a psychiatric illness. Anxiety and depression might not only be a reaction to incontinence, but may also contribute to causing it. Once the two problems coexist it is not difficult to envisage how each might reinforce the other.

Those with impaired mental function, whether because of a learning difficulty, a confusional state, or dementia, are less likely to be able to cope with the complex social requirements for continence. It may be useful to make a formal assessment of cognitive and social functioning (see Chapter 14 for a behavioural assessment of a person with learning difficulties; Chapter 11 for assessment of a confused person). In some circumstances it may be appropriate to ask a psychologist or psychiatrist to contribute to the assessment.

Social Network
An individual's social contacts will often determine how well a problem is coped with. Many incontinent people deliberately isolate themselves and refuse to participate in former social activities. A note should be made of any curtailment of these that is occasioned by incontinence. If the patient lives with others, it is necessary to find out if the incontinence is affecting them as well, and what their attitude is to the problem. Stress is often caused, whatever the age of the sufferer. Extra laundry, reluctance to go out, and the unpleasantness of incontinence can all put a strain on relationships, whether with a child, spouse, parent, friend or landlady. At times the problem can become acute and be a factor in child abuse, matrimonial disharmony, abuse of elderly people or refusal to care any longer for a dependent relative.

Sexual relationships are often disrupted because of incontinence during intercourse, poor self-image of the incontinent person, or bedwetting. The whole family is often affected if one member is incontinent. This may be because they feel unable to go away on holiday because a child wets the bed, or because they cannot go on outings because one member has to be continually stopping and looking for a lavatory. There may be a reluctance to invite relatives and friends in if heavy incontinence causes the house to smell.

Most incontinent people are not receiving any help from health or social services. Assessment should be made of whether any services would be appropriate or, if they are being provided, whether they are the most appropriate (see Chapter 12). Once someone is receiving services, their needs are often never reassessed. Any change in circumstances may indicate the need for more, less, or different services. Since the Community Care Act came into force in 1993, Community Care Assessments should be carried out. These assessments should lead to individualised packages of care which enable people to remain in their own homes for as long as possible. An accurate assessment of needs for services to help with incontinence will be crucial to successful care at home in many instances, and a nurse should ideally contribute to this assessment.

Whether in institutional care or living at home, the social environment may be such as to promote continence or encourage incontinence. Assessment should include an impression of the prevailing atmosphere in which the individual is functioning and how this might influence the situation. If carers simply accept incontinence, then little will be done to promote continence.

Environment

The importance of the environment to the individual's ability to cope with bladder function has already been emphasised. Particular note should be made of lavatory facilities and any obstacles in reaching them (e.g. stairs, long distances, cramped conditions, chairs or beds which are difficult to get out of). In institutions, good signposting (e.g. clear large letters at an appropriate height) and good lighting may help people who are disorientated or visually impaired. The lavatory itself may be the wrong height, unclean, or difficult to get onto. Privacy is important and too often neglected (Counsel and Care, 1991). The use of screens around beds or commodes in hospital or residential settings often does not give adequate privacy to the patient to prevent embarrassment.

Does the person have access to good washing, laundry, and drying facilities? How are used products to be disposed of? Unfortunately many of the people liable to be incontinent are also likely to have the poorest facilities.

The extent to which incontinence is contained or is contaminating the surroundings should be noted. In extreme cases, incontinence becomes the overwhelming factor in the environment and is so poorly dealt with that total squalor results.

Results of Physical Examination

Every incontinent person should have a full medical investigation, including neurological, abdominal, vaginal and rectal examination, with an assessment of all major body systems as a screen for other health problems. In practice this ideal is not always attained. However, a nursing assessment should also include a basic examination of the patient. Careful observation will tell the nurse much about the general state of health, mobility, confusion, and mental state. Inspection of the genital area will reveal any skin problems, an obvious vaginal prolapse, or atrophic changes in the vulva (see Chapter 11).

A digital rectal examination will indicate if there is a faecal impaction present in the rectum. If there is a history or symptoms of constipation, it may be advisable to palpate the abdomen or to request a straight abdominal X-ray. This is the case even if the rectum is empty, since impaction of soft faeces may occur higher up in the colon, above the rectum.

Where stress incontinence is suspected, it may be elicited with the patient standing with a full bladder and coughing vigorously. It is wise to protect the floor in anticipation!

Too often significant voiding problems are overlooked. A simple in-out catheter after voiding will measure post-micturition residual urine volume and should be a routine component in the assessment of incontinent people. In younger patients, residual volume is usually nil immediately after micturition, although a volume up to 50ml is generally accepted as not being significant. In the older population (over 75 years) up to 100ml is considered to be within normal limits. The patient who has a larger residual volume should be investigated for a voiding problem.

Hand-held portable ultrasound machines can be used as an alternative to in-out catheterisation to measure residual volume, but they remain expensive and their use is likely to be restricted to specialists. Only very experienced professionals can estimate residual urine with any degree of accuracy by abdominal or bi-manual palpation of the bladder.

A midstream or catheter specimen of urine should be collected for urinalysis and microscopy, culture and sensitivity screening. If a patient has an incontinence problem it may not be possible to obtain a good MSU, as he often cannot stop voiding midstream, or the volume passed may be very small. If the residual urine volume is measured by catheterisation, a catheter specimen of urine should be obtained.

Several different problems may be diagnosed from a urine specimen, such as glycosuria (possible diabetes mellitus), high specific gravity (possible dehydration), haematuria (blood), or infection.

Results from Charting

The chart is probably the single most useful nursing tool in assessing incontinence. At the same time it is often also the most misused. Charting is not an end in itself, but acts as a record to be interpreted in the light of all the other findings of the assessment, and as an aid in diagnosis and care planning. Charts are too often kept for long periods of time, even indefinitely, and either left on a clipboard at the foot of the patient's bed or filed in the back of notes, with totals columns carefully filled in, but with no action resulting from them.

The chart has two main uses: as a part of the baseline assessment of the individual's incontinence, and later as a record of progress during treatment, to monitor the effectiveness of therapy. Indeed, for bladder training programmes it forms the cornerstone of the regime (see Chapter 4).

To be useful, a chart must be kept accurately (a seemingly obvious necessity that is often ignored). When a chart is being kept it is important that all involved, including the patient, know about it and that it is clear who is responsible for it. Wherever possible, encourage patient-centred responsibility. This will obtain the patient's involvement and commitment to his own progress, especially since – if he is embarrassed – he may well not want too many people aware of the problem. On a ward, charting is usually most reliably achieved where patient allocation is practised as there is clear responsibility for individual patients. In many instances, much more responsibility could be given to the patient to fill in his own chart – he is the only person present twenty-four hours a day and it is beneficial to engage his interest in the problem at the outset. In the case of an outpatient, the patient or a relative will have to keep the chart, and many take a pride in keeping an accurate and neat chart for their doctor or nurse to examine, often doing it better than many nurses!

To be reliably accurate the chart should be filled in as events occur (rather than at the end of the day from memory). The place where the chart is kept may influence the likelihood of this happening. While always remembering that it may cause embarrassment for a chart to be on public view, it is in some circumstances best to keep the chart in the lavatory or sluice, or with the patient (in a pocket or handbag). If the patient is in a dayroom with a nearby lavatory, a chart hanging on his bed or in the nurse's office – which may be a considerable distance away – is much more likely to be forgotten, or else only filled in after a time lag.

The words 'continence' or 'incontinence' chart can be embarrassing for the patient if on view; this can be changed to 'Analysis Chart', which offers a more acceptable image.

Many different charts are available, some interchangeable, others with different functions. Before choosing a chart it is important to decide what information is needed. At its very simplest (Figure 3.1) a chart should show voidings and episodes of incontinence. This particular chart was designed to be easy to fill in and suitable for both inpatient and community use. The less information that is requested, the greater the likelihood of it being kept accurately. With bold colouring and simple instructions, most people (patients or nurses) are able to recognise easily what is expected and to fill it in accurately. Such a chart, kept for 4–7 days, gives the nurse and patient a good baseline record of the problem.

For some purposes it may be desirable to obtain more information than this chart provides. A frequency/volume chart will give an idea of functional bladder capacity (i.e., how much the bladder can routinely hold), and this is often combined with an input estimation in a 'fluid balance chart'. Measuring input will highlight both polydipsia (excessive thirst, possibly a sign of metabolic disorder such as diabetes mellitus) and low fluid intake (possibly caused by fear of incontinence, which may eventually cause dehydration, constipation, electrolyte imbalance and confusion, especially in an elderly patient). When interpreting the results, it should be noted whether the input was measured or just estimated. A simple plastic jug can be used to measure urine output. It is important that the patient understands that he must note *all* voids, even those that could not be measured (e.g. while out), or a very inaccurate picture can be obtained.

Some charts do not specify times but are left blank, to be filled in as necessary. This means that times can be recorded more accurately than to the nearest hour. The assessment chart shown in Figure 3.2 (overleaf) also incorporates information about the patient's behaviour. This requires a nurse's signature, especially useful where patient allocation is not practised, since whoever supervised the episode can be easily

Continence Chart

Week commencing _____ Name _____

Please tick in LEFT column each time urine is passed

Please tick in RIGHT column each time you are wet

	Monday		Tuesday		Wednesday		Thursday		Friday		Saturday		Sunday	
6 am														
7 am														
8 am														
9 am														
10 am														
11 am														
12 pm														
1 pm														
2 pm														
3 pm														
4 pm														
5 pm														
6 pm														
7 pm														
8 pm														
9 pm														
10 pm														
11 pm														
12 am														
1 am														
2 am														
3 am														
4 am														
5 am														
Totals														

Special Instructions

Figure 3.1   *Continence chart.*

CONTINENCE ASSESSMENT CHART

Name...

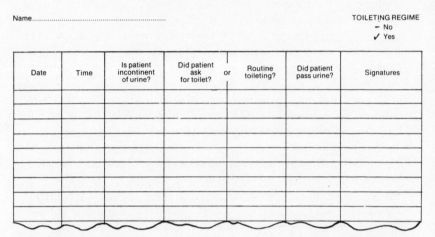

Date	Time	Is patient incontinent of urine?	Did patient ask for toilet?	or	Routine toileting?	Did patient pass urine?	Signatures

Figure 3.2 *Continence assessment chart* (courtesy of Longmore Hospital, Edinburgh).

identified. This chart is obviously designed for use by a nurse or carer, where the patient is unable to be self-caring. It would reveal the patient's pattern of continence and incontinence, his ability to indicate needs, and the success of any toileting programme already being used. It is also useful in distinguishing between whether toileting was requested (i.e. patient-initiated) or nurse-initiated.

If toileting does not result in urine being passed, this may mean either that it is being done at the wrong time, or that sensation is inaccurate (if the patient asked), or possibly that, in the case of a demented patient, the realisation of what a lavatory is for has been lost. If a patient is toileted without result and is subsequently wet within a short period, this may indicate confusion about the social meaning of a lavatory, or possibly that the patient was inhibited from emptying the bladder by lack of privacy, or by being rushed, and is suffering 'respite micturition' when relaxed back in the chair or bed.

Some charts use letters, ticks or dots or other symbols. It must be ensured that instructions as to the use of the symbols are written on the chart, and that staff or the patient have been given adequate teaching to use the symbols with accuracy. Symbols can increase the amount of information which can be gathered in the same space. However, they may also cause confusion if too many different ones are used, or if they are too similar and may be misread.

For some patients it may be useful to record events occurring simultaneously with incontinence, for example, a cough, or severe urgency. It may be useful to have an indication of how wet the patient was, as 'incontinent' may mean anything from a few drops to a bladderful. This might be achieved by indicating when a pad was changed (but remembering this does not always necessarily mean that it was soaked), by indicating 'size of wet patch', or how far it spread (pants only, pad wet, clothes wet, leaked onto floor, bed or chair). However, the only completely accurate assessment of volume entails weighing pads.

Some patients can maintain a 'diary' of events and this can be helpful, especially when external influences are thought to be affecting the overall problem.

When assessing confused patients, it may be useful to record behavioural assessment information on the chart: what the patient was doing prior to the incontinence; what indication, if any, was given that incontinence had occurred (e.g. verbal or activity); and what were the subsequent results, such as how did staff/carers or others around react in response to incontinence? A record showing what happens when the patient voids continently, and how he is responded to when dry, would also be useful (see Chapter 11).

An assessment chart kept for four to seven days will give an accurate picture of the current problem and will help to put the problem into perspective. Indeed, sometimes the mere act of charting actually reduces the incontinence, possibly by focusing the patient's or the staff's attention on the problem (patients who were previously forgetful being more likely to remember to visit the lavatory regularly). It also often happens that a problem which seemed random and out of control is in fact not so bad as was supposed, and the chart shows that the incontinence is reasonably predictable.

SUMMARY OF PROBLEMS

What conclusions may be drawn from the information gathered during this assessment? A detailed picture should have been built up of the individual as well as of the problems causing and caused by incontinence. Table 3.2 (overleaf) summarises the most common relationship of symptoms to medical problems, likely exacerbating factors, and underlying bladder dysfunction. However, it cannot be over-emphasised that many people do not have a simple problem and that any combination of factors may exist. This assessment should

Table 3.2 Relationship of Symptoms to Bladder Dysfunction
(Note – This Table gives broad generalisations only)

PATIENT'S MAIN SYMPTOMS	MOST LIKELY BLADDER DYSFUNCTION	COMMONLY ASSOCIATED MEDICAL PROBLEMS	FACTORS LIKELY TO EXACERBATE SYMPTOMS
Urgency, urge incontinence, frequency, nocturia, nocturnal enuresis	Unstable detrusor	Upper motor neurone lesion, e.g. CVA, multiple sclerosis dementia; or may be 'idiopathic'	Immobility or other physical disabilities Poorly-designed environment Anxiety
'Stress incontinence (leakage upon physical exertion)	Genuine stress incontinence (urethral sphincter incompetence)	Vaginal prolapse Atrophic vaginitis Past obstetric difficulties Post-prostatectomy	Chronic cough Obesity
Dribbling incontinence and/or difficulty voiding	Under-active bladder or outflow obstruction leading to retention with overflow	Lower motor neurone lesion, e.g. diabetic neuropathy Spinal injury Obstructed: prostatic hyperplasia	Faecal impaction
Passive incontinence without warning or apparent reason	Any of above, or no specific bladder dysfunction	Often mental impairment e.g. dementia, confusion, mental handicap	Disorientation, strange surroundings Carers unaware of individual's needs Institutionalisation or poor motivation

have enabled identification of the most likely bladder dysfunction, factors affecting bladder function, and factors affecting the individual's ability to cope with it. In the light of these findings, realistic aims or goals can be set for each individual and a plan of action formulated. A date should be set to review the outcome of planned management.

It is important that wherever possible the nurse has medical support and cooperation, as medication may be required to complete the treatment.

A computerised history-taking and assessment programme has been developed and run by continence advisers. Patients are asked to respond to a structured series of questions. The programme then generates suggestions for further investigations and advice (Dawes et al., 1990).

Where symptoms are mixed or ambiguous, where surgery may be offered, or where treatment of presumed causes has not resulted in continence, further investigation by urodynamic studies may be indicated. While urodynamic studies are by no means essential for every incontinent patient, they are invaluable in contributing to a difficult or doubtful diagnosis.

If no urodynamic investigation facilities are available locally, when indicated, patients should be referred by the general practitioner to the relevant urologist or gynaecologist, or to consider referral further afield. Conversely, urodynamics alone will often not be able to determine why a particular individual is incontinent. The results from such tests must be interpreted in the light of findings from the total assessment.

URODYNAMIC STUDIES

Urodynamic investigations study the pressure, volume and flow relationships in the lower urinary tract. Although such measurements have been made for decades, the science is still emerging and techniques and interpretation of results are not yet universally agreed, although the Standardisation Committee of the International Continence Society has gone a long way towards establishing a common framework (Andersen et al., 1988). The clinical significance of many of the findings remain open to debate, especially in the more sophisticated areas of investigation. This discussion is confined to the simpler and generally accepted findings from urodynamic studies. (For a more detailed discussion of techniques see Chapple and Christmas, 1990, or Mundy et al., 1984).

There are now over 200 centres where urodynamic facilities are available, covering most areas of the UK. The investigation department may be run variously by a urologist, gynaecologist, geriatrician, radiologist or physicist, depending upon local interest and expertise. Often several of these specialists collaborate. Obviously, not every incontinent person is within easy reach of a urodynamic clinic and many have to travel considerable distances to reach one. In many instances the effort is well justified. It is to be hoped that urodynamic clinics will continue to spread so that eventually every health authority will have at least one centre for urodynamic studies (recommendation of the Incontinence Action Group, 1983).

Three investigations form the basis of urodynamic studies: measurement of urinary flow rate, cystometry, and urethral pressure profile.

Flow Rate
The rate of urinary flow during micturition can be measured simply and non-invasively by use of a flow meter (Figure 3.3). The rate at which urine is passed is measured by a weight transducer under the receptacle, an electronic dipstick or by a revolving disc inside the commode itself. A flow rate is expressed in millilitres of urine passed per second. The patient, whose bladder should be comfortably full, is asked to pass urine in privacy (women seated, men usually standing) into the flow meter. The flow rate is recorded on a chart which plots rate against time.

A flow rate is interpreted by rate and pattern. Figure 3.4 shows a normal flow curve. The flow starts promptly, builds up to a good peak rapidly, and then drops again smoothly. When the volume of urine passed is over 200ml, a normal flow rate is at least 15ml per second. Figure 3.5 (overleaf) shows some typical abnormalities.

A flow rate alone has been found to be adequate investigation for nearly half of men with uncomplicated prostatic outflow obstruction (Chapple and Christmas, 1990). Where no flow meter is available, it is possible to get some of the same information by direct observation of urinary flow (but always remembering the possibility that flow may be inhibited during the presence of an observer).

Cystometry
Cystometry, or the performance of a cystometrogram (CMG), is the key investigation in urodynamics. The patient is catheterised, immediately after voiding, with two catheters: one will be used to fill

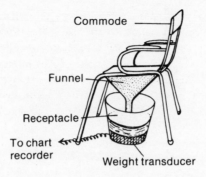

Figure 3.3 *Weight transducer flow meter (may also be dipstick or rotating).*

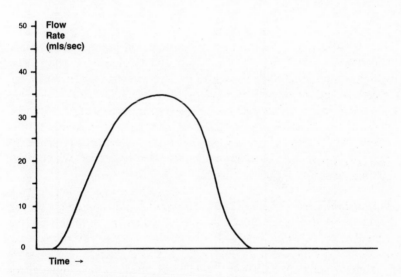

Figure 3.4 *Normal flow curve.*

the bladder, the other to measure bladder (intravesical) pressure. A catheter is also introduced into the rectum (or vagina) to measure abdominal pressure. The bladder-filling catheter is connected to a reservoir of fluid. The two pressure catheters are connected to a chart recorder via pressure transducers (see Figure 3.6, page 60, for diagrammatic representation). A note is made of any residual urine volume in the bladder and any unusual difficulty or sensitivity in passing the catheters.

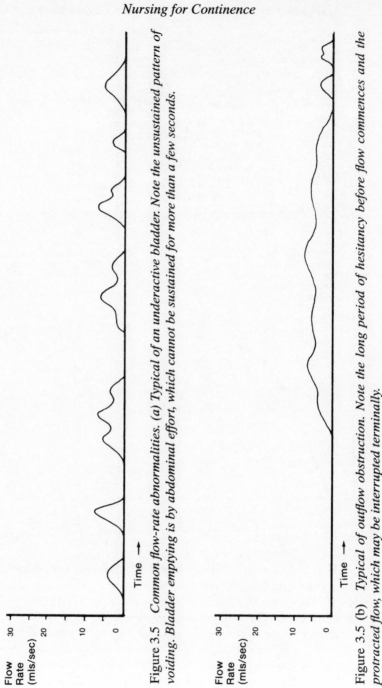

Figure 3.5 *Common flow-rate abnormalities. (a) Typical of an underactive bladder. Note the unsustained pattern of voiding. Bladder emptying is by abdominal effort, which cannot be sustained for more than a few seconds.*

Figure 3.5 (b) *Typical of outflow obstruction. Note the long period of hesitancy before flow commences and the protracted flow, which may be interrupted terminally.*

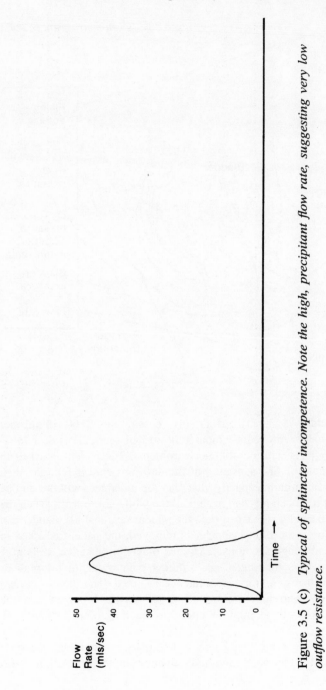

Figure 3.5 (c) *Typical of sphincter incompetence. Note the high, precipitant flow rate, suggesting very low outflow resistance.*

Figure 3.6 *Cystometrogram schema.*

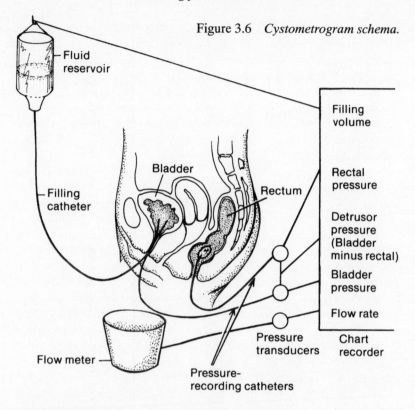

The bladder is then filled rapidly, commonly at 60–100ml per minute, usually with room-temperature normal saline. A slower fill is used for patients with neurological problems. The patient is asked to indicate when the first sensation of the desire to void is felt, and then when the maximum capacity that can be tolerated without undue discomfort has been reached, trying all the while not to leak. When the subjective capacity is reached (i.e., the patient says that his bladder can hold no more), the filling catheter is removed, the patient is asked to stand up and cough vigorously. Various other 'provocative' tests may be tried, such as running a tap, drinking cold water, or jumping or walking on the spot. Any incontinence is noted. The patient is then instructed to void into a flow meter, as above. In midstream the patient is asked to attempt to interrupt the flow, and then void to completion.

The purpose of the rectal line is to monitor abdominal pressure. Because the bladder is an intra-abdominal organ, the pressure inside it reflects both actual bladder activity and general abdominal pressure changes. All movement and activities affect total bladder pressure, but these pressure changes are not necessarily the bladder itself doing anything. If bladder pressure alone were measured, it would be very difficult to distinguish a bladder contraction from, say, the patient straining. The rectal pressure is measured to take account of these general abdominal pressure changes, and the chart recorder subtracts rectal pressure from total bladder pressure to give a reading of bladder activity alone – that is, *detrusor pressure.*

Figure 3.7 (overleaf) shows the trace from a normal cysto-metrogram. Residual urine should be zero. The pressure rise during filling of the bladder should be minimal. The bladder expands to accept urine without the intravesical pressure rising very much. First desire to void is usually felt at about half of capacity, and total comfortable volume is usually 400–600ml. Even at capacity the bladder should be stable and not contract. Vigorous coughing and provocative tests should not cause incontinence or bladder contractions. When the patient is instructed to void, the bladder should contract smoothly (with a pressure around 30–40cm H_2O for women, 50–60cm H_2O for men), and the flow start very soon afterwards. The patient should be able to interrupt flow promptly, initially by closing the sphincter and then by inhibiting the contraction, and be able to re-start at will. The bladder should empty completely.

It is usually possible to conduct a cystometrogram with minimal embarrassment and discomfort to the patient. Great care should be taken to explain the procedure fully, both before the test and while it is in progress. Every effort should be made to maintain the maximum privacy possible. Where feasible, it is usually preferable that someone of the same sex as the patient should perform the catheterisation and supervise the procedure. If the patient is very anxious or frightened the results of the tests are often difficult to interpret, as it may be difficult to distinguish between inhibited voiding and a genuine voiding difficulty.

Figures 3.8 to 3.12 show several of the most common abnormalities to be diagnosed by cystometrogram. Figure 3.8 (pages 64–5) shows an unstable detrusor. The patient is unable to inhibit contractions during filling, and bladder capacity is usually lowered. Incontinence may occur if bladder contractions are high enough. Contractions or a pressure rise more than 15cm H_2O are taken by some researchers as the threshold for diagnosing an unstable detrusor, although this figure is no longer recognised by the International Continence Society. Figure 3.9

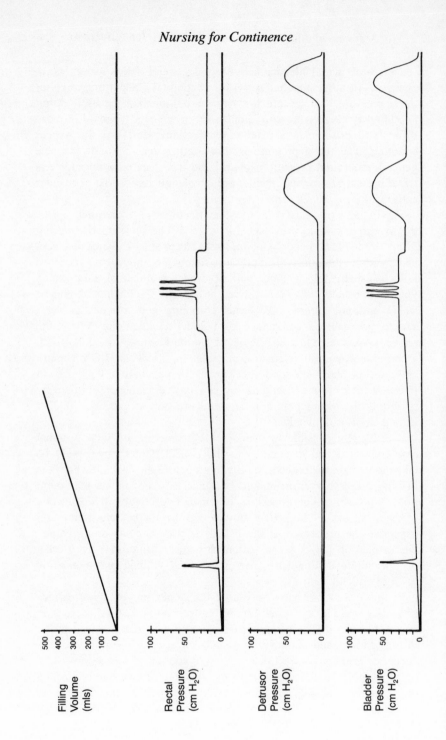

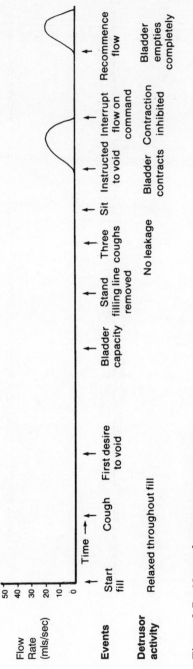

Figure 3.7 *Normal cystometrogram trace.*

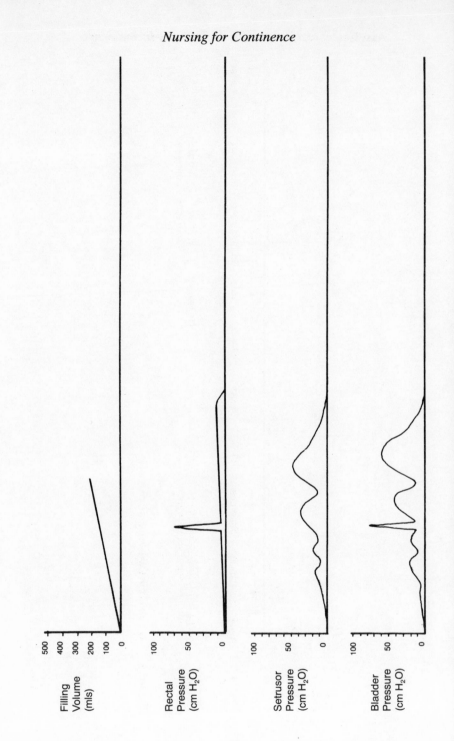

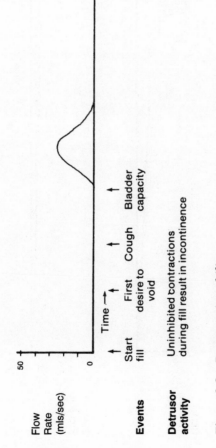

Figure 3.8 *Detrusor instability.*

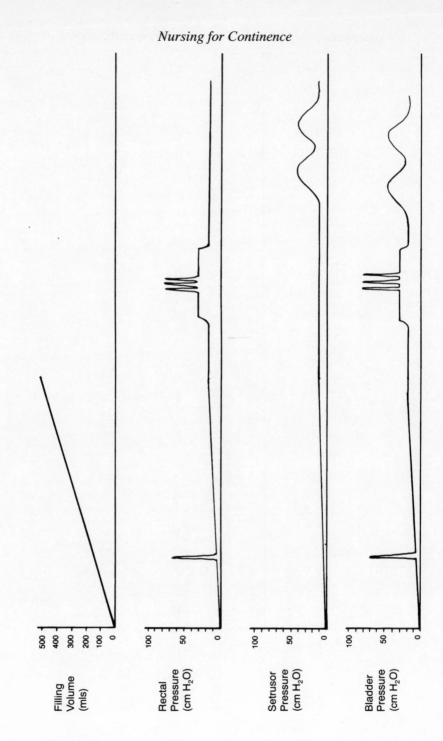

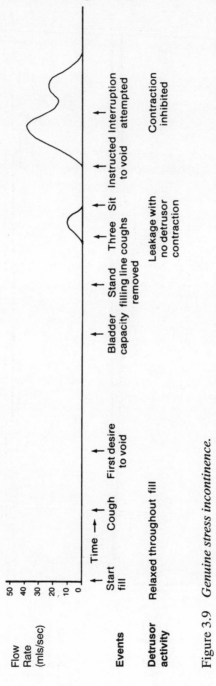

Figure 3.9 *Genuine stress incontinence.*

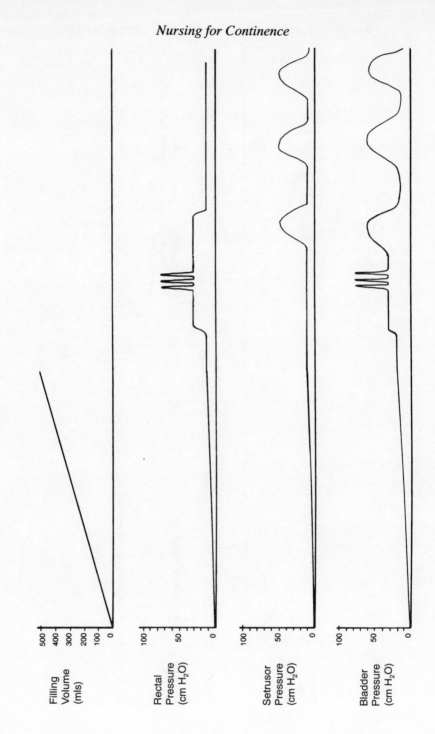

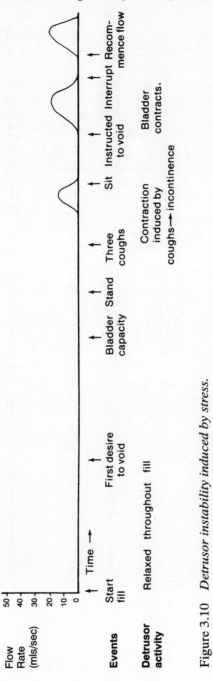

Figure 3.10 *Detrusor instability induced by stress.*

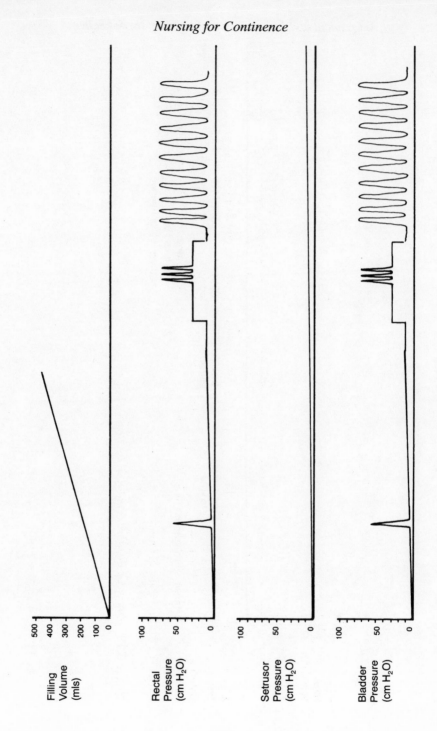

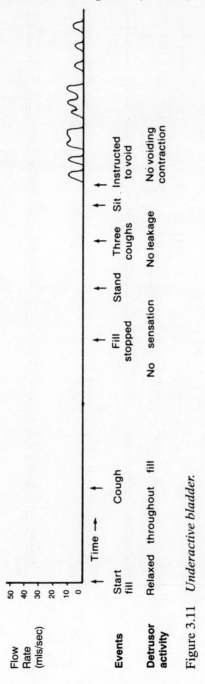

Figure 3.11 *Underactive bladder.*

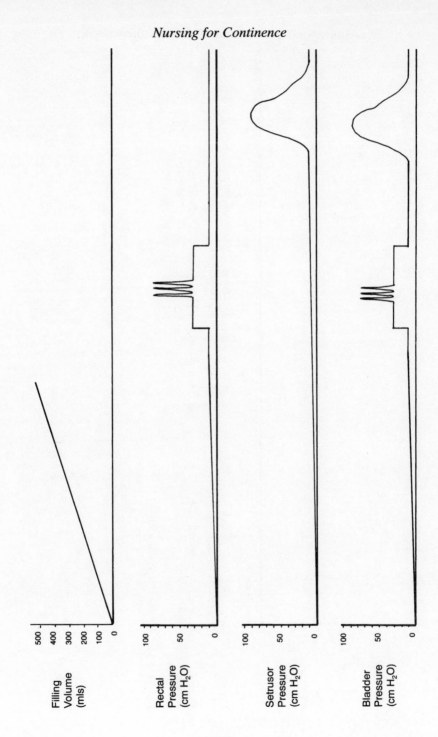

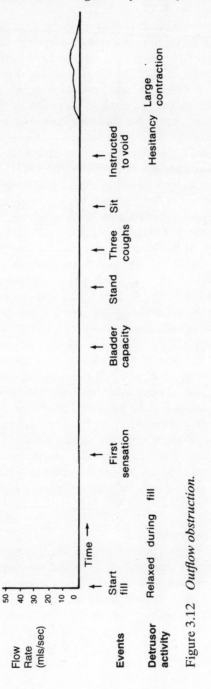

Figure 3.12 *Outflow obstruction.*

(pages 66–7) shows genuine stress incontinence – essentially normal bladder function with incontinence during coughing and usually a high flow rate, low voiding pressure, and often impaired ability to interrupt flow. Figure 3.10 (pages 68–9) shows an unstable detrusor mimicking stress incontinence. This is an easily missed diagnosis as incontinence does occur with effort, but as a result of the cough triggering a bladder contraction and not because the sphincter is incompetent. Figure 3.11 (pages 70–71) shows an underactive bladder with a large residual urine volume, an increased capacity, delayed or absent sensation, and no voiding contraction – any voiding which occurs is achieved by pelvic floor relaxation or abdominal effort. Figure 3.12 (pages 72–3) shows outflow obstruction. Voiding pressure is high in an attempt to overcome outflow resistance, but the resultant flow is poor.

Thus the physiological bladder dysfunctions described in Chapter 2 can be accurately differentiated by cystometrogram. Increasingly, the results of urodynamic studies are being recorded directly onto computer programmes which can analyse an ever-widening number of parameters and relationships. Added sophistication can be gained by performing cystometry under X-ray control (video-cystourethrography). The bladder is filled with X-ray contrast instead of saline, and may be visualised during filling, coughing and voiding. This is especially useful in distinguishing bladder-neck abnormalities and in locating the site of an obstruction. Bladder diverticula, reflux of urine into the ureters, and various other abnormalities may be revealed. More recently, technological advances have led to 'ambulatory urodynamics', with equipment to continually monitor detrusor pressure over a period of hours, even in a mobile patient. This has become a useful research tool. It also appears that a proportion of patients have an unstable detrusor which is not manifest on static CMG, but which will be revealed by ambulatory monitoring over a longer period.

Urethral Pressure Profile
Intra-urethral pressure can be measured by using either a water-filled or a microtransducer catheter, which is withdrawn slowly along the urethra with the patient in a supine or semi-recumbent position. A recording is obtained of urethral pressure from the bladder neck to the external meatus as the catheter is gradually withdrawn. A cough profile may be obtained by asking the patient to cough repeatedly during withdrawal of the catheter. Leaving the catheter static in mid-urethra may record abnormal pressure falls in urethral pressure ('urethral

instability'). At present this investigation is mostly used as a research tool, and the full significance of many of the findings remain open to debate.

Electromyography

Electromyography (EMG) studies the electrical potentials generated by the depolarisation of the striated muscle of the urethral sphincter. Needle or skin surface electrodes may be used. The results need skilled interpretation. EMG is mostly used with patients with neuropathic problems or as a research tool.

REFERENCES AND FURTHER READING

Andersen, J. T., Abrams, P., Blaivas, J. G., Stanton, S. L., 1988. The standardisation of terminology of lower urinary tract function. *Scandinavian Journal of Urology and Nephrology*, Supplement, 114: 5–19.

Bernard, M. A., 1994. Urinary incontinence in elderly females. *Journal of Oklahoma State Medical Association*, 87: 217–24.

Brocklehurst, J. C., 1990. Urinary incontinence in old age: helping the general practitioner to make a diagnosis. *Gerontology*: 36: 3–7.

Chapple, C. R., Christmas, T. J., 1990. *Urodynamics made Easy*. Churchill Livingstone, Edinburgh and London.

Counsel and Care for the Elderly, 1991. Not such private places. Counsel and Care, London.

Dawes, H., Small, D., Glen, E., 1990. Adding computers to the armoury. *Nursing Times*, 86, 46: 68–9.

Duffin, H., 1992. Assessment of urinary incontinence. In: B. H. Roe (ed). *Clinical Nursing Practice: The Promotion and Management of Continence* (1st edn), 1–16. Prentice-Hall, Hemel Hempstead.

Incontinence Action Group, 1983. Action on incontinence. Kings Fund Centre, London.

Joseph, A., 1992. Joseph continence assessment tool. *Urologic Nursing*, 12, 4: 144–6.

McFarlane, J., Castledine G., 1982. *A Guide to the Practice of Nursing Using the Process of Nursing*. Mosby, St. Louis (Chapter 4).

Mundy, A. R., Stephenson, T. P., Wein, A. J. (eds), 1984. *Urodynamics: Principles, Practice and Application*. Churchill Livingstone, Edinburgh and London.

Norton, C., 1982. The effects of urinary incontinence in women. *International Rehabilitation Medicine*, 4: 9–14.

Roper, N., Logan, W. W., Tierney, A. J., 1990. *The Elements of Nursing*. Churchill Livingstone, Edinburgh and London.

Chapter 4

Treating and Managing Urinary Incontinence

Christine Norton, MA, RGN

Clinical Nurse Specialist (Continence),
St Mark's Hospital, Harrow, Middlesex

The principles involved in treating or managing urinary incontinence which are relevant to any incontinent person are covered in this chapter. Later chapters cover aspects relevant to specific client groups, so the present chapter should be considered in conjunction with as many of the later chapters as apply to any individual.

All interventions must be planned in the light of information gathered during the assessment and investigation of the individual's incontinence, as outlined in Chapter 3. The aim of treatment is to alter those factors which have been found to be causing incontinence. Management is aimed at ameliorating the effects of being incontinent upon the individual and carers. Obviously treatment, aimed at 'cure', and management, aimed at improved quality of life and coping, cannot be completely separated, and usually both will be implemented at the same time.

Sometimes one single intervention is indicated. This tends to be the case for the younger, otherwise fit, incontinent person where the sole cause is a bladder dysfunction. In other cases a complex interrelated package of interventions, involving several different team members, will be needed. There are very few people for whom any attempt at cure is inappropriate, usually only critically or terminally ill people and those with profound dementia. For the majority, cure or considerable improvement is possible and should be attempted. However, it is certainly likely in the foreseeable future that there will be a substantial minority who cannot regain total continence. For these people, efficient and appropriate management methods are essential if incontinence is not to be a handicap in its own right.

THE MULTIDISCIPLINARY TEAM

In a well-integrated multidisciplinary team, each member has a role to play in helping incontinent people. Although the strict differentiation of roles is artificial, and in practice they often overlap, each profession has a sphere of expertise which may be of use to a particular patient.

The nurse has a key role in giving advice and support to the incontinent individual and his family or carers, whether the problem is being treated or has been found to be intractable. Minimising the effect of incontinence upon the patient and surroundings means that most people can lead a relatively normal life despite their incontinence. Wherever the nurse is advising the patient or relatives about the condition, the basic principles of teaching should always be remembered. If information is to be retained, it should be imparted in small amounts and repeated often. Written information is useful, as this can be read later. (See Appendices 1 and 2 for organisations which provide information leaflets and Appendix 4 for useful patient books.) It will often be a nurse who takes a lead role in a bladder training programme and in advising on the most suitable products to use.

The role of the nurse and doctor overlap to a considerable extent. Much of the advice described below, and bladder training (pages 87–92), might equally well be initiated by a nurse or doctor. Many specific drug and surgical treatments, aimed at remedying the underlying bladder dysfunction, may also be initiated by doctors.

The physiotherapist, whether in hospital or community, can assess the patient's mobility and dexterity, and implement a treatment plan if these could be usefully improved. Extending the range and strength of movements may make it easier for the patient to get to, or on to, the lavatory. A demonstration of safe lifting techniques may prevent accidents or strains in cases where an assistant is involved in aiding transfers. Where a walking-aid or wheelchair is used, the physiotherapist can ensure that these are optimal for the individual's needs. For stress incontinence a patient may be referred for pelvic floor exercises (with or without electrical stimulation, Chapter 6).

The occupational therapist is skilled in helping the individual towards independence in the activities of daily living, including personal hygiene and toileting. Techniques may be used to improve function, or aids provided to maximise the abilities present. Modifications to clothing, alternatives to the lavatory, and implements to aid washing or dressing can all be tailored to the specific needs of the individual.

Social workers have extensive knowledge of local facilities and can mobilise and coordinate resources in the community. It may be possible to arrange modifications to the home, attendance at a day centre or luncheon club, home care assistants or laundry services, voluntary services and financial assistance, according to the individual's needs (Chapter 12). A social worker will often be the 'key worker' in mobilising community care packages.

A psychologist can be of particular help to patients who have psychological problems or learning disabilities and where incontinence is felt to be a behavioural problem. A detailed psychological assessment will enable a treatment plan to be made to meet the needs of the individual. The psychologist may also be involved in treating psychologically disturbed patients and in counselling patients, families, and other staff members. In the community, the community psychiatric nurse may fulfil this role. The community nurse for learning disabilities works closely with clinical psychologists and special schools (Chapter 14).

Where appropriate, a variety of other professionals may become involved with an incontinent person. The chiropodist can make a great difference to mobility. The optician may help to improve the patient's vision and make mobility safe. The dietitian or dentist may be involved in ensuring that the patient can eat a healthy diet.

The nurse must be aware of the potential contribution of all of these professionals and know when referral is appropriate. Often restoration of continence is only one aspect of a comprehensive rehabilitation programme designed to achieve maximum possible independence for each patient.

EXPLAINING THE PROBLEM

Many people lack knowledge about how the body functions, and understanding of incontinence is often based on misconceptions. A clear explanation of the working of the lower urinary tract and why it has gone wrong will help the patient to participate in therapy. The patient who understands the cause can be a much more active participant in tackling problems, yet the tendency of many health professionals is to remove that responsibility from the individual by not imparting sufficient information. Where the patient is unable to learn, the rest of the family can usually benefit from teaching (Norton, 1983).

Information will also help the patient and his family to come to an informed decision about treatment options, if alternatives exist. For instance, if surgery is suggested the patient has the right to know what is involved, what the chances of success are, and what risks or side effects there may be. Although the surgeon would discuss these, it is often the nurse to whom the patient turns for detailed information. Many people are reluctant to ask what they feel might be 'obvious' questions or to reveal their fears or ignorance, and the nurse must allow time and offer appropriate prompts to help the patient to make a decision. It must be up to the individual to decide how far treatment is to be pursued.

PSYCHOLOGICAL SUPPORT

The nurse's attitude and approach towards a person with continence problems should demonstrate that incontinence is not seen as something to be ashamed of, but as a symptom to be dealt with. The guilt, shame and embarrassment felt by many incontinent people (and their relatives on their behalf) can be eased by a nurse who treats the individual with respect. This is vital, as so many incontinent people lose all self-esteem and confidence and become pessimistic about the possibilities of improvement. The nurse must feel comfortable and unembarrassed about discussing intimate details if the patient is to be able to express all his fears and worries. It may be tempting to brush away unfounded fears quickly, but a brusque 'of course you don't smell', or 'nobody thinks you are a baby', or 'of course your husband/wife/partner still finds you attractive' will do little to reassure. It may also lead the nurse to fail to understand the real problem – what constitutes a problem to the patient may not be obvious to the nurse. Unless a close and trusting relationship is developed, the nurse may never be able to empathise with the patient and realise what help is needed.

Support may take different forms. Sometimes just listening is enough. A sounding-board for the expression of feelings, especially frustration and anger, can be useful in defusing tensions within a family. Often, the individual can be helped to reach his own solutions by a nurse who listens, encourages, and prompts full expression of the problems, rather than by a nurse who talks continuously and leaves no space for any response.

Improving the incontinent person's self-image is an essential element to enable coping with incontinence (Gartley, 1987). If interpersonal or sexual relationships have suffered because of the incontinence, considerable encouragement is often needed before there is any attempt to resume normal relationships. Fear of rejection is powerful and restricting.

Relatives who are caring for a heavily incontinent person at home are in as much need of support as the patient. It is not difficult to see how relatives might come to feel inadequate and hopeless, guilty that they are not doing all they could, especially if comparing themselves with a nurse who appears very competent and able to cope. The district nurse visiting under such circumstances may usefully spend as much time reassuring and listening to the carer as giving nursing care to the patient.

Some incontinent people are in need of more formal psychological help, and where the nurse does not have the appropriate training or expertise it may be better to consider referral to a counsellor, psychiatrist, psychologist or sexual dysfunction clinic, rather than attempt to support the patient alone. The nurse must recognise her own limitations and be able to recognise the point at which another professional would be of greater help to the patient.

TREATING URINARY INCONTINENCE

There is an ever-expanding range of therapeutic options for treating urinary incontinence. Most are specific to a given cause of incontinence, which is why assessment and diagnosis is so crucial. Unless the cause is known, it is extremely difficult to select the most appropriate treatment.

Table 4.1 summarises the major options and indicates in which chapter of this book they are dealt with.

Table 4.1   *Treatment Options for Urinary Incontinence Caused by Bladder Dysfunction*

DIAGNOSIS	CONSERVATIVE	DRUG	SURGERY
Genuine stress incontinence	Pelvic floor exercises (6) Cones (6) Electrotherapy (6) Pessaries (6)	Oestrogens (11) Alpha stimulants (6)	Vaginal (6) Suprapubic (6) Endoscopic (6) Neourethra (6) Artificial sphincter (7)
Unstable detrusor	Bladder training (4) Enuresis alarm (5) Alternative therapies (4) Electrical stimulation (4)	Anticholinergics (4)	Clam cystoplasty (4) Neurectomy (4) Ileal conduit (4)
Outflow obstruction	Indwelling catheter (9) Appliance (15) Intermittent catheter (8) Disimpact (10)	Alpha Blockers (7) 5-alpha reductase inhibitors (7)	Prostatectomy (7) Urethrotomy (7) Stent (7)
Underactive bladder	Intermittent catheter (8) Voiding techniques (8)	Carbachol Bethanechol Distigmine (4)	Electrical implant (4)
Severe intractable (any cause)	Pads (15) Appliance (15) Catheter (9)		Artificial sphincter (7) Ileal conduit (4) Continent diversion (4)

(Numbers in brackets refer to the chapter which deals with each treatment.)

Note: It is not uncommon for a patient to have more than one condition coexisting, in which case the predominant problem should usually be treated first.

Drug Therapy

Many different drugs are prescribed to help people with urinary incontinence. There is certainly no 'wonder drug' for any type of incontinence. However, considerable progress has been made in recent years and there are some drugs which may be useful for carefully selected and accurately diagnosed patients. Table 4.2 lists those most commonly used.

Table 4.2   Drug Therapy for Urinary Incontinence

CONDITION	DRUG	MODE OF ACTION
Unstable Detrusor		
	Oxybutynin hydrochloride	Antispasmodic/ anticholinergic
	Imipramine hydrochloride	Anticholinergic + ? central
	Propantheline bromide	Anticholinergic
	Flavoxate hydrochloride	Antispasmodic
Genuine Stress Incontinence		
	Phenylpropanolamine hydrocholoride	Sympathomimetic
	Ephedrine hydrochloride	Sympathomimetic
	Oestrogen replacement	Oestrogenisation
Outflow Obstruction		
	Prazosin hydrochloride	Selective alpha-1 blocker
	Indoramin	Selective alpha-1 blocker
	Phenoxybenzamine hydrochloride	Non-selective alpha blocker
	Finasteride	Selective 5-alpha reductase inhibitor
Underactive Bladder		
	Bethanechol chloride	Cholinergic
	Carbachol	Cholinergic
	Neostigmine bromide	Anticholinesterase
	Distigmine bromide	Anticholinesterase
Bedwetting		
	As unstable detrusor	See above
	Desmopressin	Antidiuretic

Unstable Detrusor

The control of unstable bladder contractions and urge incontinence, by using a drug to relax the detrusor muscle or inhibit reflex contractions, seems to offer one of the most promising areas for drug therapy. Most have side effects if given in high enough doses to be effective, and this can be so troublesome as to make the treatment unacceptable.

In trials, a placebo effect has been found to be considerable. It seems likely that the general advice, concern and bladder training which usually goes with the prescription of these medications may often be as important as the drug itself. This is not to say that drugs cannot be very useful, especially in the initial stages of treating a patient with urge incontinence or nocturnal enuresis. Their effect can help with the introduction and acceptance of a bladder training programme. For some people the drug alone will be effective in curing incontinence, although there is a tendency for relapse if medication is withdrawn. Used in combination with a retraining programme, the patient can often be weaned from the medication once a normal bladder pattern has been attained. Oxybutynin is probably the most acceptable first choice for therapy, combining reasonable success rates with few side effects if used in low doses. Imipramine is also useful. New drugs with greater specificity for the bladder and therefore fewer side effects are under development.

Because the purpose of all these drugs is to reduce bladder contractions, they should be used with great care with patients who have a voiding difficulty, since urinary retention may be precipitated. Careful prior assessment will have included a measurement of residual urine; drug therapy should be introduced with great caution in cases where the volume is over 100ml.

Genuine Stress Incontinence

Drugs have been used in an attempt to treat stress incontinence by increasing urethral tone. Phenylpropanolamine and ephedrine are the most commonly used, especially in children, and are thought to act on the alpha receptors in the urethra.

Oestrogen replacement therapy can improve urinary symptoms in the presence of an atrophic urethra (see Chapter 11).

Outflow Obstruction

Drug therapy may be used to relieve outflow obstruction. Phenoxybenzamine is the most commonly used but may have very troublesome side effects (tachycardia and postural hypotension), and must be used with great caution. 5-alpha reductase inhibitors and alpha-blocking agents may reduce obstruction due to benign prostatic hyperplasia. Chapter 7 discusses this in more detail.

Underactive Bladder
Where the bladder will not contract sufficiently to ensure complete bladder emptying, drug therapy may be tried to improve the force of the voiding contraction. Carbachol, bethanechol and distigmine bromide have all been used, with limited success. All may produce unacceptable side effects if used in effective doses.

Bedwetting
Antidiuretic hormone, as desmopressin, can be used for adults or children with night-time wetting. Although not curative, it will give symptomatic relief to a high proportion of people (Chapter 5). The same drugs as used for an unstable detrusor may also be helpful.

Other Drugs
Other drugs may be useful in treating factors influencing bladder function, for instance appropriate antibiotics to treat a urinary tract infection or laxatives to treat or prevent constipation. Many drugs may exacerbate a tendency to incontinence, and the physician should be aware that drugs prescribed for many conditions may be adversely affecting bladder function (see Table 2.2, pages 26–7).

A policy of choosing medication with minimal effects on continence should be pursued, where possible, with all people vulnerable to incontinence. For example, a slow-acting diuretic, in a divided dose, may allow those with urgency to avoid urge incontinence. An analgesic may be preferable to night sedation for those who wet the bed at night and need pain relief.

Surgery for Urinary Incontinence
Urinary incontinence is unfortunately sometimes the result of surgery, usually urological or gynaecological, but also major pelvic or spinal operations. This iatrogenic incontinence may be caused by neurological or mechanical damage, leading to any of the bladder dysfunctions.

As with drug therapy, surgery designed to remedy incontinence is best considered according to the bladder problem it aims to solve. Table 4.3 summarises the most common surgical options.

Table 4.3   Surgery for Urinary Incontinence

CONDITION	SURGICAL OPTIONS	CHAPTER
Genuine Stress Incontinence	Stamey or Raz	6
	Colposuspension	6
	Sling	6
	Collagen injection	6
	Artificial sphincter	7
Unstable Detrusor	Phenol injection	4
	Sacral neurectomy	4
	Clam ileocystoplasty	4
Outflow Obstruction	Prostatectomy	7
	Stent	7
	Urethrotomy	7
	Urethral dilatation	7
Underactive Bladder	Electrical implant	
Severe Intractable Incontinence	Ileal conduit	4
	Continent diversion	4

Genuine Stress Incontinence
Where stress incontinence is caused by an incompetent sphincter mechanism in women, the experienced surgeon can offer either suprapubic or, generally less successfully, vaginal surgery (Chapter 6). In men a damaged sphincter may be repaired by a prosthesis (Chapter 7). These are the most commonly performed operations for the treatment of incontinence and, if diagnosis and surgical technique are correct, excellent results are usual.

Unstable Detrusor
None of the several surgical approaches which have been tried to treat the unstable bladder has gained widespread use. In experienced hands surgery can be effective, but the condition tends to recur and it is difficult to envisage general acceptance. Cystodistension (stretching the bladder under general anaesthetic), phenol injection into the sympathetic pelvic nerves, bladder transection and selective sacral neurectomy are all presumed to act by disturbing the neurological pathways which control uninhibited contractions (Murray and Mundy, 1989). They are most used where the instability has a neuropathic origin (detrusor hyperreflexia).

The 'clam' ileocystoplasty (Figure 4.1) is a major procedure used to treat a severely intractable unstable detrusor. The bladder is split in half and opened up like a clam. A segment of ileum, isolated with its own blood supply, is then sewn onto the bladder as a patch to augment bladder capacity and absorb unstable contractions. However, the bowel segment continues to produce mucus, which can cause problems in the bladder; a mucus plug can even cause retention. Many patients have difficulty emptying the bladder completely after this operation, and some need to use intermittent self-catheterisation. Metabolic imbalance may occur and the long-term risk of bowel malignancies developing in the bladder is unclear. However, it can produce good results for a person who would otherwise be incapacitated by very severe frequency and urge incontinence.

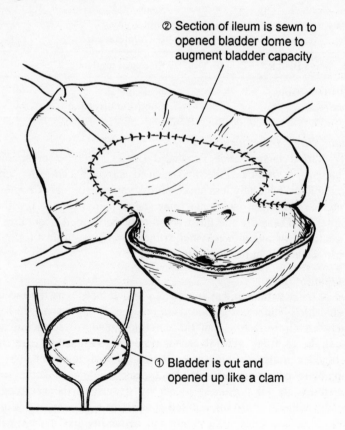

② Section of ileum is sewn to opened bladder dome to augment bladder capacity

① Bladder is cut and opened up like a clam

Figure 4.1   *Clam ileocystoplasty.*

Outflow Obstruction
Surgery may be used to relieve outflow obstruction, for example, to remove an enlarged prostate gland (Chapter 7), divide a stricture or widen a narrow urethra (urethrotomy). If any of these procedures are performed by an inexperienced surgeon there is a risk of rendering the patient incontinent.

Severe Intractable Incontinence
Some people with severe intractable incontinence which has failed to improve, despite all treatment efforts, may wish to consider major surgery to correct this. For those with a damaged urethra, a neourethra can be constructed from a bladder flap, or else an artificial sphincter can be inserted (Chapter 7). Occasionally a whole new bladder is constructed from bowel anastamosed to the trigone of the bladder. In some instances a urinary diversion into an ileal conduit with a stoma can bring tremendous benefits, especially for women (who do not have the option of using an incontinence appliance). Although a seemingly drastic solution, a stoma is often much easier to cope with than an incontinent urethra, because an effective appliance will contain the urine. Extensive pre-operative counselling is essential for people considering this option, and wherever possible an experienced stoma care nurse should become involved with the patient and family.

More recently, a 'continent diversion' has been devised. The ureters are diverted into a pouch constructed from bowel (Koch's pouch), with a continent stoma, which can be catheterised intermittently. Alternatively, with a Mitrofanoff procedure the bladder may be retained, the bladder neck closed surgically and a narrow conduit inserted between the bladder and the skin (using, for example, the appendix or a piece of ureter). The conduit is then used as a channel for intermittent catheterisation. The long-term results of continent diversion have yet to be proven. Some patients experience fluid and electrolyte disturbances, stone formation and even metabolic acidosis.

Bladder Training
'Bladder training' or 'retraining' is a much misused and misunderstood term in nursing. Nearly every nurse who has incontinent patients will, if asked, claim to be practising 'bladder training'. It is very common to read in nursing care plans: 'Problem – incontinence; planned action – bladder training'. There is rarely any elaboration on what is meant by the term, how such training is to be carried out, or what the ultimate goal may be (other than a very general 'the patient will regain

continence'). Bladder training has come to be seen as a panacea for incontinence, a treatment which is universally applicable. In practice, the 'training' often amounts to nothing more than reminding the patient or taking him to the lavatory every two hours.

Cheater (1991) has highlighted the inconsistencies in the understanding of terms and criteria for patient selection, even amongst continence advisers. The differences between the methods are far from clear-cut, and there remains an urgent need for standard definitions so that results can be validly compared.

Bladder training is indeed a useful nursing tool, but only when used appropriately by a nurse who understands the technique and knows how to select a programme appropriate to the individual's needs. Success is highly unlikely if every incontinent person is treated identically. It is important that any other factors contributing to the incontinence have already been diagnosed and are being treated – for instance, a urinary tract infection or constipation – as these will certainly impair the success of a programme.

Bladder training programmes are most suitable for people with the symptoms of frequency, urgency and urge incontinence (with or without an underlying unstable detrusor), and for those with a non-specific incontinence which they are unable to account for and which seems to 'just happen'. Elderly patients in institutional care very often have this non-specific incontinence. Programmes for elderly mentally infirm people and people with learning disabilities are covered in Chapters 11 and 14 respectively.

Patients with a bladder dysfunction other than an unstable bladder are less likely to benefit from bladder training. A woman with an incompetent urethral sphincter, and consequent stress incontinence, will seldom be able to regain continence by manipulating her lavatory visits, although there is some evidence that retraining may help (US Department of Health, 1992). She may be able to keep the bladder relatively empty so that only a little urine is in it, but her underlying sphincter weakness will remain. Even if she has just passed urine, the next time she coughs she is likely to leak. Similarly, the person with urinary retention and overflow incontinence will seldom be helped by training. This emphasises the importance of thorough assessment and accurate diagnosis prior to the implementation of any treatment programme.

Bladder Retraining for Urge Incontinence

The aim of bladder retraining is to restore the patient with frequency, urgency and urge incontinence to a more normal and convenient micturition pattern. The objective is that voiding should occur only every three to four hours (or even longer), without any urgency or incontinence. When the bladder is known or thought to be unstable, drug therapy is often combined with the bladder training.

The key to success is accurate record-keeping and frequent professional contact and support. Retraining may be used with success with inpatients or outpatients. Occasionally patients may be admitted to hospital specifically to undergo a retraining programme (gynaecologists in particular may use inpatient programmes, Frewen, 1978; Jarvis and Millar, 1980).

The patient must fully understand this treatment and enthusiastically participate in it – there is no doubt that it can be very demanding for the patient. A lot of time must be spent at the outset explaining the programme in detail, emphasising that only the patient's own willpower can make it a success. Initially, a clear description of normal bladder function and why and how it has gone wrong should be given. If, for whatever reason, the patient cannot or will not cooperate, there is little point in attempting this type of bladder retraining.

It should be explained that the bladder for some reason (usually unknown or because of some neurological disease) has become 'overactive' and 'over-sensitive'. The individual may have experienced urge incontinence. The natural reaction to this embarrassing experience is to try to prevent it happening again. Usually the patient will develop a habit of rushing to the lavatory at the first hint of bladder filling, in order to preempt an accident. Since the bladder fills continuously (and most people can sense some urine in the bladder if they think about it), it is not difficult to see how a vicious circle of passing urine more and more frequently can develop. The person anxious about incontinence is likely to interpret any slight bladder sensation as an urgent need to pass urine, and immediately interrupt activities to seek a lavatory. Anxiety or worry merely enhances the sensation of urgency.

In extreme cases, someone's life may become completely ruled by the need to pass urine every ten to fifteen minutes. Few people get to this unhappy state, but many visit the lavatory every hour or half-hour throughout the day. In spite of this level of frequency, they may also experience urge incontinence, especially if they have an unstable bladder. If someone gets up and rushes to the lavatory while the bladder is contracting, incontinence is very likely. Women are more vulnerable than men, because of a lower urethral resistance. 'Key-in-the-lock' incontinence may develop. The person can hang on while rushing urgently home, but wets on the front doorstep while fumbling to get the door unlocked, or gets to the lavatory but is incontinent while trying to remove clothing.

Bladder training aims to restore the individual's confidence in the bladder's ability to hold urine, and to re-establish a more normal pattern of voiding. Initially the patient should keep a baseline chart for three to seven days, recording how often urine is passed and when incontinence occurs. This is then reviewed with the nurse or doctor supervising the programme, and an individual regime is devised. The purpose is gradually to extend the time interval between visits to the lavatory, encouraging the patient to practise hanging on, rather than to give in to the urgency. Initially the times chosen should not be too difficult to achieve.

The times may be at set intervals throughout the day (e.g. every hour or two hours), or variable, according to the individual's pattern as shown by the baseline chart. For example, someone taking diuretics in the morning might need to go hourly in the morning, every hour-and-a-half in the middle of the day, and two-hourly in the evening. Someone who has fixed time commitments (e.g. working, or taking children to school) might need times to fit in with travelling or meal breaks. Every attempt should be made to make the programme as convenient as possible, as it is then much more likely to be followed. If the baseline chart reveals a definite pattern to the incontinence it may be possible to set toileting times to anticipate this. If someone is always wet at 3.30 p.m., a good time would be 3 p.m.

The patient is therefore set a pattern of toileting times throughout the day. Usually no times are set at night, even if nocturia or nocturnal enuresis are problematic. The patient is instructed to pass urine as necessary at night. Sometimes it is useful to set an alarm clock to anticipate a known peak wetting time. This is often unnecessary, because nocturnal problems will often resolve once daytime frequency has returned to normal.

The patient is asked to pass urine at the set times and to attempt to hang on in between. Sometimes the provision of a suitable pad or appliance will add to confidence and mean that if incontinence does occur, the results will not be too disastrous. If urgency is experienced, the patient must sit or stand still and try to suppress it, rather than rush immediately to find a lavatory. A normal fluid intake is encouraged, as the aim is to enable the patient to be continent and able to drink whatever is wanted. However, many people with an unstable detrusor find that it is helpful to avoid caffeine (see also page 99).

As the patient achieves the target intervals, without having to go prematurely or leaking urine, the intervals should gradually be lengthened. The speed of progress in this is very individual and will depend on many variables, such as initial severity of symptoms, motivation, and the amount of professional support. Outpatients will often need to remain at one time interval for one to two weeks before this is extended at the next clinic visit. Inpatients may have their programmes reviewed much more often, even daily in some cases. It is usual to increase the time interval by fifteen minutes to half-an-hour at a time, but again this will vary considerably and some people will manage leaps of an hour at a time. Any times which seem particularly difficult should be adjusted to suit individual needs, e.g. someone who habitually drinks four mugs of tea at breakfast will probably never achieve a four-hourly voiding interval in the morning. An intelligent patient who understands fully the purpose of the programme will often adjust the time intervals independently and be able to progress considerably between clinic visits.

Once the target of three- to four-hourly voiding without urgency has been achieved, it is useful to carry on keeping the charts and set times for at least another month to prevent relapse. Some people take several months to achieve this, whereas others may need only a few weeks. There seems to be no way of predicting how long bladder training is likely to take for each individual. Filling in the charts consistently is vital in assessing progress, and gives the patient useful feedback that results are positive.

An alternative to bladder training by pre-set time intervals is to instruct the patient gradually to extend the time interval between the first sensation of urgency and actually passing urine. Instead of setting a pattern to aim for, the patient tries to hang on for ever-increasing intervals after feeling the need to go, and so gradually spaces out toilet visits. For example, someone with severe urgency might be asked to count to ten slowly before starting for the toilet. Once this is achieved without incontinence, the count should be raised to twenty, then thirty, then sixty. If urgency is less severe, the patient might start by waiting ten minutes, then twenty minutes, then half an hour. The highly motivated patient will often see how the ticks on the chart are gradually spacing out, and set a new target to aim for. Some patients may also be taught to control precipitancy (inability to delay) once actually at the toilet, by getting into position and then deliberately delaying starting the stream. This can be exceedingly difficult for someone with urgency, but if it can be mastered it will do a great deal to boost self-confidence in the ability to be in control. Again, it is best to start with small achievable targets (e.g. count to ten), and then gradually extend the delay.

Some people find that practising pelvic floor exercises (Chapter 6) helps to suppress urgency. Pressure on the perineum (such as sitting on a heel or a beanbag) may also be helpful. It is important not to underestimate how difficult it is to ignore the sensation of urgency if you know that you might wet yourself.

Many patients will be tempted to give up the bladder retraining or refuse to push themselves. Bladder retraining may contradict other advice they have been given. For example, many children are taught that it is bad to hold on for too long. However, it is one of the best hopes that people with urge incontinence have of regaining continence, and every attempt must be made to encourage and support their efforts. Jarvis and Millar (1980) found that over 80% of women treated with inpatient retraining were symptom-free six months later. Fantl et al. (1991) report that amongst elderly women, 12% regained continence and three quarters had at least 50% reduction in the number of incontinent episodes. More use could be made of mutual support between patients, in the form of groups, than is currently practised.

Habit Retraining
Habit retraining attempts to match voiding intervals to an individual's own natural voiding pattern, usually in a long-term institutional context. A baseline chart is kept to determine the individual's pattern of continence and incontinence. A programme of toileting times is then worked out to anticipate incontinence. Times are therefore worked out for each individual, rather than treating all patients or residents the same. Once continence is achieved, the time intervals may then be lengthened. In practice such a programme is much more likely to keep patients continent than set-interval toileting for all, and may retrain some bladders (Hu et al., 1989; Engel et al., 1990). Possibly the biggest benefit, certainly to long-stay patients, is to 'retrain' the staff to recognise individual toileting needs, rather than taking everyone at the same time.

Timed and Prompted Voiding
Much of what goes under the name of 'bladder training' in fact does nothing to train the bladder, and consists solely of reminding or taking a patient to pass urine at set intervals. This is most commonly practised

in residential homes and long-stay hospitals. The intervals chosen may be time-related (e.g. every two or four hours) or else be related to events (e.g. before or after taking meals, drinks, or drugs). Often such programmes are applied indiscriminately to all residents, or at least to all those who are incontinent. As everyone's bladder functions differently, such a programme will at best catch some incontinence before it occurs. Usually it is completely unrelated to individual needs. Hopefully, with the advent of more individualised patient care, such a rigid regime for a whole group will be recognised as both ineffective and time-consuming.

However, set patterns are useful for selected patients. Those with a very poor memory, who tend to simply forget about the bladder until it is too late, may benefit from fixed time interval reminders or a standing instruction always to visit the lavatory after meals. Sometimes an alarm clock or a set interval timer may serve as a reminder if there is no one around. Patients with impaired bladder sensation may also need to be instructed to pass urine by the clock, rather than waiting for sensation, if they are to avoid overflow incontinence. Patients with advanced dementia, for whom all attempts at continence have failed, may be kept dryer by set interval toileting (see Chapter 11).

Prompted voiding attempts to teach a confused person to discriminate their own incontinence status. By regular monitoring, prompting to use the toilet and positive reinforcement for the desired outcome (e.g. continence or passing urine appropriately), some patients may improve continence (Schnelle, 1990). This is most successful for people who have lower natural voiding frequencies and some self-toileting skills.

Biofeedback

Biofeedback can be used as a sophisticated form of bladder training for patients with detrusor instability. The patient must be reasonably intelligent and motivated, and the treatment is generally only available in urodynamic clinics. By connecting the patient to the urodynamic equipment, as for a cystometrogram (as described in Chapter 3), filling the bladder slowly and showing the patient what is happening to bladder pressure, many patients are helped in learning to inhibit their unwanted bladder contractions (Cardozo et al., 1978). It has been found useful as part of an inpatient treatment package for patients with an unstable detrusor (Millard and Oldenberg, 1983). Usually six to ten one-hour sessions are needed with a skilled therapist, so the treatment is expensive and time-consuming.

Biofeedback has also been used for treating unstable bladder in children, as well as for teaching coordinated voiding to children with incomplete bladder emptying – when cystometric feedback may be combined with EMG (Hellstrom, 1990). Further research is warranted to define optimum treatment protocols and bring this technique to greater numbers of people. It may be that the technology which has enabled the development of ambulatory urodynamics will also make it possible to have self-administered biofeedback at home.

Biofeedback of pelvic floor contractions (usually using a perineometer) is also a useful adjunct to pelvic floor exercises (see Chapter 6).

Complementary Therapies for Urinary Incontinence

Many different 'complementary' therapies have been advocated in recent years. As yet, very few options have been subjected to well-designed research. Freeman (1982, 1985, 1989) has found hypnotherapy helpful for women with an unstable detrusor. Patients were given suggestions under hypnosis that they could hold more urine and void less frequently. Over half became symptom-free after twelve sessions, although there was some relapse with time.

Pigne (1985), Philp et al. (1988), Chang (1988) and Kelleher et al. (1993) have all found that symptoms from an unstable detrusor can be lessened by acupuncture. Psychotherapy has likewise been found helpful (Macaulay et al., 1987). Homoeopathy has been reported to improve symptoms, especially frequency (Krahulec and Dvorakova, 1994). The possibilities of reflexology, aromatherapy and other complementary therapies warrant investigation.

Electrical Stimulation

Electrotherapy is increasingly used as an adjunct to pelvic floor exercises for stress incontinence (Chapter 6). Electrical stimulation has also been used to inhibit unstable bladder contractions. Vaginal or anal electrodes can be connected to an external battery operated stimulator (Plevnik, 1989). Implantable stimulators are in development.

MANAGING INTRACTABLE INCONTINENCE

Skin Care

Good skin care is essential for anyone who is incontinent. Regular incontinence can be associated with dermatitis, and in conjunction with a factor such as friction, with the development of pressure sores in vulnerable individuals. Both urine and faeces can cause direct skin irritation. They also provide a damp and warm environment which is ideal for the proliferation of potentially pathogenic micro-organisms. However, it must be said that the majority of incontinent people do not have sore perineal skin for most of the time, and only a minority develop significant soreness, infection or pressure sores. Even an immobile person with double incontinence does not inevitably suffer skin problems. Skin health depends to a large extent on general health, especially upon a balanced diet and adequate fluid intake. Those who are very sick, debilitated or immobile are much more vulnerable to skin breakdown. The nurse can offer much useful advice on diet and general health care to help prevent or treat skin problems.

The most important element of skin care is thorough cleansing of the entire genital area (and any other skin in contact with urine or faeces) at least twice a day. Ideally a bath or shower should be taken daily. This is not always practicable and a good wash must sometimes suffice. Warm water and a mild soap should be used. Heavily scented soaps may provoke a skin reaction and may cause discomfort if the skin is already sore. After washing, the skin should be gently but thoroughly dried with a soft towel. Healthy skin should not require any creams or lotions. If the skin is known to be vulnerable, a simple barrier cream such as zinc and castor oil may be used. Any cream should be used sparingly as too much may make the skin surface soggy and actually increase the risk of problems. It can also make any absorbent product used less efficient, as the cream may form a barrier to urine absorption. Skin should be patch-tested before using a proprietary cleansing or barrier product, as so many people are sensitive to one or more of the many different substances contained in these products. If it is unclear whether soreness is due to incontinence or to the cream supposedly used to protect the skin, the product should be applied to a separate area of skin (for example, on the back) and observed for skin reaction over several hours. Where the skin is already sore, a cream with combined barrier, analgesic and healing properties is often found to promote healing. Talcum powder is best avoided as it can irritate, especially if strongly perfumed, and tends to form lumps when dampened by urine or sweat, causing encrustations in the groin skin folds.

If the skin is becoming sore, factors other than the incontinence should not be forgotten. An aid or pad may be the cause. A pad may have a rough surface, or an appliance be too tight-fitting. Plastic in contact with wet skin is an especial source of trouble, and plastic pants should be avoided. Some patients' skin may be sensitive to the materials of a pad or appliance, and inflammation may be caused by an allergic reaction (such as to the latex of a penile sheath). Pressure or friction is often more significant than urine. In elderly women, a sore vulva may be the result of atrophic vaginitis rather than incontinence.

If the skin has become very sore and the surface has broken down, sometimes the only viable method of healing it is by using an indwelling catheter to control the incontinence. This should never be used solely for nursing convenience (see Chapter 9), but may be unavoidable for people with severe skin problems.

Controlling Odour and Soiling

Odour is one of the greatest fears of incontinent people (Norton, 1982). People may restrict their activities and social contacts, not because of obvious leakage, but because they are worried about the possibility of odour. In Western society, natural odours have become taboo, and vast amounts of money are spent on disguising everyday smells in the home and on the body. If perspiration is considered unacceptable how much more is this true of excreta? Modern man (or woman) does not like to be reminded of bodily necessities. People who smell of urine or faeces are considered socially unacceptable, and are avoided. Most people assume that those who smell must neglect themselves and be unclean in their habits.

For most incontinent people the worry is unfounded, as no unpleasant odour is apparent. This does not prevent worrying, and repeated reassurance is often needed. Freshly voided urine has only a faint odour, provided that it is not too concentrated and is not infected. If adequate attention is paid to personal hygiene even regularly incontinent people should not have an odour problem. Only if urine is allowed to linger does odour become offensive, and this is because of the breakdown of the constituents of urine upon contact with air. Ideally, soiled pads and clothing should be changed as soon as possible after incontinence has occurred.

Appliances usually present less of an odour problem because urine is contained in a bag, as long as the patient is able to wash a reusable appliance effectively. Washing the skin is not usually necessary or feasible after each episode of incontinence, but it must be done regularly (see 'Skin Care', above). Faecal incontinence represents a more difficult problem (see Chapter 10).

If urine is particularly offensive, the patient should be encouraged to increase fluid intake and the urine must be tested for infection. One of the most effective methods of preventing odour is to ensure that the incontinence is well contained by a good pad or appliance, and that clothing and the environment are protected from contamination. When a pad is removed it should be put immediately into a sealed container such as a plastic disposal bag with twist seal, or a bin with a well-fitting lid. Appliances should be washed thoroughly each day.

Soiled clothes, beds, chairs or carpets are often the source of a lingering smell. Some materials (notably wool) seem to exacerbate the problem. Furniture can be difficult to clean effectively if soiled. Boric acid (5%) can help to remove smell from carpets. Often this is overcome by using a waterproof mattress or cushion cover, and a washable floor surface rather than carpet. However, this can make the bed or chair uncomfortable and many people do not wish to live in an environment where everything is plastic-covered. This is true both in the person's own home as well as in an institutional setting. It may be difficult to strike a balance between adequate protection and an aesthetically pleasing environment. Some fabrics have been developed which look normal but are in fact waterproof. This can dispense with the need to use plastic, especially on the bed.

There is some evidence which suggests that, the more normal are surroundings, the less likely incontinence becomes. Shrubsole and Smith (1984) found a 30% reduction in incontinence amongst adults with profound learning disabilities by environmental improvements alone, without any specific toileting programme. Confused people may be less likely to be incontinent on a homely sofa than on an institutional plastic chair with an underpad on it.

Probably the best answer is to minimise the risk of contamination by using the best available continence products (Chapter 15). Odour can become very offensive if clothes or furniture are not noticed to have been soiled and thus are not cleaned. Slippers are often a particular source of smell. Well-fitting shoes which can be wiped easily are usually preferable to soft carpet-slippers, which are difficult to clean properly. Not all incontinent people are able to maintain high standards of hygiene, especially those who live alone at home and also have a disability. Even a good wash may be impossible for many people without help. In some areas help with bathing can only be given weekly, or even fortnightly. This is obviously insufficient to prevent odour. Some people have great problems in washing soiled clothes and bedding. A home care assistant or laundry services may be able to help (see Chapter 12), but some people are obliged to just dry soiled items without first washing them. The nurse can advise that this is not a good idea, but without adequate social services there may be no other solution. The problem may be eased by advising the patient to buy clothes or bedding made of materials which are easy to launder and quick to dry. Dark coloured clothing also tends to show wet patches less and so reduces embarrassment.

Some people have very poor standards of personal hygiene and seem unconcerned about odour or cleanliness. The nurse may be in the difficult position of receiving complaints from those around the patient, while the individual is oblivious of any problem. Sometimes the nurse has either to discuss this frankly with the patient, or risk his being banned from activities or ceasing to have visitors. Incontinent people may be sacked from work, stopped from going to a luncheon club, or no longer be invited to visit relatives because of a smell that they themselves appear to be unaware of.

In some instances, odour comes to dominate the incontinent person's environment, whether at home or in an institution. Sometimes the only answer is to cleanse everything completely, often discarding carpets and mattresses, and start again. In severe cases the Environmental Health Department may be called in to fumigate the home. The tell-tale odour that used to be associated with elderly care wards is becoming less common, but may still be encountered, especially where high-quality products are not used. The main focus of the nurse's attention should be control of the incontinence rather than the smell it causes. Several proprietary deodorants are available for use where smell is a problem.

Fluid Intake
The fluid balance of incontinent people is often disturbed. Most adults drink between one and two litres of fluid in twenty-four hours, but this may be considerably increased with exercise, heat or sociable drinking. It is necessary to produce a minimum of 500ml of urine in twenty-four hours to permit the adequate excretion of waste products. Many incontinent people restrict their fluid intake in an attempt to control incontinence. If taken to extremes, this can lead to dehydration and even to electrolyte imbalance and confusion, especially for elderly people. Others suffer almost continuous thirst, which can become most unpleasant. Extreme fluid restriction should be discouraged, and the individual advised to drink as he feels the need or desire.

It is possible that fluid restriction may actually be counter-productive, for several reasons. A very low urine production, if combined with frequent voiding, will mean that the bladder is never expanded to its full capacity. While this is unlikely to physically reduce bladder capacity, it is likely to lower bladder sensitivity to a smaller habitual volume. In those prone to cystitis, a urinary tract which is only irregularly and infrequently emptied and flushed out may encourage re-infection. Low fluid intake will worsen any tendency to constipation. It is also possible that very concentrated urine may actually irritate the delicate mucosa of the bladder trigone and aggravate feelings of urgency and frequency.

Incontinent people should be encouraged to consume a reasonable fluid intake (between 1 and 1.5 litres per day). However, the times at which this is taken are unimportant, so timing can be manipulated. If the patient is most troubled by incontinence while out in the daytime, it may be wise to drink the bulk of the intake after returning home. If nocturia and nocturnal enuresis are the main problem, some fluid restriction may be advisable in the evening. However, this does not justify the extremes that some people (including nurses) practise – for example, no fluids after afternoon tea for anyone with nocturnal enuresis. This is both inhumane and frequently ineffective. All too often it becomes a 'ward policy' and is continued unthinkingly, even if it has never been proved effective, and even if the patient is still wet every night.

Certain fluids may create special problems for some individuals. Some people find that either tea or coffee has a rapid diuretic effect for them and is better avoided. Caffeine sensitivity is probably far more common than is realised, and caffeine can actually trigger unstable bladder contractions. Others say white wine is fine but red wine is not. It is usually a matter of trial and error to discover these idiosyncrasies, giving up each type of drink in turn and watching for improvement.

Some people may seem to be drinking excessively. This often follows advice, from medical or lay sources, on avoiding cystitis. At times people are discovered habitually drinking more than five litres per day. This will obviously make incontinence more of a problem. People on antibiotics should avoid excessive fluid intake as this will dilute the effect of the antibiotic. Anyone with a voiding difficulty will exacerbate their symptoms if they drink a lot. Women with stress incontinence may benefit from moderate fluid restriction, especially prior to planned exercise.

Incontinence Products
The nurse will usually be the person to advise the incontinent person on the appropriate use of products to control or cope with incontinence. This subject is discussed in Chapter 15.

Bowel Management
Poor bowel function may affect bladder control and is often the major problem in faecal incontinence. The nurse must help the individual to establish and maintain a good bowel habit. Chapter 10 discusses bowel management and faecal incontinence.

The Environmental and Physical Abilities
An environment adapted to the individual's needs, especially if he has a physical disability, will often enable incontinence to be avoided. Chapter 13 includes suggestions as to how the environment might be modified to improve continence, and ways in which the individual's physical abilities may be maximised to enable coping with bladder and bowel function.

REFERENCES AND FURTHER READING

Cardozo, L., Stanton, S. L., Hafner, J., Allen, V., 1978. Bio-feedback in the treatment of detrusor instability. *British Journal of Urology*, 50: 250–4.

Chang, P. L., 1988. Urodynamic studies in acupuncture for women with frequency, urgency and dysuria. *Journal of Urology*, 140: 563–6.

Cheater, F., 1991. Continence training programmes: need for standardisation. *Nursing Standard*, 6, 8: 24–7.

Engel, B. T., Burgio, L. D., McCormick, K.A., et al., 1990. Behavioral treatment of incontinence in the long-term care setting. *Journal of the American Geriatrics Society*, 38, 3: 361–3.

Fantl, J. A., Wyman, J. F., McLish, D. K., et al., 1991. Efficacy of bladder training in older women with urinary incontinence. *Journal of the American Medical Association*, 265, 5: 609–13.

Freeman, R. M., 1989. Hypnosis and psychomedical treatment. Chapter 10 in: Freeman, R., Malvern, J. *The Unstable Bladder*. Wright, London.

Freeman, R. M., Guthrie, K. A., Baxby, K., 1985. Hypnotherapy for idiopathic detrusor instability: a two-year review. *British Medical Journal*, 290: 286.

Freeman, R. M., Baxby, K., 1982. Hypnotherapy for incontinence caused by the unstable detrusor. *British Medical Journal*, 284: 1831–4.

Freeman, R., Malvern, J., 1989. *The Unstable Bladder*. Wright, London.

Frewen, W. K., 1978. An objective assessment of the unstable bladder of psychosomatic origin. *British Journal of Urology*, 50: 246–9.

Gartley, C., 1987. *Managing Incontinence*. Souvenir Press, London.

Hadley, G. C., 1986. Bladder training and related therapies for urinary incontinence in older people. *Journal of the American Medical Association*, 256, 3: 372–9.

Hellstrom, A-L., 1990. *Dysfunctional Bladder in Children*. Gothenberg University, Sweden.

Hu, T. W., Igou, J. F., Kaltreider, D. L., et al., 1989. A clinical trial of a behavioural therapy to reduce urinary incontinence in nursing homes: outcome and implications. *Journal of the American Medical Association*, 261, 18: 2656–62.

Jarvis, G. J., Millar, D. R., 1980. Controlled trial of bladder drill for detrusor instability. *British Medical Journal*, 281: 1322–3.

Kelleher, C. J., Filshie, J., Burton, G., Cardozo, L. D., 1993. Acupuncture and the treatment of irritative bladder symptoms. *Proceedings of the 23rd Meeting of the International Continence Society*, Rome.

Krahulec, P., Dvorakova, M., 1994. Homoeopathic therapy of urinary frequency and urgent urinary incontinence. *Proceedings of the 24th Meeting of the International Continence Society*, Prague.

Macaulay, A. J., Stanton, S. L., Stern, R. S., Holmes, D. M., 1987. Micturition and the mind: psychological factors in the aetiology and treatment of urinary disorders in women. *British Medical Journal*, 294: 540–3.

Millard, R. J., Oldenberg, B. F., 1983. The symptomatic, urodynamic and psychodynamic results of bladder re-education programmes. *Journal of Urology*, 130: 715–19.

Murray, K., Mundy, A. R., 1989. Surgery for intractable detrusor instability. In: Freeman, R., Malvern, J. *The Unstable Bladder*. Wright, London.

Norton, C. S., 1982. The effects of urinary incontinence in women. *International Rehabilitation Medicine*, 4, 1: 9–14.

Norton, C. S., 1983. Training for urinary continence. In: Wilson-Barnett, J. (ed), *Patient Teaching*. Churchill Livingstone, Edinburgh and London.

Philp, T., Shah, P. J. R., Worth, P. H. L., 1988. Acupuncture in the treatment of bladder instability. *British Journal of Urology*, 61: 490–3.

Pigne, A., DeGoursac, C., Nyssen, C., Barrat, J., 1985. Acupuncture and the unstable bladder. *Proceedings of the 15th Annual Meeting of the International Continence Society*, London.

Plevnik, S., Vodusek, D. B., Janez, J., 1989. Electrical stimulation treatment of bladder instability. Chapter 11 in: Freeman R., Malvern, J. *The Unstable Bladder*. Wright, London.

Roe, B. H., 1991. Benefits of bladder re-education. *Nursing*, 4, 39: 11–13.

Schnelle, 1990. Treatment of urinary incontinence in nursing home patients by prompted voiding. *Journal of the American Geriatrics Society*, 38, 3: 373–6.

Shrubsole, L., Smith, P.S., 1984. The effects of change in environment on incontinence in profoundly mentally handicapped adults. *British Journal of Mental Subnormality*, 30: 44–53.

Stanton, S. L., Tanagho, E. A., 1980. *Surgery of Female Incontinence*. Springer Verlag, Berlin.

US Department of Health and Human Services, 1992. Urinary incontinence in adults. Clinical practice guideline. Agency for Health Care Policy and Research, US Dept of Health and Human Services. Rockville, USA.

(See also Appendix 4 for books which review treatments.)

Chapter 5

Childhood Enuresis

Penny Dobson, MSc, CQSW, RGN

Director, Enuresis Resource and Information Centre, Bristol

Achieving bladder control is an important developmental milestone for children. Once past that crucial age at which continence is expected, it is no longer acceptable to crouch in a gutter or pass urine against a wall in public view. What was once viewed as 'quaint' behaviour become 'incontinence' as the toddler approaches school age. Children begin to realise that it is considered shameful to lack bladder control. Parents may react with anger in an attempt to disguise their own feelings of failure, guilt or embarrassment – and, as a result, the child may become shy, anxious and withdrawn.

Children who have achieved dryness often see themselves as 'grown up' and may mercilessly tease their less fortunate peers. Parents too do not always show tolerance and understanding to each other. Most schools *are* enlightened, but sometimes strict routines that only allow toilet visits during official breaks may result in an accident. Dirty lavatories with no doors, or doors that do not close properly, can also cause anxiety about toileting.

Some nursery schools will not take children until they are reliably dry during the day, and sometimes children with physical or learning difficulties are obliged to attend special schools, not because of their intellectual abilities or emotional or physical needs, but because they are incontinent.

'Enuresis' is the term used to describe an otherwise normal child who lacks bladder control at an age when control is to be expected. It is defined as the 'involuntary discharge of urine by day or night or both, in a child aged five years or older, in the absence of congenital or acquired defects of the nervous system or urinary tract', (Forsythe and Butler, 1989). 'Nocturnal enuresis' is lack of night-time bladder control, or bedwetting. The term diurnal enuresis is sometimes used to describe daytime wetting.

TOILET TRAINING

It is likely that 'training' does more to teach the child socially acceptable toileting behaviour, and to recognise the permitted places, than to train the bladder itself. The complex neuromuscular control necessary for continence and voluntary micturition cannot be 'taught' by a parent. Natural maturation of the musculature and central nervous system is the most important factor in acquiring control. It is likely that even with no training at all children will eventually control micturition, although they may not necessarily use the 'correct' receptacle.

Adults take continence so much for granted that it is easy to forget how many different skills are involved. The child must learn to consciously perceive the need to micturate and to be able to 'monitor' the state of the bladder while both awake and asleep. Once the need is appreciated, micturition must be postponed until an appropriate receptacle is reached. It is not always easy to know what an acceptable place is, especially if the surroundings are unfamiliar. For example, boys must learn to recognise a urinal and a lavatory as appropriate, but a bidet as inappropriate. Girls must learn to pass urine behind a closed, preferably locked door, except in the countryside when they can go behind a bush! Boys can go in front of other boys, but not in front of girls, and must defaecate in private. Children must be able to read signs on public conveniences. They must learn to open doors, remove clothing, start the stream voluntarily, use toilet paper, flush the lavatory, and wash their hands. Not until all these skills have been mastered can the child be independent at toileting.

The Process of Micturition

The process of micturition consists of a complex chain of reflexes, some of which are under voluntary or conscious control, others are not. The first stages, filling and storage, are *not* under voluntary control. At the filling stage, the detrusor muscle of the bladder wall gradually expands to allow filling, with little increase in the internal pressure.

The next stages – postponement of urination until a toilet is reached and the act of micturition itself – are both under voluntary control and are the result of a complex chain of messages between the bladder and the brain. Chapter 2 gives a detailed description of the mechanism of continence.

The Development of Bladder Control

There is broad agreement on the sequence and approximate age at which the majority of children develop bladder control. This has been summarised by Bettison (1978) as follows:

1) Reflex micturition in infancy.
2) At 1–2 years – gradual awareness of the sensation of a full bladder.
3) At 3 years – able to tense the muscles of the pelvic floor and 'hold' urine for prolonged periods, thereby increasing the bladder capacity.
4) At 3–4 years – able to initiate the urine stream from a full bladder when seated on the toilet.
5) At 4 years – able to stop the urinary stream at will.
6) At 6 years – able to start urination at almost any degree of bladder filling.

The above should be used as a very approximate guide. Many children fall quite normally outside these age bands.

One consequence of neuromuscular immaturity is that continence at birth is impossible. Parents who start potty-training at three months may 'catch' some urine in the pot, but this will be purely by chance. Even attempting some sort of toilet training by the infant's first birthday is far too early, often causing anxiety and a prolonged battle.

The optimum time to attempt training is probably around the second birthday, depending upon the child's general development. Ideally he or she should be able to walk and follow simple instructions, and have some speech and basic feeding skills. At this point the training is more likely to be easy and rapid.

Most children are toilet trained without professional intervention. However, many nurses are asked for advice, either officially as a health visitor, district or practice nurse, or socially as a relative or friend. The best advice is to wait until the child is ready and then to train fairly intensively, choosing if possible a time when little else is going on (e.g. avoiding Christmas, or family holidays). This is preferable to random and premature attempts over a long period. The child should be taken out of nappies and put into dry pants, so that he or she learns to appreciate the difference between wet and dry. Clothing and under-wear should be easy for the child to remove independently. Choose moments which are stress-free and always be encouraging but clear, with explanations of what is required. If the potty is successfully used, always praise – and this can be linked with a physical reward. If not, be 'matter of fact' or give a mild rebuke. Never punish – this is counter-productive as it raises anxiety, thereby decreasing the potential for learning. It may be useful to temporarily increase fluid intake as a means of increasing the number of learning opportunities.

Some very intense toilet-training methods have been devised, for example, *Toilet Training in Less than a Day* (Azrin and Foxx, 1974). These need experienced professional supervision to succeed.

If a planned attempt at an appropriate time fails, it is best to put the child back into nappies and try again after an interval of two to three months, while reassuring the parents that there is unlikely to be anything wrong and that the child is not stupid or naughty.

If repeated attempts fail, keeping a chart to monitor progress can help to put the problem into perspective. Buying a new pot or using a different room, or having a different person doing the training can also provide a fresh start, and a parent or sibling can assist by demonstrating appropriate toilet behaviour. Confidence and optimism, with an emphasis upon achievements rather than failures, is the general message.

DAYTIME WETTING

Daytime wetting, although less common than bedwetting, is often more stressful for the individual child. It is also more likely to have an organic association, the most common cause being an unstable detrusor. There is therefore some debate as to whether the term 'enuresis' (as defined on page 102) is a correct description for the problem of daytime wetting. The term 'daytime wetting' is used in this chapter.

Prevalence
Children usually become dry during the day between the ages of two and five years, although some may become dry earlier than this. Wetting episodes during the day do not usually become a problem until the age of five years, when the child starts school.

Daytime wetting is experienced by more girls than boys (Fielding et al., 1978). 1.0%–1.1% of girls aged 4–7 years regularly wet during the day; 0.3%–0.8% of boys aged 4–7 years regularly wet during the day. Many, but not all, children who are wet during the day are also wet at night.

Severity

Meadow (1990) grades daytime wetting into three grades, according to severity and effect. This helps both the assessment, and the recording and evaluation of progress:

Grade 1: Damp pants and underclothes, but urine does not seep through to the outer clothing.

Grade 2: Wetting does seep through to the trousers or skirt, making a visible wet patch.

Grade 3: A wet puddle on the seat or floor.

Most children with daytime wetting have a mixture of Grade 1 and Grade 2 incidents, with a sizable proportion having no Grade 2 or 3 wetting at all.

Presenting Symptoms and Associations

The most common symptom of day-wetting is urgency (sometimes linked with frequency). One of the most common associations, particularly in girls, is between daytime wetting and urinary tract infections (Berg et al., 1977). Each seems to contribute to each other. A midstream urine test is therefore advisable.

Most urodynamic studies of children with daytime wetting alone show that at least half of the children have unstable detrusor contractions during the filling phase (Borzyskowski and Mundy, 1987). This finding contrasts with children with nocturnal enuresis, most of whom do not have unstable bladders (Whiteside and Arnold, 1975). The strong bladder contractions associated with urgency and the reactive voluntary contraction of the urethral sphincter *may* give rise to reflux (backward passage of the urine up the ureters). Although rare, there is a risk that this may cause kidney damage.

A fairly common cause of damp pants, particularly in girls who are overweight, is urine seeping back into the vagina during micturition. If the child is in too much of a hurry this can flow out later, dampening the pants.

There seems to be no clear association between daytime wetting and emotional or psychological 'disturbance'. Also, as little is known about the general emotional effects of wetting it is difficult to separate cause and effect.

Assessment

Many children will quite naturally become dry without any formal intervention. However, because of the social effects and the possibility of an underlying physical cause, a medical assessment is advised once the child reaches the age of five years. All children are examined by the school medical officer when they commence infant school.

If a nurse is involved with the family, the assessment should be a joint exercise between nurse and doctor. Medical assessment is usually carried out by the school medical officer, general practitioner or a general paediatrician, paediatric urologist or nephrologist. This is likely to include a general examination, examination of the perineum and a test for urinary tract infection. If there is infection, an abdominal X-ray and ultrasound of the urinary tract is likely to be requested.

The nurse can helpfully initiate a 'baseline' recording of the frequency and severity of the wetting. One way of doing this is to divide the day into four or five periods and to note the state of the pants at the end of each of these periods (Meadow, 1990). Over a 2–4 week period this can provide useful information on when the 'risk periods' are and perhaps find ways to prevent a wetting episode. Sometimes the recording reveals only slight staining of the pants – well within the normal – and counselling a parent who may be over-anxious is therefore indicated, rather than treating the child. Recording can also provide a useful basis for reviewing progress once treatment has started, and is most effective if the child takes responsibility for filling in the chart.

The nurse can also establish whether the child is able to 'recognise' the signals that the bladder is full. A simple diagram of the urinary tract can help (Dobson, 1992). If the parent persistently neglects to respond to the child's request to use the potty or toilet, or the child persistently ignores the signals, then 'recognition' is either delayed or else not acquired. It is also important to find out whether the child is able to 'hold on'. For those children with urgency (and adults too), the urge to void can be reduced by adopting special positions, such as sitting with the heel pressed up against the perineum ('Vincent's curtsey sign'), or crossing the legs. In addition, establish whether the child does completely empty the bladder (or has to go to the toilet again a few minutes later) and *can* undress and visit the toilet independently. Sometimes difficult straps, braces or a stiff zip can cause difficulty, particularly at school.

It is important to ask the child how he or she feels about being wet and what the good things might be about being dry. Sometimes gentle questioning can reveal a particular worry; it can also allow the nurse to assess what the child's motivation might be to undergo a training programme.

Treatment

A positive, energetic and sympathetic approach is essential to engage a child and family, who are all likely to be feeling depressed and demoralised by the time that they seek help. Advice about washing carefully, and using a bacteriostatic/fungicidal dusting powder on the pants, can reduce the smell of stale urine. Helping the parents to liaise with the school in a positive and discreet way can also reduce tension, and the school nurse has an important role in this. It is also important to prepare the child and family for the first visit to the GP or paediatrician.

Following medical assessment, a bladder training regime may be considered appropriate – for children who are old enough to carry this out (suggested minimum age seven years). This is often supervised by a doctor, but can equally well be carried out by an experienced nurse. The most effective regime for the problem of urgency is one that encourages the child to go to the toilet more regularly and frequently. The child is encouraged to go to the toilet every hour, with the aid of a wristwatch or alarm clock. Once the holding period of an hour (or a shorter period, if necessary) has been achieved for one week with no wetting incidents, the time between visits can be lengthened by ten minutes. In week 2, therefore, the timing between toilet visits should be one hour and ten minutes. In week 3, this is increased to one hour and twenty minutes and so on, until the child can confidently manage six visits a day: rising; mid-morning; lunchtime; mid-afternoon; teatime; and bath/bedtime.

This regime is more likely to be successful if the child takes responsibility for it, rather than the parents or a teacher. School holidays may be the most convenient time to start bladder training.

A chart should be kept to monitor progress – and to give the parents and professional adviser opportunities to praise the child for each small step forward. Small achievable rewards can provide an extra incentive. They can be given for achieving dry periods of two or three hours or a whole day. However, some accidents should be expected and tolerated.

If the child wets 5–10 minutes after visiting the toilet, it is possible that he or she is unable to fully empty the bladder. In this case, teach the child to visit the toilet twice in quick succession. A regime of retention-control training (delaying micturition once the sensation is felt) – has proved to be less helpful than a timed micturition programme for children with urge incontinence (Fielding et al., 1978).

For children who have difficulty 'recognising and responding' to the sensation of a full bladder the mini- or body-worn alarm may prove useful (see page 114). However, unlike its use for bedwetting, there are few trials which have recorded or evaluated the effectiveness of an alarm for daytime wetting. It can of course only be used at home, and preferably during the holidays.

Success has also been reported using biofeedback techniques to treat both an unstable detrusor and voiding difficulties with children (Hellstrom, 1990).

Daytime stress incontinence is less common. This leakage upon physical exertion is thought to be caused by a congenital weakness of the collagen component of the urethral sphincter mechanism. The treatment of choice is pelvic floor exercises, described in detail in Chapter 6. The child should be taught to interrupt the urine flow midstream and then to practice pelvic floor contractions regularly through the day. A few girls seem to be born with a congenitally weak or open bladder neck. This resolves spontaneously for most at puberty, but corrective surgery is occasionally required if incontinence is troublesome.

Some girls suffer 'giggle micturition', whereby they start to leak when they laugh, then wet themselves completely until the bladder is empty. This is probably a combination of stress incontinence and an unstable detrusor, and can be treated by combining a bladder training programme with pelvic floor exercises.

Antibiotic medication will be necessary if a urinary tract infection is found. For children with an unstable detrusor, where bladder training has failed, an anticholinergic drug such as oxybutynin may be considered. This drug, taken orally, has an antispasmodic action on the smooth muscle of the bladder as well as an anticholinergic action. But as Meadow (1990) concludes, 'There is no convincing evidence that any drug therapy is effective for children with day-wetting. Many drugs have been used, but most have not been subjected to satisfactorily controlled trials.'

BEDWETTING (NOCTURNAL ENURESIS)

Most children have gained daytime control by the age of three years. Night-time control usually takes a little longer and girls often achieve this earlier than boys, probably because they tend to develop generally faster than boys. It is quite normal for children as old as four years to still be wetting the bed, and accidents may occur from time to time for a number of years.

Parents can encourage their child to take that 'first step' towards dryness by replacing nappies with pants, leaving a nearby light on and keeping a potty beside the bed. Praise for smaller wet patches or dry beds can help to build up confidence, but progress may be erratic and may take a number of months to achieve. A 'matter of fact' approach towards wet beds is essential, and if they persist over a three-week period (or any period that is causing undue stress within the family), it may be advisable to return to nappies and try again in three to four months time.

Prevalence
For one in six five-year-olds, achieving night-time dryness is not straightforward. Bedwetting, or nocturnal enuresis (as defined on page 102), affects over half a million children in the UK between the ages of five and sixteen years (out of a population of seven million in this age group). It affects:

15–20% of 5 year olds (1 in 6)
7% of 7 year olds (1 in 14)
5% of 10 year olds (1 in 20)
2–3% of 12–14 year olds (1 in 30)
1–2% of 15 year olds and over (1 in 50–100)

(Pierce, 1980; Rutter et al., 1973). *Note:* The above figures are based on an average of two wet nights per week.

Approximately twice as many boys as girls suffer from bedwetting, although this difference becomes less from thirteen years onwards (Fielding et al., 1978).

Effect upon Child and Family
From the many letters from children received by the Enuresis Resource and Information Centre (ERIC), feelings of isolation and 'aloneness', with the problem and fear that others might find out, seem the most pressing reactions. Loss of social life is also a major concern, with bedwetting often resulting in restrictions to staying overnight with friends or going on school camps or other holidays.

For parents, the greatest concern is the emotional and social effect on the child's life, followed by the concern about the extra washing and cost (Butler et al., 1986). For a number of parents, bedwetting can cause stress and conflict within the family. One study reported 30% of mothers scolded or beat their bedwetting child (White, 1971). Benjamin (1971) in a study of 90 parents who brought their children for a routine paediatric visit, found that night-training was retarded by the use of negative reinforcers, such as shaming, spanking, rejecting and name-calling.

For the estimated 100,000 young adult sufferers in their twenties, bedwetting can seriously inhibit their social and sexual lives. Some people writing to ERIC have not mentioned the problem to a prospective partner, and are often prepared to break off the relationship rather than face the embarrassment of disclosure and the risk of rejection.

Contributory Factors

Mothers rate heavy or deep sleep as the major cause of bedwetting, followed by emotional factors and family history (Butler and Brewin, 1986). However, there is as yet little scientific evidence to confirm the 'deep sleep theory'. Wetting episodes seem to occur at all stages of sleep (with the exception of the dreaming stage). In addition, there is nothing to prove that children who bedwet are any more difficult to rouse than non-bedwetting children. On the other hand, it is clear that stress can be a factor, particularly in situations when a child re-starts bedwetting after a period of a year or so of being dry (secondary wetting). There is no evidence that children who bedwet are any more emotionally disturbed than the non-bedwetting population.

Studies have indicated a strong familial link in bedwetting (Devlin, 1991; Bakwin, 1971). More recent research has made progress towards isolating the gene relating to primary nocturnal enuresis (Eiberg et al., 1995).

A small but significant number of mothers give the child being 'not bothered' as a cause, although the indications are that bedwetting is very rarely due to laziness or lack of willpower.

Finally, parents often worry that their child has a 'small bladder'. It is true that children who bedwet *are* likely to have a smaller functional bladder capacity than those who are dry (Fielding, 1980); however, it is uncertain whether a small bladder capacity *causes* wetting or is a consequence of wetting. Neither is it known why some children with a small bladder capacity are able to wake up to pass urine and stay dry at night, and some are not.

Assessment

Assessment of nocturnal enuresis should include all the ingredients of the assessment for daytime wetting (see page 106); however, there is usually less need for further investigations, such as abdominal X-ray or ultrasound of the urinary tract.

In addition to a baseline recording (see record chart, Table 5.1), it is important to find out how much the child drinks during the day. Restricting fluids does not help, as the bladder will 'adjust' to less fluid and therefore will hold less before a feeling of fullness occurs. It is important to find out *what* is drunk. Drinks such as tea, coffee and fizzy drinks have diuretic properties and can 'trigger' a bedwetting episode. Details of the night-time routine may reveal clues for change. For example, the child may forget to go to the toilet before going to bed, or leave a wet bed to creep into his parent's dry one, thus 'rewarding' the wetting behaviour!

It is important to assess the parents' attitudes to the bedwetting before embarking upon a programme, as these will affect the commitment to change. Three studies to date have confirmed that maternal intolerance predicts drop-out from treatment (Morgan and Young, 1975; Wagner et al., 1982; and Butler et al., 1988). If this is a problem it is best, where possible, to relieve the pressures on the family first,

Table 5.1   Baseline Night Record Sheet for Parents to Complete (with the help of the child)

Please check whether the bed is wet or dry:
1) Before going to bed yourself; 2) In the morning.
Put W if wet and D if dry.

	Week One			Week Two		
	Night	Morning	Any additional wet episodes	Night	Morning	Any additional wet episodes
MON						
TUES						
WED						
THURS						
FRI						
SAT						
SUN						

(Reproduced from: Blackwell, C., 1989 with permission of ERIC.)

perhaps by arranging medication for temporary relief, or organising more adequate bedding protection. The attitudes and feelings of the child are also important, as resistance to becoming dry is linked to a poor response to treatment, and to relapse (Butler et al., 1990(b)). Exploring the child's views and feelings may also reveal fears such as fear of the dark or 'monsters' in the corridor leading to the toilet. A simple remedy such as leaving the light on can sometimes solve the bedwetting.

Treatment

A confident and positive attitude is essential to inspiring confidence and hope – essential ingredients to success. Reassuring the child and family that they are not the only one in the world with a bedwetting problem is vital, as is giving the facts about bedwetting. Practical advice on bedding protection, keeping warm at night and access to the toilet are also important.

Asking the child what he or she has tried, and what he thinks would help, is an essential part of the process of engaging the child in a jointly agreed treatment programme. The child should be responsible for the programme and the recording, with the parents or carers acting as the support team.

If the child seems either not bothered or reluctant to work towards change, it is best to leave a programme until he or she is older. In the meantime, the self-help book for 7–14 year olds – *Eric's Wet to Dry Bedtime Book* (Butler, 1989) may educate and inspire!

Most children and parents have tried a number of methods before asking for help. The most common of these is *lifting*, with parents taking the child to the toilet on their way to bed. This may prevent a wet bed, but does not help the child to recognise the sensation of a full bladder, and either to wake up or hold on. Lifting may be counter-productive if the child comes to expect it or if he or she is not fully awake, therefore in effect being taught to pass urine in his sleep! If lifting is used, it is important to vary the time of lifting and to make sure that the child is fully awake.

Simple incentive or reward schemes, if used carefully, can be a source of encouragement, particularly for children in the 5–7 year age range, and some respond well. However, to be more helpful than discouraging there are a number of basic rules. Always negotiate with the child goals that are *achievable*, such as going to the toilet before bed-time, or telling the parent when the bed is wet. A dry night is for some too difficult as a first goal. Build up the goals gradually. The rewards must be something that is valued by the child. Always link a tangible reward with praise. Give the reward immediately and consistently for the specific, desired behaviour. Do not punish, or put a black mark or a sad face on the chart, if the goal is not achieved.

Medication for Bedwetting

Medication such as desmopressin (Desmospray), imipramine (Tofranil) and amitriptyline (Tryptizol) are commonly used as short-term measures to reduce bedwetting, either to give the child a break during holiday periods or to relieve stress within the family. They are also sometimes prescribed to give children the experience of being dry, and for adults they provide a lifeline to a normal existence.

Neither desmopressin nor the tricyclic antidepressant group of drugs provide a cure. They are effective for the majority of children (about 70%), but approximately 80–85% will relapse once the medication is withdrawn.

Desmopressin is a synthetic analogue of the naturally occurring anti-diuretic hormone (ADH) and is produced in the form of a nasal spray or tablet. It has an effect on bedwetting because it reduces urine output at night to a level more manageable to the child. It is not fully understood how or why either desmopressin or the antidepressant group of drugs work.

The disadvantage of the tricyclic antidepressants such as imipramine and amitriptyline are their unpleasant side effects – irritability, dry mouth, loss of appetite, headaches, difficulty in concentration and constipation (Shaffer, 1979). There is also, of course, the risk of fatal overdose if the medicine is left within reach of younger children.

Enuresis Alarms

If the bedwetting does not respond to simple measures, and if the family circumstances are supportive, the enuresis alarm or buzzer could be considered. This is a conditioning device that prompts the child to make the connections between the bladder and brain. It is effective in 60–80% of cases, although the theory of *how* it works seems unclear. It is effective for children aged seven years or older, providing they are keen to become dry, are willing (with parental support) to take charge of the device, have a bed of their own (and if they share a room, a sympathetic room-mate) and are clearly instructed and supported by a nurse or other medical adviser. It is important to point out from the outset that the alarm is hard work, that it may take up to four months to achieve the initial success of fourteen consecutive dry nights and, once achieved, relapses are common – but containable!

There are two types of alarm – the bedside alarm, otherwise known as the 'buzzer' or 'bell and pad', and the mini- or body-worn alarm. With both types there is a detector plate, containing a pair of electrodes, connected to a control or alarm unit. Urine bridges the gap between the two electrodes, causing the alarm to sound. In the bedside alarm the detector plate is in the form of a single plastic mat or two gauze mats in which the electrode strips are embedded (Figure 5.1).

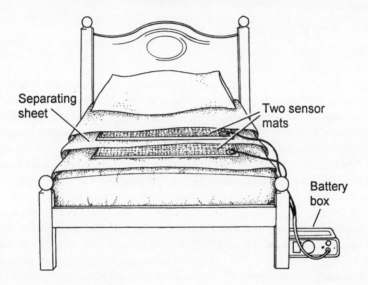

Separating sheet

Two sensor mats

Battery box

Figure 5.1 *Bedside alarm.*

With the body-worn alarm, the detector plate is smaller and can be worn inside an absorbent disposable pad (this can be the 'panty shield' type), or for boys, between two pairs of pants. The alarm unit is pinned to the upper pyjamas (Figure 5.2, overleaf).

Both types of alarm can be bought with a vibrator unit in the alarm box. This can be useful for children with hearing difficulties, children who fail to respond to the alarm, or in situations when the alarm needs to be used discreetly, such as in a boarding school dormitory. The mini-alarm is also available with a flashing light instead of an auditory signal.

The purpose of all enuresis alarms is to 'alert and sensitise the body to respond quickly and appropriately to a full bladder during

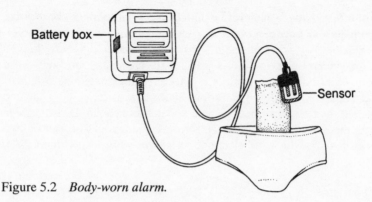

Battery box

Sensor

Figure 5.2   *Body-worn alarm.*

sleep' (Butler, 1994). As urination begins, the child generally reacts to the noise of the buzzer by tightening up the muscles of the pelvic floor, thus stopping the urine flow, and waking up. Gradually the child begins to tighten up and wake up to the sensation of a full bladder without the alarm.

There is little difference in the performance between the two types of alarm; however, as many children, particularly older children and adults, prefer the mini-alarm, the professional adviser should be able to offer a choice.

It is also vital that the alarm is demonstrated to the child and family in advance and that they are given the opportunity for a trial run before using it on their own. Similarly, common initial difficulties, such as not waking to the alarm or overcoming fear of the noise, should be discussed. Frequently, parents have to rouse the child when the alarm goes off, often for the first two weeks, but it is important that the *child* then switches the alarm off, goes to the toilet, changes the pants or bed and resets the alarm. Problems such as false alarms (often due to perspiration) can be overcome by reducing the bedding and ensuring that sheets are cotton rather than nylon. Parents and children may find two guides published by ERIC on how to use an enuresis alarm useful: *You and Your Alarm* (for children) and *Your Child's Alarm* (for parents), (Adams, 1990).

To emphasise the gains rather than failures it is important that a record of progress is kept (see Table 5.2, 'Child's Record Chart', to be kept while using the alarm).

Table 5.2   Child's Record Chart, to be Kept While Using the Alarm

	'D' if dry	'S' if small wet patch	'W' if wet patch	Woke up by self to alarm and went to toilet	What time(s) did the alarm go off?	No. of times
MON						
TUES						
WED						
THURS						
FRI						
SAT						
SUN						

Signs of progress are:

- Smaller wet patches in the bed or pants
- More urine 'finished off' in the toilet
- Better waking to the alarm
- Wetting occurring later in the night, indicating an increase in holding capacity
- More dry nights

The professional adviser should see the child and parents at least weekly for the first two weeks, then fortnightly, both to provide encouragement and support and to provide early advice in overcoming common difficulties.

Relapse after Alarm Treatment
It can be reassuring to the child and family to explain at the outset that relapses often occur, but that there are steps that can be taken to reduce the risk, and overcome them. The high-risk groups for relapse seem to be children with a history of secondary enuresis and children who are not concerned about their bedwetting (Butler et al., 1990(a)). Approximately one in three children will relapse after having achieved fourteen

dry nights. The term 'relapse' is usually defined as 'more than two wet nights in two weeks' (Butler, 1991). This rate can be lowered to approximately one in ten children by using a method called 'over-learning' (Blackwell, 1989). Once the child has been dry for fourteen consecutive nights he or she should deliberately drink one or two pints of extra fluid, or as much as the child can comfortably drink, before setting the alarm and going to bed. This will often result in wetting re-occurring for a few nights, but the child usually becomes dry again and now has a 'margin of error'. Once two dry weeks on the high fluid intake have been achieved the extra fluid and the alarm are discontinued. However, if wetting does not start to diminish after using over-learning for two weeks, it is best to return to the usual fluid intake with the alarm, until fourteen dry nights have been achieved again. The child may prefer to keep the alarm nearby, but not switched on, for a further week or two before taking it away altogether.

It is important to maintain contact with the family for the next six months, as this is the risk period for relapse. If relapse does occur, this does not mean the alarm will not work a second time. The child who has relapsed once does in fact have the same chance as 'first timers' of becoming completely dry. The term 'continued success' is defined as 'no relapse in the six months after initial success' (Butler, 1991).

CONGENITAL ABNORMALITIES

Certain congenital abnormalities of the urinary tract may be the underlying cause of incontinence in childhood. Minor abnormalities may well be overlooked unless a careful physical examination is carried out on a child presenting with continuous or very frequent wetting day and night. Occasionally, congenital deformities are not picked up in childhood and persist undiagnosed into adult life.

Epispadias and Hypospadias (Figure 5.3)
Epispadias is a condition where the urethra opens on the upper surface of the penis. It can vary from an abnormally wide meatus to a complete split of the penis. The more extensive the abnormality, the more likely is incontinence. It is rare in females, where the clitoris and pubic bone are split. Treatment is surgical repair, but only one-half of boys achieve complete continence.

Hypospadias, an opening of the urethra on the undersurface of the penis, is much commoner, affecting 1 in 600 boys. The boy tends to

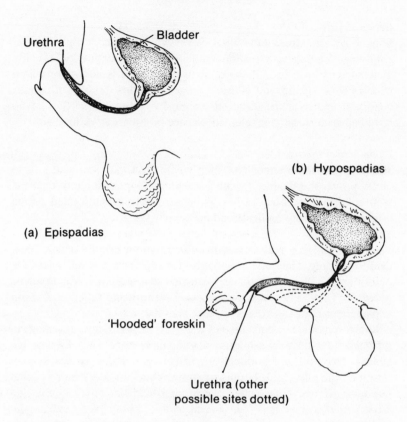

Figure 5.3   *Congenital abnormalities.*

have a 'hooded' foreskin, no normal erections, and a urinary stream which is passed backwards, between the legs. Again, treatment is surgical and usually gives good results in both continence and sexual function.

Ectopic Ureter
The ureter, instead of inserting into the bladder at the trigone, may enter the urethra directly. If this is below sphincteric level, a continuous dribbling incontinence will result. Sometimes this is associated with duplication of the upper urinary tract, with one ureter in the correct place and the second being ectopic. In this case the child will be able to pass urine normally, but will also suffer dribbling.

Urethral Valves
Some boys are born with urethral valves which prevent proper bladder emptying, leading to retention with overflow incontinence. Usually diagnosed early in life, the baby often presents in renal failure with a poor urinary stream and a urinary tract infection. This is a serious condition and must be corrected surgically. Occasionally, boys who have had such surgery develop continence problems at a later date.

Exstrophy of the Bladder
This is a rare and obvious condition where the abdominal wall fails to develop over the bladder, which consequently opens directly onto the skin at birth. The bladder has to be surgically reconstructed or the ureters diverted into an ileal conduit.

Parents of children with congenital abnormalities usually need a great deal of support. They often feel guilty for somehow having caused the deformity. They are usually very worried that the child will never be 'normal'. They may fear for later sexual identity and function. Careful explanations and realistic reassurance are vital.

Some repairs are done in several stages, involving the child in repeated hospital admissions at a vulnerable age. The child or his siblings may suffer emotionally, whether or not the parents stay in hospital with the child. If the condition is not urgent, repair is often left until he can cope better psychologically, e.g. after school age. However, this may result in several years of both incontinence and feeling abnormal. Although long-term physical results are often excellent, the nurse has an important contribution in ensuring that the patient adjusts psychologically to the fullest possible extent.

REFERENCES AND FURTHER READING

Adams, J., 1990. *Your Child's Alarm* and *You and Your Alarm*. Enuresis Resource and Information Centre, Bristol.

Azrin, N. H., Foxx, R. M., 1974. *Toilet Training in Less Than a Day*. Simon and Schuster, New York.

Bakwin, H., 1971. Enuresis in twins. *American Journal of Disease in Childhood*, 121: 222–5.

Benjamin, et. al., 1971. Night-training through parents' implicit use of operant conditioning. *Child Development*, 42: 963–6.

Berg, I., Fielding, D., Meadow, S. R., 1977. Psychiatric disturbance, urgency and bacteriuria in children with day and night wetting. *Archives of Disease in Childhood*, 52: 651–7.

Bettison, S., 1978. Toilet training the retarded child: analysis of the stages of development and procedures for designing programmes. *Australian Journal of Mental Retardation*, 5: 95–110

Blackwell, C., 1989. *A Guide to Enuresis*. Enuresis Resource and Information Centre, Bristol.

Borzyskowski, M., Mundy, A. R., 1987. Video-urodynamic assessment of diurnal urinary incontinence. *Archives of Disease in Childhood*, 62: 128–31.

Butler, R. J., Brewin, C. R., 1986. Maternal views of nocturnal enuresis. *Health Visitor*, 59: 207–9.

Butler, R, J., Brewin, C. R., Forsythe, W. I., 1988. A comparison of two approaches to the treatment of nocturnal enuresis and the prediction of effectiveness using pre-treatment variables. *Journal of Child Psychology and Psychiatry*, 19, 4: 501–9.

Butler, R., 1989. *Eric's Wet to Dry Bedtime Book*. Nottingham Rehab, available from the Enuresis Resource and Information Centre, Bristol.

Butler, R. J., Brewin, C. R., Forsythe, W. I., 1990a. Relapse in children treated for nocturnal enuresis. Prediction of response using pre-treatment variables. *Behavioural Psychotherapy*, 18: 65–72.

Butler, R. J., Redfern E. J., Forsythe, W. I., 1990b. The child's construing of nocturnal enuresis. A method of enquiry and prediction of outcome. *Journal of Child Psychology and Psychiatry*, 31: 447–54.

Butler, R. J., 1991. Establishment of working definitions in nocturnal enuresis. *Archives of Disease in Childhood*, 66: 267–71.

Butler, R., (Dobson, P. (ed)), 1993. *Enuresis Resource Pack*. Enuresis Resource and Information Centre, Bristol.

Butler, R. J., 1994. *Nocturnal Enuresis: The Child's Experience*. Butterworth-Heinemann, Oxford.

Devlin, J. B., 1991. Prevalence and risk factors for childhood nocturnal enuresis. *Irish Medical Journal*, 84: 118–20.

Dobson, P., 1991. *A Guide for Teenagers*. Enuresis Resource and Information Centre, Bristol.

Dobson, P. M., 1992. *Bedwetting – a Guide for Parents*. Enuresis Resource and Information Centre, Bristol.

Eisberg, H., Berendt, I., Mohr, J., 1995. Assignment of dominant inherited nocturnal enuresis (ENURI) to chromosome 13q. *Nature Genetics*, vol 10, part 3: 354–6.

Fielding, D. M., 1980. The response of day and night wetting children and children who wet only at night to retention control training and the enuresis alarm. *Behaviour Research and Therapy*, 18: 305–17.

Fielding, D. M., Berg, I., Bell, S., 1978. An observational study of postures and limb movements of children who wet by day and by night. *Developmental Medicine and Child Neurology*, 20: 453–61.

Forsythe, W. I., Butler, R. J., 1989. Fifty years of enuretic alarm: A review of the literature. *Archives of Disease in Childhood*, 64: 879–85.

Hellstrom, A.-L., 1990. *Dysfunctional Bladder in Children. Studies in Epidemiology and Urotherapy*. Department of Paediatrics, University of Gothenburg, Sweden.

Meadow, S. R., 1990. Day wetting. *Paediatric Nephrology*, 4: 178–84.

Morgan, R. T. T., Young, G. C., 1975. Parental attitudes and the conditioning treatment of childhood enuresis. *Behaviour Research and Therapy*, 13: 197–9

Morgan, R. (Dobson, P. (ed)), 1993. *Guidelines on Minimum Standards of Practice in the Treatment of Enuresis*. Enuresis Resource and Information Centre, Bristol.

Pierce C. M., 1980. Enuresis. In: Kaplan, H. I., Friedman, A. M., Sadock, B. J., (eds). *A Comprehensive Textbook of Psychiatry* (3rd edn), Williams and Wilkins, Baltimore.

Rutter, M., Yule, W., Graham, P., 1973. Enuresis and behavioural deviance: some epidemiological considerations. In: Kolvin, I., MacKeith, R. C., Meadow, S. R. (eds), *Bladder Control and Enuresis*, 137–50. William Heinemann Medical Books, London.

Shaffer, D., 1979. Enuresis. In: Rutter, M., Hersov, L., (eds). *Child Psychiatry: Modern Approaches*. Blackwell, Oxford.

Wagner, W. G., Johnson, S. B., Walker, D. et al., 1982. A controlled comparison of two treatment methods for nocturnal enuresis. *Journal of Paediatrics*, 101: 302–7.

White, M., 1971. A thousand consecutive cases of enuresis: result of treatment. *Child and Family*, 10: 198–209.

Whiteside, C. G., Arnold, E. P., 1975. Persistent primary enuresis: a urodynamic assessment. *British Medical Journal*: 364–7.

Chapter 6

Female Urinary Incontinence

Valerie Bayliss, MSc, DipSoc, RN
Continence Adviser, Loddon NHS Trust, Basingstoke

While both men and women suffer urinary incontinence for all the reasons outlined in Chapter 2, there are some conditions specific to the female which are described in greater depth in this chapter.

All nurses have an important role in teaching preventive measures and in teaching, counselling and giving care to women with continence problems. It may often be a nurse who teaches and supervises a programme of pelvic floor exercises. For women who are undergoing surgery, pre- and post-operative care and support are major contributory factors to a successful outcome. The midwife and health visitor will encounter many women with continence problems, or potential problems, in pregnancy and immediately after childbirth. Practice nurses and family planning practitioners have many opportunities (e.g. well women or family planning clinics), both to identify incontinent women and to give preventive advice and education.

GENUINE STRESS INCONTINENCE

Stress incontinence is particularly common amongst women, and indeed is the commonest continence problem (Thomas et al., 1980). There is considerable confusion over the term 'stress incontinence', and it can in fact be used to describe a sign, a symptom or a medical diagnosis.

The *sign* of stress incontinence describes visible leakage of urine at the time of a rise in abdominal pressure, such as a cough, during clinical examination. As a *symptom* it denotes the experience of leaking urine upon physical exertion – the 'stress' describes the physical stress upon the sphincter and pelvic floor muscles, and has nothing at all to do with emotional stress.

As a *diagnosis* it refers to incontinence caused by incompetence of the urethral sphincter – a failure of the urethra to maintain continence when stressed by raised intra-abdominal pressure. The International Continence Society recommends the term 'genuine stress incontinence' to describe this urethral sphincter incompetence.

The sign, symptom and diagnosis do not always coincide in the same person. Leaking upon exertion may sometimes be caused by an unstable detrusor, where a cough may provoke a bladder contraction, mimicking an incompetent sphincter. Likewise, people in retention may experience overflow incontinence upon effort. Conversely, a patient whose underlying bladder problem is an incompetent sphincter may complain of symptoms more suggestive of bladder instability, including frequency and urge incontinence. More than one condition may, of course, coexist in the same person. It is for these reasons that assessment must be carried out most carefully. Even so, the history may be misleading in diagnosing the true cause of the incontinence, and urodynamic investigation may be required (see Chapter 3).

In the remainder of this chapter, the term 'stress incontinence' is used to refer only to incontinence caused by a weak or incompetent urethral sphincter, i.e. 'genuine stress incontinence'.

Stress incontinence usually occurs immediately and coincidentally with the onset of effort, and ceases promptly when the activity ceases. It may be mild, only occurring with extreme physical exertion, such as playing squash or trampolining. It can be severe, with very minor effort such as walking, talking, or standing up from a chair causing leakage.

Mechanism

There are many different theories as to the causation of genuine stress incontinence and it seems likely that more than one mechanism is involved. Women with seemingly identical symptoms may actually have different causes for stress incontinence underlying the problem. In some instances a woman may have more than one reason for her stress incontinence.

One of the most widely accepted theories is that stress incontinence in women is caused by an altered anatomical relationship between the bladder and urethra and their muscular supports, notably the pelvic floor.

Figure 6.1 shows the normal relationship. The bladder and proximal urethra sit well supported above the pelvic floor. The intravesical (bladder) pressure is below maximum urethral pressure at rest – a pressure gradient maintains continence. As the bladder is situated inside the abdominal cavity, any rise in intra-abdominal pressure (e.g.

with a cough) raises intravesical pressure, tending to squeeze urine out of the bladder. However, the upper (proximal) urethra is well supported; it is also inside the abdominal cavity and therefore subject to the same rise in pressure as the bladder. The rise in pressure therefore tends to squeeze it shut and the pressure gradient is maintained (Figure 6.2). As long as urethral pressure is above bladder pressure at some point along the length of the urethra, continence is maintained.

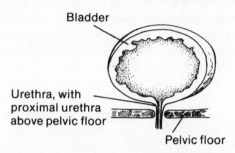

Figure 6.1 *Normal anatomical relationship of bladder, urethra and pelvic floor: at rest.*

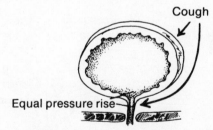

Figure 6.2 *Normal anatomical relationship of bladder, urethra and pelvic floor: during a cough.*

Figure 6.3 shows the relationship of bladder and urethra to the pelvic floor in a woman with stress incontinence. The bladder has prolapsed down through the pelvic floor. At rest this woman will be continent, because urethral pressure is above bladder pressure. Bladder pressure is raised when she coughs, but transmission of this pressure rise to the urethra is at best partial, at worst nil (Figure 6.4). If the rise in intra-abdominal pressure is high enough, or the urethral pressure low enough for the pressure gradient to be lost, incontinence is the inevitable result.

It is possible that the relationship of the urethra to the pubic bone is also important to continence. A urethra which is firmly supported up behind the pubic bone is likely to have transmission of intra-abdominal pressure rises augmented by reflection from the bone (Figure 6.5). This theory remains unproven.

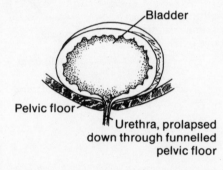

Figure 6.3   *Relationship of bladder, urethra and pelvic floor in a woman with stress incontinence: at rest.*

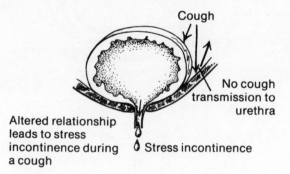

Figure 6.4   *Relationship of bladder, urethra and pelvic floor in a woman with stress incontinence: during a cough.*

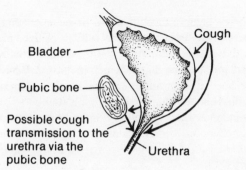

Bladder

Cough

Pubic bone

Possible cough
transmission to the
urethra via the
pubic bone

Urethra

Figure 6.5   *Possible cough transmission to the urethra via the pubic bone (side view).*

The pelvic floor itself contracts reflexly as abdominal pressure is raised (Figure 6.6). This again adds to urethral closure pressure at the crucial time. If, however, the pelvic floor is at an oblique rather than a right-angle to the urethra, the efficiency of this extra margin for continence is impaired (Figure 6.7).

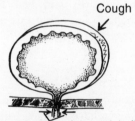

Cough

Reflex contraction of the pelvic floor

Figure 6.6   *Normal contraction of the pelvic floor with raised abdominal pressure.*

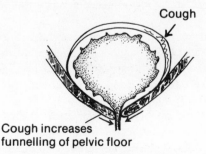

Cough

Cough increases
funnelling of pelvic floor

Figure 6.7   *Contraction of the pelvic floor with stress incontinence.*

The role of collagen and connective tissue in maintaining urinary continence in women is currently the subject of debate and research. There is some evidence that women with stress incontinence *without* significant prolapse or descent of the pelvic floor may have abnormally low collagen density. This might explain a lack of support around the urethra and consequent urinary leakage upon stress.

There is evidence that vascularity is an important component of urethral closure pressure, maybe contributing up to one third of the total closure pressure. Vascularity increases with muscle use and decreases with age.

Stress incontinence tends to be worse in pre-menopausal women in the week before a period, as resting urethral pressure falls with oestrogen withdrawal and a rise in progesterone levels. Likewise, post-menopausal women whose oestrogen level is falling experience an increased tendency to stress incontinence. This is discussed in detail in Chapter 11.

Some females are born with a congenitally weak sphincter mechanism and even an open bladder neck at rest. This may be the cause of incontinence in girls who wet themselves when they laugh – 'giggle incontinence'. For some this may resolve at puberty, but a few women will never know what it is like to have a good laugh without getting soaked.

Causes

The fact that stress incontinence as described above does not occur in men (who may however have sphincter incompetence caused by direct trauma to the sphincter, e.g. post prostatectomy) highlights the vulnerability of the female anatomy. With such a short urethra and a relatively weak sphincter mechanism, women are very susceptible to stress incontinence. Indeed, some surveys suggest that over half of all women experience stress incontinence at some time during their lives (Wolin, 1969).

Many women with stress incontinence are too embarrassed to consult their doctor about it, and for some it leads to considerable social restriction. They are unwilling to dance, go to aerobic or exercise classes, are fearful of laughing and come to dread colds, hay fever or even carrying shopping.

There can be little doubt that childbirth is the single most important risk factor underlying stress incontinence. The incidence rises sharply after childbirth and again after a fourth child. The crucial factors seem to be the length of the second stage of labour and type of delivery. Particularly at risk are women who have a very quick or very prolonged second stage, an obstructed delivery leading to the use of forceps, and those who have had large babies (over 4kg). Any combination of these may lead to tearing or over-stretching of the pelvic floor musculature. The relative role of episiotomy and perineal tears in protecting against or contributing to stress incontinence is as yet unclear.

These same obstetric risk factors can lead to damage to the nerve supply of the pelvic floor (pudendal nerve damage), in addition to direct muscle damage (Snooks et al., 1984). This nerve damage may improve with time with re-innervation. However, it may be progressive in some women (Snooks et al., 1990).

During and after the menopause, many women experience atrophy and sagging of the pelvic musculature. This is in part due to the fact that oestrogen levels drop, and as oestrogen strengthens collagen fibres, the muscles thin out laterally and become less effective. It is likely that this laxity, combined with an existing weakness from previous childbirth, will allow the bladder and urethra to prolapse down through the pelvic floor. The uterus may also prolapse.

Other factors have been implicated in the causation of stress incontinence, none with totally convincing evidence. Obesity may aggravate it and some women will experience an improvement in their symptoms with weight loss, but the underlying weakness of the pelvic floor still exists. Chronic constipation and straining at stool can cause eventual prolapse or nerve damage. A chronic cough, possibly due to smoking, may put repeated stress on the pelvic floor, as may a job which involves repeated heavy lifting. Advancing age leads to a generally decreased muscle density and strength, as well as decreased vascularity and general activity levels, which may in turn lessen the effectiveness of urethral closure and the pelvic floor. However, the fact that slim young nulliparous women can experience stress incontinence suggests a basic 'design fault' in the female anatomy.

Prevention
The most effective preventive measure is probably regular pelvic floor exercise for all women. Ideally this should be started in schools and continued throughout life as a natural part of a general fitness and exercise programme.

Many women do not appreciate, or are not properly taught, the risk to their continence associated with childbirth. Many obstetric units now have a physiotherapist with an additional qualification in obstetrics and gynaecology (Association of Chartered Physiotherapists in Women's Health), and place great emphasis on pelvic floor education post-natally. Where there is no such physiotherapist, the nurse, midwife and health visitor must take on responsibility for teaching and reinforcing the importance of these exercises. Immediately post-natally it can be difficult for the new mother to perform the exercises, as the area will be very tender and pain may inhibit contraction of the pelvic floor. Later, and in the excitement of having a new baby, the mother may well forget or abandon all thoughts of exercise. Here it is imperative for the health visitor to reinforce the teaching started in hospital. Indeed, with increasingly early discharge, some women are missing out altogether on teaching in hospital.

It may be that greater health awareness will also help to prevent stress incontinence in more general ways. More regular bowel habits, aided by a well-balanced high fibre diet, regular exercise, a general interest in fitness and an increased demand for hormone replacement therapy may all lead to future generations of women suffering less from stress incontinence than their mothers did. Some keep-fit and aerobics classes now routinely teach pelvic floor exercises.

There is a generally poor awareness of the pelvic floor, and every opportunity should be taken to promote preventive measures. Many women are totally unaware that they have these internal muscles and that, like any other muscle, the pelvic floor needs to be used or it will atrophy. About one-third of women are unable to voluntarily contract the pelvic floor upon request, without further explanation or teaching. This contrasts with some Eastern cultures, where mothers teach their daughters to use the pelvic floor muscles for sexual stimulation of a partner. Modern pedestal lavatories also mean that women do not have to bother to control the direction of urinary flow; more 'primitive' facilities, where the stream has to be directed into a small hole in the ground, may in fact be more beneficial to the pelvic floor, as well as providing a much more natural posture for defaecation.

Women on prolonged bedrest for any reason should also be encouraged to practice pelvic floor exercises. Immobile women are likely to experience a degree of atrophy of these muscles, in the absence of everyday activities which stimulate pelvic floor contractions.

General exercise, as well as specific pelvic floor exercise, has been found to be important in pelvic floor strength. Women with a weak pelvic floor, or those at risk (e.g. post-partum) should be encouraged to undertake regular general exercise as well as pelvic floor exercises.

Assessment

Clinical history and examination will give a working diagnosis in many instances. When this is in doubt, or if surgery is contemplated, this should always be verified by urodynamic studies (see Chapter 3). If a woman with an unstable detrusor is misdiagnosed as having genuine stress incontinence and given an operation, there is a risk of her symptoms being made worse instead of better.

When pelvic floor exercises are to be used, a more detailed assessment of the pelvic floor will be needed (see below).

Treatment

The ideal time to start treatment for stress incontinence is as soon as the problem arises. Unfortunately, many women tolerate their symptoms for considerable length of time and do not seek help until it becomes really troublesome. Public health education could do much to make women realise that they should not expect to leak after having a baby or as they get older, and that they should seek help for this curable condition. Women do not as a rule volunteer any information about stress incontinence, and need to be asked if they have any continence problems.

All adult women should be asked as a matter of routine, particularly at female-orientated clinics such as family planning, well woman or cervical smear sessions. Questioning will need to be gentle and sensitive – asking if she ever has a leak when she coughs or sneezes will gain a much better response than asking if she is incontinent.

The choice of treatment will depend on the severity of the symptoms, the degree of concomitant uterine prolapse, and individual personal preference.

Pelvic Floor Exercises (PFE)

Strengthening of the pelvic floor muscles by regular exercise is the best form of therapy for mild to moderate stress incontinence, in the absence of marked prolapse of the anterior vaginal wall. To achieve a successful outcome, it is imperative that the patient is well motivated and sufficiently mentally alert to carry out the exercise programme. Pelvic floor exercises have historically been taught largely by physiotherapists, but may be taught by a knowledgeable nurse.

There is not as yet a consensus on the best way of teaching or practising pelvic floor exercises, and insufficient research has been done to describe a definitive treatment plan. Physiotherapists themselves are not agreed on the optimum therapeutic regime (Mantle and Versi, 1991; Laycock and Wyndaele, 1994).

There are three groups of muscles comprising the pelvic floor: the levatores ani, the urogenital diaphragm and the outlet group of muscles. For the purposes of this exercise, the most important are the levatores ani (Figure 6.8). These have three components, the pubococcygeus, the ileococcygeus and the ischiococcygeus.

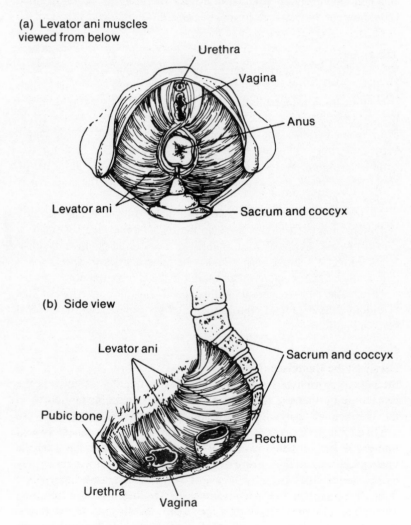

(a) Levator ani muscles
viewed from below

Urethra

Vagina

Anus

Levator ani

Sacrum and coccyx

(b) Side view

Levator ani

Sacrum and coccyx

Pubic bone

Rectum

Urethra

Vagina

Figure 6.8 *Muscles of the pelvic floor.*

The pubococcygeus forms a sling with an anterior gap through which the urethra, vagina and rectum pass. This striated muscle forms an important component in the voluntary control of both bladder and bowel emptying.

Preventive and remedial exercises are essentially identical, although remedial exercises must be performed more frequently and persistently. Before starting the exercises a careful assessment should be made and a thorough explanation of the exercises given. To be suitable for PFE the patient must be able to understand the instructions, and be motivated to try this self-help method.

It may be useful to describe the pelvic floor as a hammock which is suspended between the pubic and tail bones. When the muscle is young and healthy it stays well toned and taut and keeps all the body's openings firmly closed. After childbirth or menopause the hammock sags and can no longer hold the openings so tightly closed, especially when any additional strain is put on it. When the patient coughs, it gives way and lets a little urine out. The aim of the exercises is to get the hammock back to where it should be. Using two cupped hands can illustrate this explanation very clearly.

Ideally, the patient should then be examined vaginally. In practice, this may not happen, often because the nurse has not been taught how to perform the examination properly. There is obviously no point in subjecting a patient to an internal examination if the examiner does not know what to look for, and if the result of the examination will not make any difference to management anyway.

The patient should be examined in a supine position with her knees bent up and abducted laterally. The presence of any cystocele (prolapse of the anterior vaginal wall) or rectocele (prolapse of the posterior vaginal wall) should be noted. If either of these is severe, or if there is any degree of uterine descent, the chances of success from the exercises may be diminished. They may still be worth a try, especially if the patient is keen and would in any event have to wait for surgery. Even if surgery is eventually needed, exercise will improve the tone and blood flow locally, thus improving post-operative healing.

The pelvic floor should then be palpated using a gloved, lubricated finger. The bulk of the muscle can be assessed by feeling all around the vagina, approximately 3–5cm inside the introitus. Two fingers can be used to assess the strength, endurance and coordination of the pelvic floor. The patient is asked to 'squeeze, lift, hold and relax' (Laycock, 1992). The examiner should feel the fingers being gripped and pulled inwards. Many women cannot do this at the first try, or tend to bear down or contract the buttocks or abdominal muscles. The muscle tone should be carefully assessed, and ideally the examiner should persist until the patient is able to identify the correct action or at least stops using the wrong muscles. Some women find it easier to identify the back portion of the pelvic floor than the front, by imagining controlling flatus or severe diarrhoea.

Laycock (1992) has proposed a grading score for assessing the strength, length and number of contractions that the patient can achieve. Note should also be made of endurance (how many seconds she can hold maximal contraction for) and how many times this can be repeated before the muscles become fatigued.

A less invasive method of helping a patient to identify her pelvic floor is to sit her forward on a hard chair, with her legs apart and feet flat on the floor, leaning forward as far as she can with her head and arms just drooping. The instructor stands slightly to one side with a hand on the patient's back. Ask the patient to relax completely – to 'flop' – and then, concentrating only on the pelvic floor, to pull up and in. This position stretches the buttocks and makes it harder to tense them erroneously, and the instructor's hand on the woman's back will enable her or him to feel if the back muscles are tensing. Carefully observe the woman's head for any movement – if she is using incorrect muscles her head will tend to move slightly.

Often patients are nervous and tense when receiving instruction, and a few simple relaxation exercises to start with can obtain a much better outcome.

Asking the woman to attempt to stop passing urine midstream is useful in helping identification of the correct muscle action for PFE. It used to be advocated for a woman to stop midstream each time she voided urine. However, regular stopping midstream may interfere with the voiding mechanism in patients with detrusor dysfunction, and is now generally discouraged. During an exercise programme it is usually advised to try the stop test once each day. This both helps to remind the woman of the correct action and gives useful feedback on improvement, i.e. if she can now stop more quickly or easily.

Once the pelvic floor has been correctly identified, the exercises can start in earnest. Many women will be able to contract the pelvic floor standing or lying, but some find it easier to sit and lean forward a little until the muscle becomes stronger. If this is the case, she may be able to perform the exercise standing, but leaning forward slightly. The exercise programme must be tailored to the individual patient's abilities. If the woman experiences only a 'flicker' when trying to contract the pelvic floor, then she may commence by lifting and holding four times, trying to hold each contraction for a count of two seconds. A woman starting with a stronger muscle may start with a much more vigorous programme. Muscles will only get stronger if they are used at their limit, without however inducing undue fatigue, which will discourage further exercise. As she improves, she should increase the number and duration of contractions, ideally repeating the exercise programme hourly. The instructor will need to assess each patient carefully for her own regime. If the patient complains that the muscle aches, then her regime is too onerous. If it is simple for her to do, then she should be holding for longer, or doing more exercises. She should be warned not to expect overnight cures, but that three to six months is a realistic target.

In addition to these long, slow contractions, the woman should also practice short, sharp 'pull-ups'. She should squeeze and lift the pelvic floor as quickly as she can, as many times in succession as she can, before fatigue sets in. This will enhance the strength of the fast twitch fibres which form up to one-third of the pubococcygeus.

The exercises are not easy to remember and patients should be given advice. Again this will need to be tailored to the individual, depending on her lifestyle. It may help to link the exercises to regular activities – for example, each time she puts the kettle on, washes her hands, uses the photocopier, waits in a queue etc. The car is an ideal place to do some exercises; what else can you do while waiting at traffic lights or in a jam? A digital bleeping watch may also be useful, or a repeating cooker timer.

A woman may like to check that she is doing the exercises correctly by inserting a finger into the vagina while exercising and feeling the gentle squeeze for herself. If she does not feel happy to do this, she can either squat over a mirror and see the vagina close and perineum lift, or insert a tampon half way into the vagina and, gently supporting the end, she will feel it move when she contracts the pelvic floor. It is advisable to put some lubricating gel onto the tampon before insertion as it tends to absorb the normal secretions, making removal difficult. A woman who is sexually active can also contract her pelvic floor during intercourse.

A perineometer may be useful (Figure 6.9, overleaf). This comprises a vaginal probe with a gauge to indicate the strength of squeeze. This can tell the patient if she is exercising correctly and if her muscle power is increasing. This is very important in the phase before symptoms improve; it is always tempting to give up unless progress

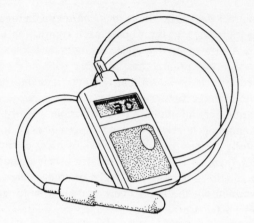

Figure 6.9 *Perineometer.*

is evident. The perineometer should not however be completely depended upon, as it may register if the patient bears down, as well as when squeezing it.

It is always important after teaching these exercises to see the patient regularly for support and advice. This will aid motivation and give an opportunity to review the exercises. Written back-up information may also be useful (see Table 6.1 for an example). Few patients will notice any improvement until they have been performing exercises for six to eight weeks. Most will have improved by three months, but some may take up to a year to achieve full benefits. Many patients can thus avoid surgery and have the satisfaction of curing themselves. As an added benefit many find that both her own and her partner's sexual enjoyment is increased as muscle tone improves.

Advice on the importance of general exercise, weight loss where indicated and avoiding constipation, should be given in addition to PFE.

Pelvic floor exercises may also help women with urgency and frequency due to an unstable detrusor. Pelvic floor contraction reflexly inhibits detrusor contraction and so regular exercise may actually help to control the problem. Once the woman has learned to contract the pelvic floor at will, this can be used during an unstable detrusor contraction, thereby both inhibiting the detrusor and increasing urethral resistance, and so making leakage less likely.

Table 6.1   Pelvic Floor Exercises (Patient Education Sheet)

Reproduced by permission of Smith & Nephew Pharmaceuticals Ltd and the
Continence Foundation.

Introduction

Physiotherapists, doctors and nurses know that pelvic floor exercises can help
you to improve your bladder control. When done correctly, pelvic floor exercises
can build up and strengthen the muscles to help you to hold urine.

What is the Pelvic Floor?

Layers of muscle stretch like a hammock from the pubic bone in front to the
bottom of the backbone (see diagram). These firm supportive muscles are called
the pelvic floor. They help to hold the bladder, womb and bowel in place, and to
close the bladder outlet and back passage.

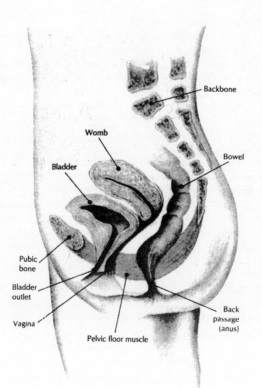

Table continued overleaf

Table 6.1   (continued)

How Does the Pelvic Floor Work?
The muscles of the pelvic floor are kept firm and slightly tense to stop leakage of urine from the bladder or faeces from the bowel. When you pass water or have a bowel motion the pelvic floor muscles relax. Afterwards, they tighten again to restore control.

Pelvic floor muscles can become weak and sag because of childbirth, lack of exercise, the change of life, or just getting older. Weak muscles give you less control, and you may leak urine, especially with exercise or when you cough, sneeze or laugh.

How Can Pelvic Floor Exercises Help?
Pelvic floor exercises can strengthen these muscles so that they once again give support. This will improve your bladder control and improve or stop leakage of urine. Like any other muscles in the body, the more you use and exercise them, the stronger the pelvic floor will be.

Learning To Do Pelvic Floor Exercises
It is important to learn to do the exercises in the right way, and to check from time to time that you are still doing them correctly.
1) Sit comfortably with your knees slightly apart. Now imagine that you are trying to stop yourself passing wind from the bowel. To do this you must squeeze the muscle around the back passage. Try squeezing and lifting that muscle as if you really do have wind. You should be able to feel the muscle move. Your buttocks and legs should not move at all. You should be aware of the skin around the back passage tightening and being pulled up and away from your chair. Really try to feel this.
2) Now imagine that you are sitting on the toilet passing urine. Picture yourself trying to stop the stream of urine. Really try to stop it. Try doing that now as you are reading this. You should be using the same group of muscles that you used before, but don't be surprised if you find this harder than exercise 1.
3) Next time you go to the toilet to pass urine, try the 'stop test' about half way through emptying your bladder. Once you have stopped the flow of urine, relax again and allow the bladder to empty completely. You may only be able to slow down the stream. Don't worry; your muscles will improve and strengthen with time and exercise. If the stream of urine speeds up when you try to do this exercise, you are squeezing the wrong muscles.

Do not get into the habit of doing the 'stop test' every time you pass urine. This exercise should be done only once a day at the most.

Now you know what it feels like to exercise the pelvic floor!

Table 6.1   (continued)

Practising Your Exercises
1) Sit, stand or lie with your knees slightly apart. Slowly tighten and pull up the pelvic floor muscles as hard as you can. Hold tightened for at least 5 seconds if you can, then relax. Repeat at least 5 times (slow pull-ups).
2) Now pull the muscles up *quickly* and tightly, then relax immediately. Repeat at least 5 times (fast pull-ups).
3) Do these two exercises – 5 slow and 5 fast – at least 10 times every day.
4) As the muscles get stronger, you will find that you can hold for longer than 5 seconds, and that you can do more than 5 pull-ups each time without the muscle getting tired.
5) It takes time for exercise to make muscles stronger. You are unlikely to notice improvement for several weeks – so stick at it! You will need to exercise regularly for several months before the muscles gain their full strength.

Tips to Help You
1) Get into the habit of doing your exercises with things you do regularly – every time you touch water if you are a housewife, every time you answer the phone if you are at the office . . . whatever *you* do often.
2) Do the 'stop test' once a day when passing urine. Stopping your urine should get faster and easier.
3) If you are unsure that you are exercising the right muscle, put one or two fingers in the vagina and try the exercises, to check. You should feel a gentle squeeze if you are exercising the pelvic floor.
4) Use the pelvic floor when you are afraid you might leak – pull up the muscles before you sneeze or lift something heavy. Your control will gradually improve.
5) Drink normally – at least 6–8 cups every day. And don't get into the habit of going to the toilet 'just in case'. Go only when you feel that the bladder is full.
6) Watch your weight – extra weight puts extra strain on your pelvic floor muscles.
7) Once you have regained control of your bladder, don't forget your pelvic floor. Continue to do your pelvic floor exercises a few times each day to ensure that the problem does not come back.

You can do pelvic floor exercises wherever you are – nobody need know what you are doing!

Do You Have Any Questions?
This Information Sheet is designed to teach you how to control your bladder, so that you'll be dry and comfortable. If you have problems doing the exercises, or if you don't understand any part of this information, ask your doctor, nurse, continence adviser or physiotherapist for help.

Do your pelvic floor exercises every single day. Have faith in them.
You should begin to see good results in a few weeks.

Vaginal Cones

Vaginal cones (Figure 6.10) may be a helpful addition to PFE. These are graded weights (20–70g) which are available in sets of either three, five or nine. One weight is inserted into the vagina for up to thirty minutes twice a day. Contraction of the abdominal or gluteal muscles will not aid retention of the cone, which must be held in place by contraction of the pelvic floor. By gradually increasing the weight of the cone the strength of the pelvic floor may be increased (Peattie et al., 1988).

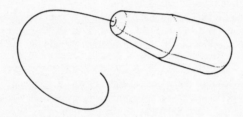

Figure 6.10   *Vaginal cone.*

Vaginal cones may be particularly useful for women with pudendal nerve damage, who may not have good sensory feedback when practising PFE. They also provide useful biofeedback – the woman knows that she is using the right muscle if she can hold the cone in, and that she is progressing if she can hold in a progressively heavier weight. Having a tangible gadget may possibly improve motivation and compliance for some women.

Careful assessment will decide which weight to start with – one that can be held in, but not too easily. The cone should be positioned just above the pelvic floor, so that the woman is conscious of the need to hold it in (Figure 6.11) (pushed in too far it may simply lie horizontally and not fulfil its desired function). The patient should use the cone while carrying out normal activities (preferably standing or walking rather than sitting). Pants should be worn to avoid toe damage if the cone does slip out!

Neuromuscular Electrical Stimulation

Neuromuscular electrical stimulation (NMS or NMES) is a technique whereby small electrical impulses applied to the body may affect nerve or muscle tissue within the field of stimulation. In muscle activation, these impulses aim to mimic bioelectrical currents produced in the

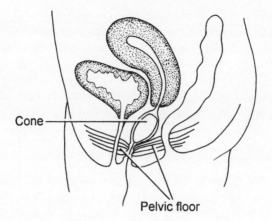

Cone

Pelvic floor

Figure 6.11   *Cone in position.*

body. Due to the perceived sensory effect (described as 'pins and needles'), current intensity is limited. This may be a disadvantage in some cases where maximum intensity is required, but may be considered as a safety factor in others.

Within the pelvic region and lower urinary tract, NMS has been shown to produce contraction of pelvic floor muscles (Erlandson et al., 1978), contraction of the underactive bladder (Katona et al., 1984), normalisation of micturition reflexes (Lindstrom et al., 1983) and pain relief in interstitial cystitis (Fall, 1987).

Traditionally, NMS was used to 're-educate' muscles. This implied that the muscles were very weak or had forgotten how to work, and so the stimulation was applied to facilitate a muscle contraction. The patient was instructed to 'join in' with the current and so learned to appreciate the feeling of a particular muscle contraction. This method applies to the pelvic floor muscles, and patients can learn to contract their pelvic floor muscles after one or two short (10 minute) treatment sessions. Muscle strengthening then continues with daily pelvic floor exercises.

However, muscle changes have been noted after prolonged stimulation periods, with low frequency (around 10 Hertz) favouring development of slow-twitch muscle fibres, and frequencies of 30 to 50 Hertz affecting fast fibre activity. As the pelvic floor is made up of approximately 70% slow- and 30% fast-twitch fibres, a combination of the above frequencies is often advocated. Two daily periods starting at 10 minutes and progressing to 1 hour of strong stimulation is said to enhance muscle development.

141

The plethora of different stimulators on the market and extravagant claims made by manufacturers can leave the clinician confused. Basically, these devices should be safe and allow for selection of a number of electrical parameters (see below).

Electrical Parameters
Intensity. NMS units must generate a current which is capable of producing a (strong) muscle contraction. This can be either a battery-operated device or mains driven.

Frequency. This relates to the number of impulses generated per second (pulses per second: PPS) and is measured in Hertz (Hz). Generally, to produce a comfortable contraction without causing undue fatigue, a frequency of 30 to 35 Hz is selected.

Pulse Width. This is the width (measured in microseconds: μs) of the individual pulses. Physiologists recommend 200 to 300 μs for muscle stimulation, and studies on detrusor instability suggest that larger pulse widths (500 μs) are more efficacious in normalising the bladder reflexes.

Duty Cycle. This describes the time 'on' (stimulation) and time 'off' (rest period); no stimulating current should be continuous. Generally, the time 'off' should be equal to, or greater than, the time 'on', e.g. 5 seconds 'on', 10 seconds 'off'. Stronger muscles require shorter rest times, and the duty cycle is designed to prevent fatigue.

Selection of the appropriate parameters may well affect treatment outcomes.

Types of Current
Traditionally, Faradism was the principle NMS current available for muscle re-education in the UK; however, this was uncomfortable and has been replaced by electronically-produced currents with many different names. Interferential therapy has been linked with the treatment of incontinence, but there is no literature to show that it is any better than any other stimulating current. Generally, any bi-phasic current will activate neuromuscular tissue, and providing the device can generate enough current and allow the clinician to modify the electrical parameters described above, such a device should be suitable for pelvic floor stimulation.

Electrodes

The efficacy of neuromuscular stimulation is only as good as the electrodes used to deliver the current to the tissues. The main impedance (resistance) to current flow is encountered at the electrode/skin interface, and for optimum effect, the electrodes should be sited as close as possible to the target tissue. In view of this, internal electrodes are generally advocated for stimulation of the pelvic floor muscles and activation of the pudendal/pelvic nerves; the vaginal mucosa offers less resistance than the skin in the perineum, and the stimulating electrodes are close to the levator ani muscles. Alternative sites for electrode placement include:

1) Two electrodes on the perineum: one anterior, immediately inferior to the symphysis pubis and one over the anus (female).
2) One over the perineal body and one over the sacral area.
3) Two small electrodes placed at 2 o'clock and 10 o'clock to the anus.
4) One electrode on the perineal body and one over the dorsum of the penis (male).

No study has shown that any position gives superior results to any other. However, internal electrodes are generally easier to apply.

Conditions

Clinically NMS is not used in isolation; when reported thus, NMS has usually been under scientific scrutiny. Generally, combination therapy is advocated. For muscle-strengthening regimens, e.g. for stress incontinence, NMS, pelvic floor exercises and biofeedback are recommended. If a home unit is available, stimulation should be applied once or twice per day for up to 2 hours (total time), at 30 Hz, using an internal electrode. If using hospital equipment, one, two or three treatment sessions per week, depending on resources, has produced good results.

Detrusor instability is best treated at maximum intensity, using internal electrodes delivering a current of around 10 Hz. Two daily sessions of 30 minutes for patients with a home unit, or one, two or three sessions per week for hospital treatment, are advisable. Bladder training and pelvic floor exercises should also be incorporated in the treatment regimen.

Contraindications

All patients undergoing NMS must be capable of understanding the treatment and the sensation it will produce, and be able to remain still during the treatment. The presence of vaginal, anal or vulval infections is a contraindication, as are pregnancy and the wearing of a pacemaker.

Surgery

Women with a moderate to severe degree of stress incontinence which has not responded to therapy often require surgery to alleviate their condition, especially if the stress incontinence is associated with moderate to severe prolapse. The choice of operation will depend on the individual surgeon and the patient's preference. It is essential that the patient undergoes urodynamic studies prior to surgery because of the poor correlation between clinical and urodynamic diagnosis.

There are a great many variations on the vaginal repair, and a vaginal hysterectomy or associated procedure may be carried out at the same time. Anterior colporrhaphy (anterior repair) used to be the most common operation for stress incontinence, but although it is an excellent operation to repair a cystocele, for genuine stress incontinence it has a failure rate of 38% (US Department of Health, 1992) and is not recommended (Stanton, 1984), except where a surgeon has a special expertise in its use.

Most gynaecologists consider the operation of choice to be a retropubic urethropexy such as the Burch colposuspension. It is an abdominal procedure where paired sutures are inserted into the paravaginal tissue on either side of the bladder neck and tied to the ileopectineal ligament on the same side, thus elevating the bladder neck (Figure 6.12). When performed as a primary procedure, the operation has a 97% success rate at one year, and 79% at five years (Stanton, 1984). Long-term complications include voiding difficulties, detrusor instability and enterocele formation. An alternative is the Marshall-Marchetti-Krantz procedure, which approximates periurethral tissue to the symphasis pubis. Overall success rates for retropubic suspension are 78% cure and a further 5% improved (US Department of Health, 1992).

Where the vagina is immobile because of scarring from previous failed operations it is often not possible to carry out a colposuspension. In this case, a sling or endoscopically guided bladder neck suspension may be performed.

The approach for a sling procedure is abdominal and is either

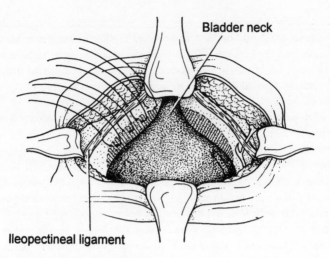

Bladder neck

Ileopectineal ligament

Figure 6.12 *Colposuspension.*

constructed so that the sling tightens every time the patient contracts her pelvic floor, or is attached to the ileopectineal ligaments, thus providing bladder neck support.

Slings may be made of organic material such as bovine rectus sheath or the patient's own rectus sheath, or inorganic material such as polyethylene. Slings are associated with a high incidence of voiding difficulty and may erode though the urethra or vagina. Infection and complications are more common if inorganic material is used, and success rates are lower (US Department of Health, 1992).

Bladder neck suspension may also be performed endoscopically (Stamey or Raz procedure). Sutures mounted on a long needle are passed either side of the bladder neck in a loop down to the vagina and tied in front of the rectus sheath under laparoscopic control. It is a more successful operation in elderly women, whereas there is a high rate of recurrent symptoms in younger patients as too much strain is placed upon the sutures. Complication rates may be higher than for open procedures (US Department of Health, 1992).

Periurethral collagen injections have also been advocated as an alternative to more major procedures. In some cases this can be done on an outpatient basis. The long-term results are not yet available.

Any type of surgery requires careful pre- and post-operative counselling. This can increase both the success of the procedure and the patient's satisfaction and adjustment. The patient must be given a full explanation of the procedure and what to expect. If hysterectomy is likely to be necessary, this is a decision which involves careful thought and discussion with partner or family. It should be made clear that none of these operations can guarantee success, and the chances of cure should be honestly discussed. Patients who are led to unrealistic expectations of total cure tend to be highly intolerant and disappointed if any symptoms, however mild, persist post-operatively.

If the patient has not yet completed her family, surgery should usually be delayed until after the final pregnancy, especially with sling operations, as vaginal delivery might both be difficult and undo the effects of the surgery. Every patient should be warned that there is a possibility of stress incontinence recurring at a later date. This is especially true if she undertakes vigorous exercise or heavy lifting. Women who only leak when they lift heavy weights, or have a heavy manual job, should probably be discouraged from opting for surgery. As the convalescent periods are different (a few weeks for vaginal procedures, up to three months for slings), women with heavy family or career commitments may prefer the former, even in the knowledge that success rates are lower.

Post-operative advice should include instructions to avoid lifting and abdominal effort for the convalescent period. The patient should also refrain from sexual intercourse for six weeks to allow full healing. Many women experience problems in returning to an active and fulfilling sex life after surgery. Sometimes the reason for this is psychological, because of a changed body image, especially after a hysterectomy. There may be physical discomfort because of incomplete healing or local infection. More commonly the actual anatomy of the vagina has been altered, and it often takes both partners a while to adjust to the new, smaller contours. Sometimes there is a ridge or kink in the vaginal wall. The woman may also be nervous or anxious in case intercourse should hurt, or the operation might be 'undone', and so be understimulated and poorly lubricated. Sometimes simple explanations, reassurance that no harm can be done, and possibly a tube of K-Y Jelly for lubrication, will resolve the problem. The lubricant can be made considerably pleasanter and more acceptable by warming the tube in a bowl of warm water before use. Occasionally it may be advisable to experiment with new positions for intercourse to overcome problems with a taut anterior vaginal wall.

In the past many women have undergone multiple operations for stress incontinence, which has either been unaffected or recurred. Sometimes this was because the original diagnosis was wrong and the woman really had detrusor instability rather than genuine stress incontinence, or the two conditions coexisted. Surgery can often make the symptoms of an unstable detrusor worse. Hopefully, the increased use of urodynamic investigations will help to avoid this in the future. The first operation has the highest chance of success. As more gynaecologists and urologists become interested and expert in incontinence surgery, and as understanding of the mechanism of successful operations increase, it is to be hoped that there will be fewer failures.

Construction of a Neourethra
In a few centres a technique has been developed for the construction of a completely new urethra from a flap of bladder muscle (Bavendam and Leach, 1987; Blaivas, 1989; Mundy, 1989). This can be used for women with congenital abnormalities, or for women with a urethra that has become scarred and dysfunctional from repeated surgery. It is too early to evaluate the success of this procedure, but it might hold hope for the future.

Drug Treatments
Drugs have been tried as a treatment for genuine stress incontinence, with rather limited success. Alpha stimulants, which should increase urethral tone, e.g. phenylpropanolamine or ephedrine, may produce some improvement for some women.

Hormone replacement therapy is useful in post-menopausal women with atrophic changes. This is discussed in more detail in Chapter 11.

URINARY FISTULA

A fistula or 'false passage' between the bladder and vagina will cause continuous, uncontrollable, passive incontinence. It is relatively uncommon in Western countries, where it is mostly caused iatrogenically as a result of a mishap during gynaecological surgery or after pelvic irradiation for tumour. It is more common in underdeveloped countries as a complication of obstructed delivery. Prolonged pressure of the baby's head causes tissue necrosis, and the resultant sloughing leaves a vesico-vaginal fistula. This is a very major problem for the unfortunate woman, who is often rejected by her spouse and family and becomes a social outcast. Many have no access to medical help nor products to deal with the total incontinence, which can be double incontinence if a recto-vaginal fistula is also present.

Fistulas caused surgically or during childbirth are usually repaired surgically. This is done vaginally six to ten weeks after the trauma, provided that the patient is in good health. Post-irradiation fistulas are often far more difficult to repair, as there is usually much scar tissue and an avascular zone in the vagina. The patient is often also in poor health.

There can be little doubt about the misery occasioned by a urinary fistula. The constant leakage of urine is extremely difficult to cope with, and there is no pad yet available that will cope reliably with this degree of female incontinence. Quality of life often becomes very poor, and the patient becomes isolated and depressed. There is no respite, waking or sleeping. Where the defect cannot be closed surgically, a urinary diversion into an ileal conduit (see Chapter 4) is strongly recommended, wherever the patient is fit enough. Even though a stoma means continuous 'incontinence', this is at least controllable with a suitable collection bag. If the patient is too unwell for this major surgery or does not want it, the best that can offered at present is one of the largest body-worn pads (see Chapter 15). These will need to be supplied freely in large quantities.

INCONTINENCE AND SEXUAL ACTIVITY

Some women experience urinary incontinence during sexual activity. One study found that 24% of incontinent women are incontinent during intercourse; two-thirds of these experienced leaking on penetration and the other one-third experienced leaking with orgasm. The mechanism is unknown, hardly surprisingly as this is very difficult to investigate. It is likely to be either mechanical pressure or a detrusor contraction underlying the problem. Sometimes treatment for a known bladder dysfunction – for example drug therapy for an unstable detrusor – will cure the incontinence.

It may be difficult for a patient to talk about this particular problem, and the nurse should provide an opportunity and give appropriate prompts to make such a discussion possible. Most women will also have bladder symptoms at other times, but for a few this is the only occasion they experience incontinence. Either way it is a potential source of distress and embarrassment, and the patient may be unable to discuss the problem with her partner. She will need a great deal of reassurance that the symptom has no pathological significance, as well as advice on learning how to live with it.

A change of position for intercourse may well alleviate the problem, particularly if mechanical pressure can be relieved, for example if penetration is from behind. The woman should be advised always to empty her bladder as fully as possible before intercourse, and it may be appropriate to protect the bed.

Some women who have difficulty experiencing orgasm find that their sexual enjoyment is improved by pelvic floor exercises. The pelvic floor contracts reflexly during orgasm, and this may be enhanced by increased muscle tone and bulk.

INCONTINENCE DURING PREGNANCY

Incontinence of urine is a common symptom during pregnancy. Probably over 50% of primiparous women and 75% of multiparous women experience some incontinence. The majority complain of increased frequency of micturition, usually starting in the first trimester, persisting and becoming more frequent until delivery.

The most likely cause is simple mechanical pressure on the bladder, which resolves automatically after the birth. Most women expect frequency during pregnancy and few are incapacitated by it.

Incontinence during pregnancy is usually experienced as stress incontinence. Sometimes this may have been present prior to pregnancy, but for many it is new. It is seldom severe but for a minority it will become a significant problem, particularly during the last trimester. Only time will resolve this, and disposable pads and plenty of support should be offered. Many women find that the stress incontinence resolves after delivery, although a minority will find that it continues to trouble them.

Pregnancy is a good time to teach and reinforce pelvic floor exercises. Exercise gives good tone to the muscle during delivery, it enhances the blood supply, promoting healing, and it is much easier to continue a regime previously learned than to try to start a new one when you are sore after the birth. Also, if problems do arise later, at least women may remember advice previously given.

It is strongly recommended that all new mothers are given a leaflet on pelvic floor exercises while in hospital – even though it may be disregarded at the time, it may be of infinite value later. In many European countries women are advised about pelvic floor exercise at a post-natal check, rather than immediately after delivery. This may be a more realistic time to start exercise – once soreness has subsided and the initial turmoil of a new baby has settled a little.

OCCLUSIVE DEVICES

Several devices are available which aim to control female urinary incontinence by occluding the urethra mechanically. Although they are most appropriate for women with stress incontinence, they can be used to control any type of leakage. The aim is to restore normal pressure and anatomic relationships by lifting and supporting the bladder neck and urethra. These devices do not treat the cause of the problem, so they should not be a first choice except if the woman is not a candidate for, or does not desire, other therapy.

Tampons

Some women find that a large menstrual tampon worn in the vagina controls mild incontinence. This method is particularly suitable for women who are accustomed to using tampons and who have only an occasional problem. For example, a woman who leaks slightly while playing sports might choose this method to control leakage. A woman who says her incontinence is better during her period should be questioned about her method of sanitary protection, because using a tampon might be the reason for this improvement. It is unwise to use menstrual tampons continuously, because their absorbent properties can make the vagina sore and dry.

A commercially produced foam tampon is available. This performs the same function as the menstrual tampon, without the drying effect on the vagina. It can therefore be worn daily.

Ring Pessary

If stress incontinence is associated with an obvious prolapse of the anterior vaginal wall, a ring pessary can be fitted by a gynaecologist (Figure 6.13). The rings come in a wide range of sizes. Insertion is usually momentarily uncomfortable, but once in place the pessary is generally comfortable if the correct size has been chosen. The ring is indwelling and will usually remain in place for several months before being changed. Some patients can learn to remove and reinsert it. Careful explanation must be given before the use of a pessary is considered; some women dislike the idea and reject it. It should be carefully established that the patient is not still sexually active, because then a ring pessary is unsuitable unless the patient is competent at removing and reinserting the device.

Some older women with vaginal atrophy and some nulliparous women have such a small introitus that a pessary cannot be inserted.

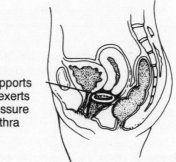

Pessary supports
cervix and exerts
forward pressure
against urethra

Figure 6.13   *Ring pessary.*

Pessaries are best used for the older woman with stress incontinence
and pelvic prolapse, who does not want or is unfit for surgery. In
some women, reduction of a large cystocele by the pessary can
actually increase incontinence. Mental and physical disabilities are not
contraindications, because little management is required by the patient
or care-giver.

REFERENCES AND FURTHER READING

Bavendam, T., Leach, G., 1987. Urogynaecologic reconstruction. *Problems in Urology*, 1, 2: 295.

Blaivas, J. G., 1989. Vaginal flap urethral reconstruction: an alternative to the bladder flap neourethra. *Journal of Urology*, 141, 3: 542.

Erlandson, B.-E., Fall, M., Carlsson, C.-A. 1978. The effect of intravaginal electrical stimulation on the feline urethra and urinary bladder. Electrical parameters. *Scandinavian Journal of Urology and Nephrology*, 44: 5–18.

Fall, M., 1987. Transcutaneous electrical nerve stimulation in interstitial cystitis – update on clinical experience. *Urology*, 24: 40–2.

Farragher, D., 1990. Trophic stimulation. *Nursing Standard*, 5, 8: 10–11.

Katona, F., Berenyi, M., Szabados, P., Balazs, M., Tunyogi, E., Vegh, I., 1984. Early electro-urodynamics and early intravesical electrotherapy. *Proceedings of the 14th ICS Meeting, Innsbruck*: 35–7.

Kegel, A. H., 1951. Physiologic therapy for urinary stress incontinence. *Journal of the American Medical Association*, 146, 10: 915–17.

Laycock, J., 1991. Pelvic floor re-education. *Nursing*, 4, 39: 15–17.

Laycock, J., 1992. Pelvic floor re-education for the promotion of continence. In: Roe, B. H., (ed), *Clinical Nursing Practice*. Prentice Hall, Hemel Hempstead.

Laycock, J., Wyndaele, J. J., 1994. *Understanding the Pelvic Floor*. Neen Healthbooks, Dereham, Norfolk, UK.

Lindstrom, S., Fall, M., Carlsson, C.-A., Erlandson, B.-E., 1983. The neurophysiological basis of bladder inhibition in response to intravaginal electrical stimulation. *Journal of Urology*, 129: 405–10.

Mantle, J., Versi, E., 1991. Physiotherapy for urinary stress incontinence – a national survey. *British Medical Journal*, 302: 753–5.

Mundy, A. R., 1989. Urethral substitution in women. *British Journal of Urology*, 63, 1: 80.

Peattie, A. B., Plevnik, S., Stanton, S. L., 1988. Vaginal Cones: a conservative method of treating genuine stress incontinence. *British Journal of Obstetrics and Gynaecology*, 95: 1049–53.

Polden, M., Mantle, J., 1990. *Physiotherapy, Obstetrics and Gynaecology*. Butterworth-Heinemann, Oxford.

Raz, S., (ed), 1983. *Female Urology*. W. B. Saunders, Philadelphia.

Raz, S., 1981. Modified bladder neck suspension for female stress incontinence. *Urology*, 17: 82.

Schussler, B., Laycock, J., Norton, P., Stanton, S. L., 1994. *Pelvic Floor Re-education – Principles and Practice*. Springer Verlag, London.

Snooks, S. J., Barnes, P. R. J., Swash, M., 1984. Damage to the innervation of the voluntary anal and periurethral sphincter musculature in incontinence: an electrophysiological study. *Journal of Neurology, Neurosurgery and Psychiatry*, 47: 1269–73.

Snooks, S. J., Swash, M., Mathers, S. E., Henry, M. M., 1990. Effect of vaginal delivery on the pelvic floor: a five-year follow-up. *British Journal of Surgery*, 77: 1358–60.

Stamey, T. A., 1980. Endoscopic suspension of the vesical neck for urinary incontinence in the female: report of 203 consecutive patients. *Annals of Surgery*, 192: 465.

Stanton, S. L., (ed), 1984. *Clinical Gynaecologic Urology*. C. V. Mosby Company, St. Louis.

Stanton, S. L., Tanagho, E. A., (eds), 1980. *Surgery of Female Incontinence*. Springer Verlag, Berlin.

Thomas, T. M., Plymat, K. R., Blannin, J., Meade, T. W., 1980. Prevalence of urinary incontinence. *British Medical Journal*, 281: 1243–5.

US Department of Health, 1992. Urinary incontinence in adults – clinical practice guidelines. Agency of Health Care Policy and Research, United States Department of Health and Human Services, Rockville, USA.

Versi, E., Mantle, J., 1989. The use of vaginal cones in the management of genuine stress incontinence. *British Journal of Obstetrics and Gynaecology*, 96: 752–3.

Wolin, L. H., 1969. Stress incontinence in young healthy nulliparous female subjects. *Journal of Urology*, 101: 545–9.

Note: The journal of the Chartered Society of Physiotherapy published a whole issue of review articles in 1994. *Physiotherapy*, 80, 3: 125–53.

Chapter 7
Male Urinary Incontinence

Jan Denning, RGN, NDNCert
*Continence Adviser, Southern Birmingham Community
Health NHS Trust*

While men can suffer incontinence for reasons outlined elsewhere in this book, certain problems affect the male exclusively and are dealt with separately in this chapter. Men seem to be especially reluctant to seek help for incontinence, which is often thought of as a 'woman's problem', and the nurse may be the first person in whom the patient confides.

BENIGN PROSTATIC HYPERPLASIA (BPH)

From the fourth decade of life onwards, all men have some degree of benign enlargement of the prostate gland (Figure 7.1). About one man in ten will experience symptoms.

It is estimated that in the UK 2.4 million men above the age of 50

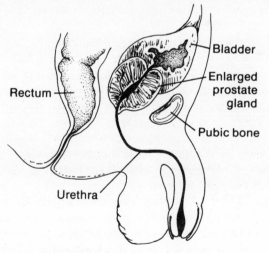

Figure 7.1   *Prostatic hyperplasia.*

years have benign prostatic hyperplasia (BPH). This amounts to 25% of men experiencing symptoms of prostate disease, which rises to 43% in the 60–69 age group, in some cases resulting in incontinence. Nowhere near this number are actually being treated for this condition (Garraway, 1991).

Prevalence studies in the general population are few and far between, because until the introduction of transrectal ultrasound there were no non-invasive techniques to measure prostate volume.

Symptoms

Symptoms caused by an enlarged prostate gland relate mostly to the outflow obstruction that this causes. Hesitancy, a slow, weak urinary stream, and terminal dribbling at the end of micturition are common. Often the bladder does not empty completely and chronic residual urine is present.

With the presence of large residual volumes there may be frequency and nocturia. Sometimes the nocturia or 'getting up' at night to void may be the first symptom to be noticed by the patient. More distressing is the symptom of nocturnal enuresis (bed wetting), which may happen if the bladder is so full that it overflows. At rest, some relaxation of the urethral sphincter may occur, due to disruption of the signalling mechanisms within the nervous control of a permanently stretched bladder. Urgency with urge incontinence or an almost continual dribbling overflow incontinence may be present. Dysuria with urgency might be present in patients in whom the residual urine becomes infected.

Sometimes rectal symptoms are troublesome – either a continuous desire to defaecate caused by prostate pressure on the rectum, or haemorrhoids resulting from repeated straining to micturate. On other occasions the first symptom the patient experiences is acute retention of urine and a complete inability to void.

Signs

The nurse may be the first person to spot the tense, distended abdomen of an elderly man who is totally unaware that his bladder is full to overflowing. If infection is superimposed, the urine may become cloudy and foul-smelling, occasionally with haematuria. A large residual volume may obstruct ureteric outflow, with consequent back pressure to the kidneys and the development of hydronephrosis. If this is the case, the patient may be confused, with anorexia, weight loss, anaemia and dehydration resulting from uraemia.

If a large residual is suspected, it will be necessary to catheterise the man to remove the residual urine. Rapid emptying of the bladder is not dangerous to the patient if done using sterile precautions and if the bladder is not allowed to become over-distended again. Any presence of blood in the urine will usually be insignificant and represents bleeding from the mucosal lining of the bladder wall. The catheter should be left in situ to allow renal function to re-stabilise. There is a possibility of a post-obstructive diuresis during the first 24-hour period. This production of copious quantities of urine follows after a period of temporary renal shut-down, caused by back pressure in the ureters from the large residual urine volume. Careful monitoring of fluid intake and output is essential during this period, and if large discrepancies are found it may be necessary to initiate intravenous fluid replacement.

Often by the time help is sought, the problem has been present for many years. If the detrusor muscle is repeatedly trying to overcome raised outflow resistance, the muscle tends to hypertrophy and may develop a secondary detrusor instability and trabeculation (weakened outpouchings between hypertrophied muscle bundles).

Investigation

A careful history will elicit many of the above symptoms, which are often aggravated by cold weather or alcohol. It is especially important to distinguish between symptoms of prostatism and those of a pure detrusor instability (instability more often presents as frequency, urgency, urge incontinence, with little or no voiding difficulty).

An unstable bladder secondary to the outlet obstruction occurs in 70–80% of men. Symptoms of an unstable bladder include frequency, urgency and nocturia. Approximately 60–75% of these bladders eventually return to normal after the obstruction has been relieved.

Symptoms of BPH tend to begin gradually and can be classified as obstructive and irritative. Obstructive symptoms are caused by the narrowing of the urethra by the enlarged prostate gland. Classically, these symptoms can be defined as hesitancy, reduction in force of urinary stream, interruption of stream and terminal dribbling. Irritative symptoms develop as the bladder reacts to having to work harder to pass urine through the obstructed urethra. These symptoms are likely to be nocturia, daytime frequency, urgency, dysuria and perhaps a sensation of incomplete voiding.

It is not generally considered to be a nursing responsibility to perform a digital rectal examination to determine the size of a prostate gland, though with the advent of nurse-led prostate assessment clinics in urology departments or in community settings, nurses are increasingly learning to perform digital rectal examinations – usually with the oversight of a doctor to lend credence. Whoever performs the examination may feel an enlarged prostate gland, although the palpable size of the gland bears no direct relationship to the degree of outflow obstruction. Even a minimally enlarged prostate can obstruct the urethra, while some relatively large glands cause no problems and that person may be virtually symptom-free.

Abdominal examination may enable palpation of the bladder, or alternatively a faecal impaction which may mimic prostatism. The perineal skin may be sore or excoriated because of urinary incontinence, but not all men with prostatic enlargement are incontinent.

Measurement of urinary flow-rate (see Chapter 3) will usually reveal a low, prolonged flow, sometimes interrupted or with a very long 'tail'. Measurement of post-micturition residual urine volume by in-out catheter should be unnecessary as a routine part of the diagnostic investigations – if all the clinical symptoms of BPH are present, including a palpable bladder, it will only serve to risk infecting a usually sterile system. Catheterisation may prove difficult to perform, anyway, if the prostate is very large or if insufficient anaesthetic gel has been instilled. Often a large volume of residual urine is present. A midstream urine specimen is analysed to see if there is blood, sugar (possible diabetes mellitus) or infection present.

A blood test (for renal function) should be routine, checking levels of urea and creatinine. Abnormal levels of these waste products indicate that the kidneys are not filtering properly. A blood test for prostate-specific antigen (PSA) can indicate possible carcinoma of the prostate, although there is debate about 'normal' values for PSA. An intravenous urogram will be performed if renal impairment is suspected.

A cystometrogram, if performed, will show a high voiding pressure with a low flow-rate and often a detrusor instability during filling. Many prostatectomies are performed without prior cystometrogram, but if the diagnosis of an unstable bladder is suspected the test is essential. A prostatectomy performed on a man with an unobstructed urethra and an unstable bladder will merely reduce his outflow resistance and make him even more likely to be incontinent.

Treatment

Roughly one half of men who experience symptoms from prostatic enlargement eventually require a prostatectomy. There are two surgical approaches commonly used to remove the prostate discussed here. A third approach via the perineum is rarely used.

Transurethral Resection of the Prostate (TUR or TURP)

A transurethral resection of the prostate is performed via a specially adapted cystoscope, and is a relatively safe operation. As no abdominal wound is involved, patients can mobilise comfortably very soon after surgery (this is important in older patients). All but the largest prostates can be removed transurethrally, but removal must be done by an experienced surgeon as it is possible to damage the external urethral sphincter, which will almost always result in incontinence (see below).

Retropubic Prostatectomy (RPP)

A retropubic prostatectomy is performed via a lower abdominal incision and the prostate is 'shelled out' of its capsule. This is in many ways a simpler operation requiring less skill than a TURP, and it can be performed for even the largest of prostates. However, it does involve an abdominal wound with its associated morbidity. Mobilisation may be delayed by abdominal discomfort, and the length of hospital stay is double that for TURP.

Complications of Prostatectomy

As with any general anaesthetic, a certain risk of mortality and morbidity is involved, especially in the older age-groups. Many urological centres are able to offer an epidural anaesthesia to those unfit for or specially at risk from a general anaesthetic.

Impotence is quite common following prostatectomy. About 7% of previously potent men will be rendered partially or totally impotent by the operation. If a man had erectile problems prior to prostatectomy, he has at least a 30% likelihood of being worse post-operatively. The majority of men are infertile following prostatectomy because of retrograde ejaculation of semen into the bladder. This is caused by surgical destruction of the bladder neck.

The most frequent complication of any approach is haemorrhage. There is the possibility of infection even with use of prophylactic antibiotics. Incontinence is dealt with separately below.

Altogether roughly 20% of men experience some complication after prostatectomy. It is important to discuss these possibilities fully with the patient prior to making a decision about surgery. Unless there are urgent medical indications, such as imminent renal failure, the patient should be encouraged to decide whether his symptoms are troublesome enough to warrant the risk of the possible complications. It should not be forgotten that an elderly man may value his fertility and potency as highly as a younger man. Good pre-operative counselling will avoid many later regrets and recriminations.

Having said this, the majority of men with symptoms of voiding difficulties or incontinence arising from prostatic hyperplasia will, if correctly diagnosed, benefit from prostatectomy, and much misery is relieved by this operation. Many men take these symptoms for granted with advancing age and suffer a restricted lifestyle and troublesome symptoms unnecessarily. There is a need for urodynamic clinics and urological surgeons to be more widely available to cope with present problems, let alone the likely increased demands of an increasingly aged population.

Alternative Non-Surgical Treatment for BPH

Over the last ten years, several new treatments have been developed that are promising alternatives to surgery for benign prostatic hyperplasia, although the majority have a lower success rate.

For those men who are unsuited to surgery because of heart, circulation or respiratory problems, or those who may be too frail for spinal anaesthesia, these options may be considered. There are also many men who reject the opportunity of surgery because of retrograde ejaculatory problems if they wish to have more children, or who feel that their symptoms are not sufficiently troublesome to warrant surgery.

Medical Treatments
There are two main types of drug treatments which are effective in reducing urinary symptoms caused by an enlarged prostate gland.

Alpha-blockers act by relaxing the smooth muscle of the bladder neck and prostate. The most widely used alpha-blocker is prazosin hydrochloride, 500mcg b.d. for 3–7 days, with dosage then adjusted according to clinical response. It should improve urinary flow rate and reduce day- and night-time frequency. Prazosin decreases peripheral vascular resistance and so blood pressure should be carefully monitored, especially for older men.

5-alpha reductase inhibitors work by actually shrinking the benign hyperplastic tissue by about 30%, so that flow rates improve. Improvement in flow rate is not usually evident until the patient has been treated for more than three months. Finasteride is given as one 5mg tablet daily.

Unlike a prostatectomy, it would seem that men who are treated with 5-alpha reductase inhibitors will be required to continue treatment for life, since the prostate will enlarge again if treatment stops. The drug appears to have few side affects and confines its activity to the prostate gland. A few men experience decreased libido as finasteride acts via androgen deprivation.

Balloon Dilatation

This is a technique of compacting the prostatic tissue by inserting a catheter through the urethra, usually under general anaesthetic (Reddy, 1988). The catheter has a balloon section which is inflated against the prostatic urethra, causing widening and improved urine flow. This is not a permanent cure and may need repeating after about six months. Poor success rates have led to decreasing usage of this technique.

Stents

Another alternative treatment to keep the urethra patent is to insert a tube through the constricted prostatic urethra. Many problems have been encountered with the use of such foreign bodies, notably infection and encrustation.

Stents may either be wire spirals or a silicone prosthesis which can be easily placed and removed, or a finely meshed wire alloy which is not easily removed. At least 10% of stents will require removal, and encrustation is seen in 25% in the long term.

The stents are valuable for men who are medically unfit for surgery, or those for whom surgery will not necessarily improve their condition, especially if there is a cerebral impairment, diabetes or Parkinson's disease. There is little to commend their use in fit men or those without retention.

Wallstents are successful for treating men with chronic urethral strictures – particularly in those men who have much urethral scar tissue present as a result of multiple surgery.

Microwave and Laser Treatment

Microwave energy from a source in the rectum or urethra may be focused in the prostate gland. Sufficient heat is produced to destroy the enlarged prostate gland, whilst not damaging any of the surrounding tissue. Newer machines may be effective using a single course of treatment, which can be given under a local anaesthetic and without the need for a catheter. Morbidity is low and results approximate to those achieved with drugs.

Recent machines deliver increased energy which destroys some prostatic tissue; thermotherapy uses temperatures over 50°C and thermoablation uses temperatures over 70°C. The long-term outcome of these treatments is as yet unknown.

Laser treatment is of two types. In one, a non-contact probe is used to vaporize prostatic tissue. There is no bleeding and the procedure can be used to carry out bladder-neck incision on a day-care basis without a catheter. The other type uses a contact side-firing laser of lower energy but greater tissue penetration, which results in necrosis of the prostate gland to a variable depth. A suprapubic catheter is inserted for 10–14 days whilst the prostate sloughs. There is little or no bleeding and, again, it can be performed as a day-case procedure under general anaesthesia.

The probes cost approximately £500 per patient (single use) but the outcome appears to be better than with microwave hyperthermia, with improvement in flow rate by up to 5 ml/sec, and up to 50% improvement on symptom scores.

CARCINOMA OF THE PROSTATE

With advancing age, the likelihood of malignant changes in the prostate gland increases. By the ninth decade, 80% of men have a prostatic carcinoma. In the very elderly this is a relatively 'benign', localised condition but it can become invasive and metastatic in younger men. The symptoms are identical with those of benign prostatic hyperplasia in 80% of cases, and for this reason alone it is worth investigating any man with symptoms of prostatism.

The gland may feel hard on rectal examination, but the only sure method of diagnosis is by ultrasonically guided transrectal or transperineal biopsy of the gland. Diagnostic techniques like transrectal ultrasound will give accurate imaging information, and are capable of detecting very small cancerous lesions without causing pain or discomfort to the patient. Regrettably, the facility is expensive and not available everywhere.

In the USA, radical prostatectomy has become a common treatment for prostatic carcinoma. This procedure carries a high risk of post-prostatectomy incontinence (see below).

Before starting any individuals on long-term medical therapy, it is advisable to obtain a prostate specific antigen (PSA) value. Although many patients with BPH have a mildly raised PSA (>4 ng/ml), a value above 10ng/ml should alert the clinician to the possibility of prostate cancer, and guided biopsy should be performed after rectal ultrasound. During long-term therapy with alpha-blockers or finasteride, PSA measurements and digital examination of the prostate should be regularly performed.

URETHRAL STRICTURE

Although urethral strictures may present in women, they are uncommon, and most occur in males. A stricture, or narrowing of the urethra, results from scarred healing after an infection (urethritis) or trauma. Figure 7.2 shows the common sites for stricture. At the external meatus it may be caused by instrumentation, especially an indwelling catheter. At the peno-scrotal junction a catheter can cause pressure necrosis and subsequent stricture. A stricture may extend along the length of the mid-urethra following a gonococcal infection.

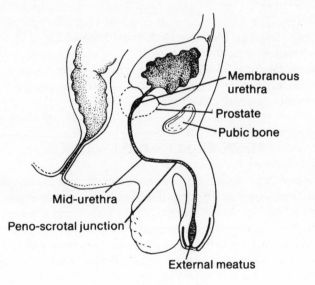

Figure 7.2 *Common sites of urethral stricture.*

A ruptured membranous urethra will often heal as a stricture. Symptoms are usually similar to prostatism: voiding difficulty, possibly with overflow incontinence and renal problems. Often a possible causative agent can be identified in the patient's history, e.g. catheterisation following major surgery or a previous urethritis. The diagnosis is made either on classical difficulty passing a catheter, or on micturating cystogram, or cystoscopy.

Treatment of a stricture involves either regular dilatation, usually under local anaesthetic using graduated bougies, or surgical division of the stricture by optical urethrotomy. The latter technique is generally undertaken with recurrent strictures. The urethra is split longitudinally through the stricture and the urethra is allowed to heal with a catheter in situ for 3–4 days. To prevent scar tissue causing a re-stenosis, these men will usually be taught to insert a self-lubricating hydrophilic catheter through the stricture site, usually just once a week. The intermittent self-catheterisation (ISC) technique for the purpose of maintaining a good urethral patency has become a regularly accepted stricture treatment since 1988; (Lawrence and MacDonagh, 1988; Robertson et al., 1991), and many men who had experienced multiple urethrotomies in past years will reduce their need for regular hospital admissions and consequent morbidity.

The nurse has an important role to play in teaching stricture patients how to perform ISC on a regular basis. Usually a weekly dilation will be sufficient. The catheter needs to be a size 18fg where possible. The use of anaesthetic gel is discouraged, so that the patient is able to gauge any difficulties in passing the catheter. The use of patient education booklets to reinforce teaching is valuable to this client group.

Chronic recurrent stricture may also be treated by the insertion of a stent to maintain urethral patency.

BLADDER-NECK OBSTRUCTION

Bladder-neck obstruction results from a lack of coordination between bladder contraction and bladder neck opening. It is most commonly idiopathic, but may occur secondarily to a neuropathic lesion of the bladder. The symptoms are, again, very similar to those arising from an enlarged prostate (voiding difficulties, with possible residual urine, overflow incontinence, and renal impairment). Classically a bladder-neck obstruction presents at an earlier age than prostatism, and the prostate is seldom enlarged. Treatment is either to attempt to relax the obstruction pharmacologically, e.g. prazosin 5mg t.d.s., or to surgically incise or resect the bladder neck. The surgical approach carries a slight risk of causing an incontinence not previously present.

POST-MICTURITION DRIBBLING

In some men incontinence takes the form of post-micturition dribbling. A small amount of urine is passed, usually without much sensation, up to several minutes after micturition is completed. This should be distinguished from terminal dribbling, which is a very slow dribbling stream at the end of the act of micturition. If clothing has been replaced, the dribble, although often only a few millilitres of urine, may be enough to soak through underpants and trousers and to leave an embarrassing wet patch, especially if trousers are lightweight or pale in colour.

Most commonly a post-micturition dribble is caused by pooling of urine in the bulbar urethra (Figure 7.3). The reason for this abnormally lax and wide bulb is unknown. If the diagnosis is in doubt, a micturating cystogram will clearly show this pool in the bulbar urethra after micturition. A simple explanation of the cause, reassurance that the problem has no significance, and instruction on emptying the urine will usually solve the problem. The patient is instructed to express the urine by firm upward and forward pressure by fingers or fist behind the scrotum at the end of micturition. The trapped urine will be 'milked out'.

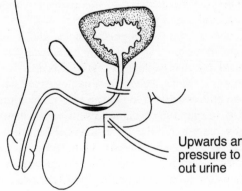

Upwards and forwards pressure to "milk" out urine

Figure 7.3   *Pooling of urine.*

Post-micturition dribble may also occur in men with prostatic enlargement and an unstable bladder, when sometimes a powerful 'after-contraction' forces out a few extra drops, or with an underactive bladder. In all of these conditions other symptoms usually coexist and suggest the cause. The man with simple pooling in the bulbar urethra will seldom have any other micturition problems.

If the problem is persistent, a dribble pouch (see Chapter 15) may be used to contain the leakage.

POST-PROSTATECTOMY INCONTINENCE

The male has two functional urethral sphincters. The proximal (internal) sphincter includes the bladder neck and prostatic urethra, which extends down to the verumontanum. The distal (external) sphincter extends from the verumontanum to the bulbar urethra and is composed of three types of muscle fibres – smooth, intrinsic and extrinsic skeletal muscle. It is the proximal urethral sphincter that is removed by prostatectomy. Where a TURP is performed, the distal sphincter must remain intact to maintain continence. Radical prostatectomy is associated with an increased risk of damage to the distal sphincter.

The incidence of incontinence associated with TURP is approximately 1 to 5%, depending upon the definition of incontinence (Worth, 1984; Chilton et al., 1978). The presence of an unstable detrusor combined with a weakened sphincter is more likely to result in post-operative incontinence. Both surgeons and patients should be aware of this condition pre-operatively, so that realistic outcomes can be anticipated.

Many men experience increased urgency and slight incontinence immediately after prostatectomy. It should be explained that time is necessary to adjust to the new weaker outflow resistance and that it should settle within a few weeks. Pelvic floor exercises are very useful at this time. The patient is instructed to interrupt micturition midstream at every void. At first he may only be able to slow rather than stop the stream. At the same time, a regime of regular pelvic floor contractions is also taught. The patient is instructed to contract the pelvic floor muscles five times per hour throughout the day. On a surgical ward with several prostatectomy patients this soon becomes part of the routine. The exercises can considerably strengthen the pelvic floor supports to the external sphincter, on which the patient is now reliant for continence. They also rapidly increase confidence in the ability to control any incontinence.

For those men with significant dribbling difficulty, the physiotherapist may use interferential therapy or faradism to stimulate greater pelvic floor awareness and activity. Many men will have relied on the bladder neck for continence and never learned the need to use the distal sphincter.

It cannot be stressed enough that the patient requires consistent education towards an understanding of what has been done and what is required of him in order to regain total continence. There are good support leaflets available for patients, and it should be the responsibility of every nurse to ensure these are available for the patient to take away with him (the Continence Foundation has a list of available leaflets). On discharge from hospital following prostatectomy, men should be aware that pelvic floor exercises should be continued until good control is established. He should also know how to obtain further help if dribbling persists, and not simply to put up with it.

Those patients who had an unstable bladder prior to prostatectomy will take rather longer to regain continence post-operatively. Instability secondary to long-standing obstruction will not disappear immediately, and it can take six to twelve months for the detrusor muscle to adjust to the new, lower outflow resistance. For a few men the instability is persistent and troublesome, causing frequency, urgency and urge incontinence. In most cases this will respond to standard therapy for an unstable bladder (usually drugs and bladder training – see Chapter 4). Explanation and reassurance and the provision of a suitable incontinence aid, for as long as needed, will help to tide the patient over this distressing post-operative phase. Few things are more depressing to a patient than an operation which leaves his symptoms unchanged or worsened. If the patient knows this is to be expected and will improve, he will often cope much better.

Surgery

In a few instances post-prostatectomy incontinence results from inadvertent sphincter damage at operation. This is more likely after TURP than RPP. If sphincter damage has been extensive, pelvic floor exercises will not effect a cure. For these men the only hope of continence is further surgery or, in some cases, Teflon or collagen injections. An implantable device may be used to correct this type of incontinence (or that caused by sphincter damage from any other source).

Periurethral and Transurethral Injections

Periurethral and transurethral collagen injections are currently being evaluated as an alternative to the implantation of mechanical devices. This procedure offers the advantage of a shorter hospital stay and fewer and less severe complications than implanted devices. The presence of an injectable material increases urethral closure pressure by bulking out the tissue and should improve continence. Injections can be repeated if necessary. Possible complications of collagen injections include urethritis and retention of urine. Until recently, Teflon was used as an injectable material with similar effects to collagen, but the use of this material has declined since adverse publicity about its migratory tendencies.

Artificial Urinary Sphincter

The AMS (American Medical Systems) Sphincter 800 consists of three parts, a cuff, pump, and reservoir, all connected by silicone rubber tubing (Figure 7.4). The cuff surrounds the urethra and is filled with fluid to exert gentle pressure, closing off the urethra. To allow micturition, the pump, located in the scrotum, is squeezed several times. (It can be used in women as well as men, in which case the pump is implanted in the labia rather than the scrotum). Squeezing transfers the fluid out of the cuff and into the abdominally placed reservoir. The pump feels flat when the cuff is empty. Urine can now flow out of the

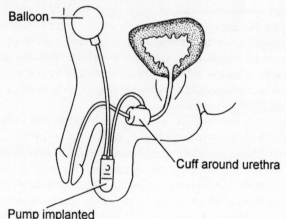

Balloon

Cuff around urethra

Pump implanted
in scrotum

Figure 7.4   *AMS artificial sphincter.*

bladder through the open sphincter. The cuff automatically reinflates within two to three minutes. No action is required on the part of the patient to accomplish this reinflation and return to continence. The reservoir has the unique ability to react to any increase in intra-abdominal pressure by transferring additional fluid into the cuff, which then increases urethral resistance and avoids stress incontinence during coughing, straining, or similar activities.

The long-term results of this device have been encouraging, but there are risks of mechanical failure, rejection, and erosion through the urethra, which are difficult to correct, especially the latter two. The number of surgeons experienced in the insertion of these devices is limited, but there is no doubt that many patients do benefit and experience few problems. Widespread use is also limited by financial considerations, as the device is expensive. However, if the alternative is a lifetime's use of absorbent products or collection devices, or a urinary diversion, a prosthesis should be considered. It may not even prove an expensive option in the long term.

Surgical implantation of an artificial sphincter is generally not considered unless a minimum of twelve to eighteen months has elapsed since prostatic surgery, and all efforts directed toward conservative treatment have failed. Treatment goals of this type of surgery include allowing the patient to return to a normal micturition pattern while being maintained without leakage between voidings. In addition, over-distension of the bladder and ureteric reflux must be prevented. Criteria for the use of an artificial prosthesis include the documentation of unobstructed urinary flow, sterile urine, adequate bladder capacity which would allow the patient to void only every two to four hours, the absence of bladder hyperreflexia, and the absence of reflux or residual urine (Furlow, 1981). Most of these can be accomplished by a surgical or pharmacological manipulation prior to implantation (Faller and Vinson, 1985).

Pre-operative nursing assessment should ensure that the patient can understand how the device functions and can learn to operate it safely and effectively. Operating the pump of the prosthesis requires finger dexterity, which should be demonstrated by the patient or care-giver before surgery. It is helpful to have a sample device available for practice sessions; the company is happy to supply this for teaching purposes. In addition, it is important for the patient's immediate family or spouse to be included in the planning and to be supportive during this time, when all the patient's energies will be focused on bladder management. The nurse can assist the patient and family to adopt realistic expectations of what will occur post-operatively and of the anticipated surgical goal. It must be stressed that pre-operative and post-operative teaching are crucial to a successful outcome.

CONTROL OF INCONTINENCE: THE PENILE CLAMP

Occasionally, penile clamps may still be found in use. They are used with the aim of controlling incontinence by external mechanical occlusion of the penile urethra. The most commonly used is the Cunningham clamp. This device is comprised of two foam-lined metal arms which fit across the penis laterally and close on a ratchet until incontinence is controlled.

The clamp is mentioned only to suggest that it must be used with *extreme* caution as it can cause considerable damage, even pressure necrosis, to the penis. A penile clamp should never be handed out as the first line of management for incontinence in the male, but if fitted properly and given with adequate instruction it can be successful in restoring the patient to continence.

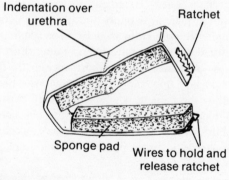

Figure 7.5   *Penile clamp.*

REFERENCES AND FURTHER READING

Absalom, M., Betts, C., (eds), 1992. *Endoscopic Urology for Nurses.* Royal London Hospital Trust, London.

Blandy, J. P., Moors, J., 1989. *Urology for Nurses.* Blackwell Scientific Publications, Oxford.

Chilton, C. P., Morgan, R. J., England, H. R., Paris, A. M., Blandy, J. P., 1978. A critical evaluation of the results of transurethral resection of the prostate. *British Journal of Urology*, 50, 7: 542.

Faller, N. A., Vinson, R. K., 1985. The artificial urinary sphincter. *Journal of Enterostomal Therapy*, 12: 7.

Furlow, W. L., 1981. Implantation of a new semiautomatic genitourinary sphincter. *Journal of Urology*, 126, 6: 741.

Garraway, W. M., Collins, G. N., Lee, R. J., 1991. High prevalence of benign prostatic hypertrophy in the community. *Lancet*, 338: 469–71.

Lawrence, W. T., MacDonagh, R. P., 1988. Treatment of urethral stricture disease by internal urethrotomy followed by intermittent 'low friction' self-catheterisation. *Journal of the Royal Society of Medicine*, 81, 3: 136–9.

Neal, D. E., 1994. Transurethral prostatectomy. *British Journal of Surgery*, 81: 484–5.

Reddy, P., 1988. Balloon dilatation of the prostate for treatment of benign hyperplasia. *Clinical Urology North America*, 15: 529–35.

Robertson, G. S. M., Everitt, N., Lamprecht, M., Brett, M., Flynn, J. T., 1991. Treatment of recurrent urethral strictures using clean intermittent self-catherisation. *British Journal of Urology*, 68: 89–92.

Worth, P. H. L., 1984. Postprostatectomy incontinence. In: Mundy, A. R., Stephenson, T. P., Wein, A. J. (eds). *Urodynamics – Principles, Practice and Application.* Churchill Livingstone, Edinburgh and London.

Books for Patients

Cunningham, C., 1992. *Your Prostate, What Every Man Over 40 Needs to Know.* Carnell, London.

Hamand, J., 1991. *Prostate Problems.* Thorsons, London.

Reynolds, R., 1993. *Coping Successfully With Prostate Problems.* Sheldon Press, London.

Chapter 8

Neurogenic Bladder Dysfunction

Maria O'Hagan, MPhil, RN, RNI, DipResMethods
Clinical Nurse Specialist, Uro-Neurology, recently at The National Hospital for Neurology and Neurosurgery, London

For many people with incontinence and other bladder problems, the underlying cause is damage to the neurological control mechanisms which regulate bladder function. As discussed in Chapter 2, continence is dependent on very long nerve pathways which are vulnerable to disease or trauma affecting the nervous system.

The problems of those with neurogenic bladder dysfunction are often exacerbated by the fact that bladder control is seldom the only impairment; many people will also have varying degrees of physical and/or mental disability. When poor bladder function and disability coexist, the problems involved in coping with micturition and incontinence are compounded. The specific problems associated with physical disabilities are dealt with in Chapter 13. The interaction of actual bladder problems and the physical ability to cope with them should be borne in mind throughout this chapter.

Damage to nerve pathways at any point between the cortical bladder centre and the bladder itself can impair continence. The range of symptoms is limited, despite the many neurological levels at which lesions can cause dysfunction (Figure 8.1).

SITES OF NEUROLOGICAL DAMAGE

Supra-Pontine Influences
The supra-pontine or higher centres which influence the pons include the medial frontal lobes and the basal ganglia. These higher centres are crucial for inhibiting detrusor contractions during the filling phase. Lesions in these areas, for example, frontal lobe tumours, normal pressure hydrocephalus and cerebrovascular accidents, will result in detrusor hyperreflexia, but with normally coordinated voiding. The presence of normal voiding is explained by the micturition reflex (in the pons) remaining intact in patients with supra-pontine lesions.

170

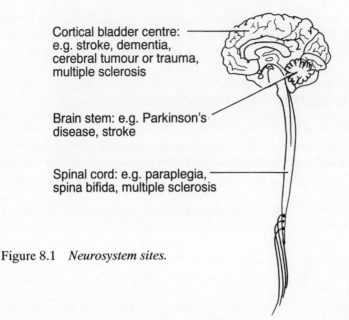

Cortical bladder centre:
e.g. stroke, dementia,
cerebral tumour or trauma,
multiple sclerosis

Brain stem: e.g. Parkinson's
disease, stroke

Spinal cord: e.g. paraplegia,
spina bifida, multiple sclerosis

Figure 8.1 *Neurosystem sites.*

Voluntary control of voiding – initiation or inhibition – may be lost, but the coordinated relaxation of the sphincter with detrusor contraction is unhindered.

Pontine Micturition Centre

The pontine micturition centre (PMC) is under the control of supra-pontine influences. During the bladder filling phase, the PMC is responsible for inhibition of the pelvic nerves. When the bladder is full, micturition is initiated following stimulation of the pons by the higher centres. The role of the pons in governing micturition has been described by Barrington (1925) and de Groat (1990). Pontine lesions are, however, rare. One consequence of pontine lesions is hesitancy of micturition and urinary retention, although the lesion may produce other life-threatening conditions.

Supra-Sacral Spinal Cord Lesions

Interruptions to the pathways between the pontine micturition centre and the sacral cord (above sacral nerves S_2–S_4) will disturb the inhibition of the detrusor muscle during the filling phase and disrupt detrusor-sphincter coordination during voiding. Symptoms experienced are therefore due to detrusor hyperreflexia (frequency, urgency and urge incontinence) and detrusor-sphincter dyssynergia (hesitancy, diminished or interrupted stream, and a feeling of incomplete emptying). Detrusor-sphincter dyssynergia is characterised by a failure of the sphincter to relax for voiding – it contracts simultaneously with detrusor contractions.

Spinal Cord Injury
The spinal shock phase that occurs following spinal cord injury is variable and may last for a few weeks, up to several months in patients with a complete supra-sacral transection. Following incomplete transection the period of spinal shock is often shorter. During this time the bladder is areflexic and the outcome is urinary retention. As the bladder recovers, there is a return of reflex detrusor contractions, which are often poorly sustained. These, in combination with inconsistent sphincter activity, either with or without bladder neck opening, cause voiding difficulties and associated residual urine volumes. The presence of detrusor-sphincter dyssynergia (DSD) means there is an increased risk of upper tract dilation and renal damage from high intravesical pressures. Established voiding patterns in upper motor neurone bladders usually consist of a hyperreflexic bladder with varying degrees of DSD.

Autonomic dysreflexia may manifest itself in patients with lesions above thoracic nerve T_5, and in particular it is those patients with cervical lesions who are most vulnerable during the period of spinal shock. It is characterised by headaches, hypertension and flushing, and sweating of the body above the level of the lesion. A distended bladder, for example caused by DSD or catheter blockage, will trigger autonomic dysreflexia, and as such is a medical emergency. Treatment involves relieving vesical distension. Bladder management should, however, be consistently aimed at preventing such a crisis.

Cauda Equina Lesions
Subsacral lesions damaging the sacral nerve S_2–S_4 roots create a lower motor neurone bladder dysfunction. If the extent of the lesion causes denervation, then sensation of bladder filling is lost and the individual is unable to initiate micturition. Examples of subsacral lesions are protrusion of lumbosacral intervertebral discs, intradural tumours, spinal metastases, possible mishaps with epidural anaesthesia, and trauma.

Perineal Nerve Injury

The perineal nerve is a branch of the pudendal nerve. Damage to this in women may occur during childbirth, whilst in men symptoms of stress incontinence may signify a lower motor neurone lesion. Extensive pelvic surgery such as radical hysterectomy and abdomino-perineal resection for rectal carcinoma can interfere with the sacral reflex arc. Denervation of the pelvic floor and sphincter causes stress incontinence. Leakage may occur during any activity that increases intra-abdominal pressure, such as coughing, laughing, straining and exercise.

Summary

Broadly speaking, bladder dysfunction in neurological disease falls into two categories – disorders of storage and disorders of voiding. Patients with a neurogenic bladder may complain of irritative symptoms such as frequency, urgency and urge incontinence and/or retentive symptoms, for example hesitancy, diminished or interrupted stream, straining to void and incomplete emptying. The two disorders should be managed separately, even if they coexist.

NEUROLOGICAL DISEASES THAT AFFECT BLADDER FUNCTION

Cerebrovascular Accident

The site of the lesion will determine the type of bladder dysfunction. Detrusor hyperreflexia is a common finding because there is a disruption of the voluntary control of the brain stem micturition centre by the cerebral cortex. Damage to the frontal lobe or internal capsule also results in detrusor hyperreflexia, and in addition to this there is uninhibited sphincter relaxation (Khan et al., 1988).

Diabetes

Diseases of the peripheral nervous system can attack the local nerve supply to the bladder. This is especially common in diabetic peripheral neuropathy, which can affect both sensory and motor pathways. Because sensation is deficient, the bladder may be allowed to become over-distended. Motor damage leads to inefficient bladder emptying and overflow incontinence may develop. Occasionally detrusor instability is detected.

Multiple Sclerosis

Multiple sclerosis (MS) is characterised by the presence of focal demyelination, particularly in the brain stem and spinal cord. Urinary symptoms feature prominently in this condition (Miller et al., 1965). It is the presence of lesions within the spinal cord which are a major determinant of impaired bladder control (Betts et al., 1993). Interruption between the sacral bladder centre and the pontine micturition centre produces symptoms of detrusor hyperreflexia. Detrusor sphincter dyssynergia (DSD) is often evidence of spinal cord disease, and the patient with MS may describe symptoms of voiding difficulty with an abnormally raised post-micturition residual urine volume.

The predisposition to upper urinary tract sequelae in MS is a subject of some debate, but it does not seem to be a common problem. It would appear that those at particular risk are men with DSD, individuals of either sex who have an indwelling catheter in situ, and patients with high intravesical pressures (Blaivas and Barbalias, 1984).

Spina Bifida and Tethered Cord

The degree of malformation to the lower part of the spinal cord and the subsequent extent of neurological deficit is variable in spina bifida. In some, the lesion may be difficult to detect (spina bifida occulta) whilst in others, the spinal cord and the surrounding nerve tissues may be exposed (myelomenigocele). The type of bladder dysfunction depends on the amount of damage to the $S_2 - S_4$ nerve pathways. Disruption of innervation to the detrusor muscle may result in a normal, flaccid or hyperreflexic detrusor muscle. Similarly, the sphincter may become flaccid or spastic or be left undisturbed. Any combination of these dysfunctions is possible, e.g. a hyperreflexic detrusor with a normal sphincter mechanism or hypocontractile bladder and a spastic sphincter.

A tethered cord is another example of a subsacral lesion. The type of bladder dysfunction associated with this includes detrusor hyper-reflexia, although some patients may demonstrate a large capacity hypocontractile bladder.

Parkinson's Disease

Parkinson's disease (PD) involves the degeneration of the substantia negra and a deficiency of dopamine. In addition to symptoms of tremor, rigidity and bradykinesia (abnormal slowness of movement), the patient with PD may complain of urinary symptoms. The exact nature and prevalence of bladder dysfunction in this patient group is not certain. Detrusor hyperreflexia and striated sphincter dysfunction have been reported. The latter has been explained as a bradykinesia of the sphincter, i.e. a failure to relax during voiding, or a pseudodyssynergia, where there is a voluntary contraction of pelvic musculature during involuntary detrusor contractions. The degree of voiding difficulty may increase as the disease advances and there is deterioration in motor function.

Multiple Systems Atrophy

Multiple systems atrophy (MSA) is characterised by central nervous system neuronal atrophy. It may present with features of Shy-Drager syndrome, cerebellar ataxia or atypical Parkinsonism. Because MSA can affect the control of micturition at several levels, the type of bladder dysfunction can alter as the disease progresses. Early on, patients may experience detrusor hyperreflexia. Later, many patients are unable to initiate micturition because of a hypocontractile detrusor which results in high residual urine volumes (Kirby et al., 1986). Previously, many people with MSA have been misdiagnosed as suffering from Parkinson's disease.

Tropical Spastic Paraplegia

Tropical spastic paraplegia (TSP) is an inflammatory process involving the lower portion of the spinal cord. This disorder has been identified in a widely distributed population which includes the Caribbean region, Central and South America and Africa. Symptoms are those of a progressive paraparesis and bladder dysfunction as a result of spinal cord involvement. Depending on the site of the lesion, urinary symptoms in TSP will be either an upper or a lower motor neurone presentation. Detrusor hyperreflexia and acontractile bladders have been reported (Eardley et al., 1991).

Causes of Urinary Retention in Women

Urinary retention can result from disease affecting the $S_2 - S_4$ roots. However, in the absence of overt neurological pathology, the condition of urinary retention in women has been attributed to hysteria. This has led to descriptions of 'psychogenic retention' in the literature. Recently, urethral sphincter electromyography (EMG) has demonstrated abnormalities in these women, which it is proposed explain the phenomenon (Fowler et al., 1987). The EMG activity has 'myotonic-like' qualities (involuntary repetitive electrical discharges) which impair sphincter relaxation and cause symptoms of obstructed voiding, and – if detrusor failure occurs – urinary retention.

INVESTIGATIONS

While the emphasis in this chapter has been on disordered bladder function resulting from neurological disease, it is worth remembering that the neurologically impaired individual may exhibit more than one pathology. It becomes essential then to exclude urological conditions which may coexist, unrelated to the neurological diagnosis. For example, the patient with multiple sclerosis or Parkinson's disease may also have symptoms of a urinary tract infection, benign prostatic hypertrophy, genuine stress incontinence, or a bladder carcinoma. The use of investigations, together with a comprehensive history and clinical examination, will contribute to a precise diagnosis.

Urodynamic studies usually include a simple measurement of urinary flow rate and a filling and voiding cystometry. If radiographic facilities are available, cystourethrography may be performed in order to visualise the bladder neck and urethra (see Chapter 3). Neurophysiological investigations such as electromyography (EMG) may be utilised to assess the degree of denervation and reinnervation to the urethral sphincter as well as the kinaesiological action of the sphincter, i.e. the timing of its activity during voiding. Additionally, this is a method that can be used to demonstrate detrusor-sphincter dyssynergia. An intravenous urogram (IVU) allows the clinician to visualise the kidneys and ureters and identify tumours, strictures and stones. This investigation is being largely replaced by renal and bladder ultrasound, which will provide similar information without exposing the patient to the hazards of radiation. A plain abdominal X-ray will identify stones and tumours in the urinary tract. Biochemical assays allow a further assessment of renal function. The measurement of post-micturition residual urine volume may be achieved during urodynamic investigations, a bladder ultrasound or a simple 'in-out' catheterisation. Urine specimens should be obtained for culture and sensitivity.

In addition to the above-mentioned investigative procedures, assessment of the patient must also extend to his or her physical and mental state (see Chapters 3 and 13). This is crucial for planning individualised and realistic outcomes of bladder management.

MANAGEMENT

The aims of management are two-fold and are directed towards (i) preservation of upper renal tract function and (ii) alleviation of urinary symptoms which may affect the individual's physical, psychological, social and sexual well-being. Clear explanations of symptoms in relation to the neurological diagnosis will contribute to the patient's understanding of the rationale for suggested treatment options.

Management of the Unstable Neurogenic Bladder

Patients with detrusor hyperreflexia usually experience an increase in daytime frequency, urgency and urge incontinence. Additional features may include nocturia and nocturnal enuresis. The severity of such symptoms may vary considerably and the completion of frequency/volume charts will assist in determining the extent of the problem. They will also prove useful in evaluating responses to treatment.

The management of detrusor hyperreflexia relies on drug therapy, specifically anticholinergic medication. This acts by 'dampening' or suppressing unstable detrusor contractions. Side effects of anticholinergics include a dry mouth, blurred vision and constipation. In addition to these, urinary retention may become evident. Patients particularly at risk of retention are those in whom detrusor hyperreflexia and symptoms of incomplete voiding coexist. A measurement of the post-micturition residual urine volume should be performed prior to commencing anticholinergics. Even if there is a negligible residual urine volume, this may need to be checked again later on, especially if the patient complains of worsening urinary symptoms and, in particular, any difficulty in voiding. Marked symptoms of voiding difficulty with a significant residual urine volume (i.e. greater than 100ml) should be managed as a separate problem.

Management of Neurogenic Voiding Difficulties

Incomplete bladder emptying can lead to a number of problems. Urinary tract infection is common if residual urine is present and, because the bladder is never completely emptied, is extremely difficult to eradicate, even with antibiotics. Re-infection and a shifting spectrum of invading organisms are common.

Residual urine often leads to overflow incontinence. It also reduces functional bladder capacity. (If the bladder capacity is 500ml, with a residual urine volume of 400ml, the functional capacity – that capacity which can be used – is only 100ml.) This will obviously increase voiding frequency. Those who have the double problem of a residual volume and hyperreflexia (e.g. some people with multiple sclerosis or spinal injury) often only have a very small margin between their residual volume and the volume at which uninhibited contractions develop. This can result in incontinence occurring very soon after voiding. Indeed, some will suffer almost continuous episodes of incontinence, since as soon as the volume in the bladder exceeds the residual volume the bladder contracts and expels the excess.

There is a variety of procedures and techniques for managing neurogenic voiding difficulties. The aim of these treatments is to achieve complete bladder emptying, thus minimising the risks associated with chronic voiding dysfunction. Intermittent catheterisation has proved to be a major contribution in this area. Whilst an overview of conservative and aggressive forms of bladder management will be given, the role of intermittent catheterisation will be considered in some depth.

Voiding Techniques

Some people with a voiding difficulty manage to find a technique that will stimulate complete voiding.

If the elements of the sacral reflex are intact but merely uncoordinated, e.g. cut off from the brain stem, it is often possible voluntarily to initiate a detrusor contraction by stimulation of 'trigger areas'. Alternatively, direct rises in abdominal pressure, especially in women, can raise intravesical pressure to the point where urethral resistance is overcome and voluntary voiding occurs (Valsalva or Crede manoeuvres, see below). If either of these can be done before overflow incontinence occurs, with the individual appropriately placed over a receptacle, continence can be achieved.

Trigger Areas. Patients without sacral damage may find a 'trigger' that will initiate a bladder contraction. Tapping the abdominal wall suprapubically is a common method. The abdomen is firmly and repeatedly tapped, usually by the tips of extended fingers of one hand, until voiding starts. Often the contraction generated is unsustained, so the tapping and voiding has to be repeated several times until the bladder is empty. Abdominal tenderness or weak fingers may be a problem. If the reflex is weak, a long period of tapping may be required before micturition starts, and it may have to be frequently repeated before the bladder is completely empty. It can therefore become very time-consuming and demoralising. However, because bladder contraction usually initiates some urethral opening, the potential for damage is low, and this method is preferable to straining, or pushing, for those who can achieve it.

Other trigger areas that work for some people are pulling pubic hairs, stroking the abdomen or interior aspect of the thighs, or digital anal stimulation and dilation (Johnson, 1980). Patients who manage their voiding difficulties in this way should experiment to discover which area works best and most easily for them.

Valsalva and Crede. Both of these techniques are only suitable for those whose sphincter mechanism is not in complete spasm – usually patients with damage at the sacral bladder centre level, when sphincteric resistance is often low and easily overcome.

The Valsalva manoeuvre (inhaling deeply and then exhaling forcefully against a closed glottis) greatly increases intra-abdominal pressure and may enable bladder emptying by straining. Alternatively, in some people this pressure rise may trigger a bladder contraction. However, this type of straining is inadvisable, certainly on a long-term regular basis. It raises intracranial pressure and impedes cardiac return, and should definitely be avoided by anyone with cardiovascular or cerebrovascular disease. Straining may eventually weaken and damage pelvic floor musculature and the bladder neck, leading to sphincter incompetence (stress incontinence).

The Crede manoeuvre, or manual bladder expression, involves applying considerable pressure, usually with the ball of the hand or a fist, suprapubically directly over the bladder. Like Valsalva, this may work to empty the bladder either by directly raising bladder pressure or by triggering a detrusor contraction. Unfortunately, if no contraction occurs the bladder neck will remain closed, and a very high pressure is needed to overcome this; eventual sphincter damage is a risk. Some people find expression uncomfortable. If sensation is deficient, great care should be taken to avoid bruising. Obese people and those with weak hands or arms also have difficulty. Sometimes someone else can be taught to apply the pressure. If reflux is suspected from the bladder to the ureters, the Crede manoeuvre should be avoided. Whether its repeated use can create reflux is unproven.

Indwelling Catheter

An indwelling catheter, urethral or suprapubic, may be indicated for patients with voiding difficulties, or a severely unstable detrusor, who fail to respond to medical treatment. When self- or assisted intermittent catheterisation is not possible, and where more aggressive forms of management are not suitable, long-term catheterisation may be the only remaining option. However, this form of bladder management is not without its own problems (see Chapter 9). The choice of an indwelling catheter should only be made after careful consideration of the advantages and disadvantages of all available treatments. Regular follow-up of these patients is essential if the risks associated with catheterisation are to be minimised.

Drug Therapy

There is little evidence to suggest that a pharmacological approach as a means of managing voiding dysfunction is successful. The use of drug therapy concentrates on either increasing detrusor contractility (e.g. bethanechol) or decreasing bladder neck resistance (e.g. phenoxybenzamine). However, these are not without side effects and are of doubtful efficacy.

Surgical Treatment

Surgical techniques are usually reserved for those patients in whom conservative forms of management have failed and where renal function is threatened. The type of surgery selected will depend on whether the objective is to improve bladder storage or to enhance bladder emptying. Bladder storage may be increased by augmentation cystoplasty or the use of an artificial sphincter, whereas an ileal conduit, continent diversion or a sphincterotomy will encourage more effective bladder emptying.

INTERMITTENT CATHETERISATION

There can be little doubt that the greatest single advance in the management of neurogenic voiding difficulties has been the introduction of intermittent catheterisation. This involves the episodic introduction of a catheter into the bladder to drain any residual urine, and then removal of the catheter, leaving the patient catheter-free between catheterisations.

Background

Recorded history shows that between the years 3000 BC to 2000 BC various civilisations, including the Egyptians and Romans, were making and using catheters of bronze, copper and gold for intermittent use. The Chinese lacquered onion stalks or coated them with linseed oil for the same purpose. A silver catheter has been discovered from the 10th century in Europe. More recently, Victorian gentlemen kept silver catheters in their top hat or walking stick, when self-catheterisation was adopted to circumnavigate urethral strictures or relieve retention caused by prostatic enlargement.

The use of intermittent catheterisation pre-dates that of the indwelling catheters, the latter only being introduced in the 1930s by Frederick Foley. It is only in the last three decades that the full potential of intermittent catheterisation has been recognised, especially in the bladder management of patients with spinal cord injuries. Sterile intermittent catheterisation was first performed by medical or nursing staff at regular intervals during the period of spinal shock (Guttmann and Frankel, 1966).

In hospital, or anywhere where catheterisation is being performed by a doctor or nurse, risks of cross-infection are high and it is always best to maintain a strict aseptic technique. For single use a Jaques or Nelaton plastic catheter, size 10 or 12 f.g., is the best and cheapest (Figure 8.2).

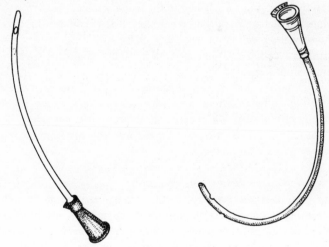

Figure 8.2   *Jaques or Nelaton catheters.*

In the past two decades, the technique of intermittent non-sterile, 'clean', self-catheterisation has become widely adopted for the long-term management of people with persistently large residual urine volumes. Most work has been done with children suffering from spina bifida (Kaye and Van Blerk, 1981) and spinal injury patients whose spinal shock does not resolve sufficiently to leave efficient voiding reflexes (Pearman, 1976). More recently its use has spread to all categories of people with incomplete bladder emptying. Many people of all ages, both sexes, and with a wide range of physical abilities have been taught to self-catheterise. Where this has proved impossible, a relative or regular carer has often been taught instead.

A Clean Technique

The clean technique was introduced by Lapides and his colleagues in the USA in the early 1970s (Lapides et al., 1972). Much to the surprise of many professionals brought up on theories of the importance of strict asepsis in catheterisation, patients using a clean rather than a sterile technique do not tend to encounter frequent problematic urinary tract infection. In fact, many who previously have had chronically infected residual urine find that infection decreases from its former incidence when intermittent catheterisation is introduced, as the focus for infection (the residual urine) is removed. It is likely that complete regular emptying of the bladder is an important factor in preventing infection becoming established in the urinary tract.

Many nurses are perturbed when they first encounter this procedure, and worry about infection risks, especially with clean rather than sterile intermittent catheterisation, as well as the dangers of trauma to the urethra from repeated catheter insertions. In practice the risks are slight, certainly nothing approaching the problems associated with indwelling catheterisation, and very few patients have to abandon intermittent catheterisation because of problems, provided of course that the procedure is correctly taught and the programme is closely supervised in the initial stages.

Criteria for Intermittent Catheterisation

Obviously, not all patients with urinary symptoms are suitable candidates for self- or assisted intermittent catheterisation. Physiologically, there are two essential requirements. These are (i) a good-capacity bladder (where residual urine volumes are persistently greater than 100 ml) and (ii) an adequate sphincter mechanism (Lancet, 1979). The rationale for this is that reasonable volumes of urine need to be retained between catheterisations for it to constitute an effective form of treatment.

Patients may present with a history of marked symptoms of voiding difficulty – hesitancy, straining to void and possibly overflow incontinence – and investigation will usually demonstrate a significant post-micturition residual urine volume. Some individuals may in fact be unaware that the bladder is not emptying, and this emphasises the importance of checking for the presence of residual urine.

Patient Selection
For self-catheterisation to be successful, four key factors have been identified, namely: motivation, mental alertness, mobility and manual dexterity.

It is natural for patients to feel anxious about learning any new technique, particularly something as invasive as clean intermittent self-catheterisation. This should be acknowledged by the nurse undertaking the teaching programme and every effort must be made to alleviate anxiety. The majority of patients cope well (including children as young as 5 years) if they have a clear understanding of the cause of the bladder dysfunction and the rationale for choosing intermittent catheterisation as a strategy for managing their symptoms. The concept of intermittent catheterisation needs to be sold with an enthusiastic approach by healthcare professionals.

Patients need to be alert enough to assimilate information regarding this technique. Those with severe learning difficulties, cognitive dysfunction or memory impairment may be more appropriate for assisted rather than self-catheterisation.

Limited mobility often presents a problem for people who are neurologically impaired. Women especially may encounter greater difficulties in identifying the urethral orifice, because of problems with balance, hip abduction, etc. However, there are strategies for dealing with most of these difficulties. These may include a careful choice of catheter as well as seeking the advice of other disciplines, for example, physiotherapy and occupational therapy.

A fairly accurate indication of whether a patient has the manual dexterity for intermittent catheterisation is whether or not they are able to cut up food and feed themselves, and how well they can write. There are catheters available for women with impaired manual dexterity (Figure 8.3, overleaf).

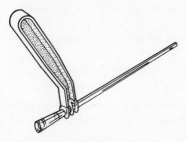

Figure 8.3   *Female intermittent catheter with handle (Intex).*

Teaching the Technique

The technique of intermittent catheterisation should be fully discussed with the patient as a preliminary to teaching the method. Many patients are initially worried at the idea of using a catheter, and will wish to discuss the possibilities of causing damage to themselves, and what the long-term effects will be. A few, especially women, are embarrassed at the idea of touching the genitals and (rarely) some people reject the technique completely for this reason. It is important that whoever is teaching the patient, whether nurse or doctor, approaches the subject in a very down-to-earth fashion, imparting optimism that the patient will both be able to do it and will benefit. The alternatives, including voiding techniques, indwelling catheter, surgery or drugs, and continuing with the voiding difficulty and overflow incontinence, should be outlined, with the advantages and disadvantages of each. Intermittent self-catheterisation will not be successful without the patient's full and intelligent cooperation, and cannot be started unless the patient is willing.

People vary greatly in their aptitude for self-catheterisation. Teaching should always take place in a relaxed, private and unhurried environment. If several different members of staff are involved with the patient it is a good idea to have a written, consistent policy, so that he or she is told the same thing by everyone. First a full and detailed explanation of the local anatomy is given, usually with the aid of diagrams (Figure 8.4). Few men or women have an accurate idea of important facts such as the length of the urethra, or the relationship of the various genital organs. Many have fears – for example, that the catheter might get lost inside, or that they could puncture the bladder if the catheter goes in too far.

The patient is then catheterised in the semi-recumbent position and a detailed commentary given. Usually the teacher (doctor or nurse)

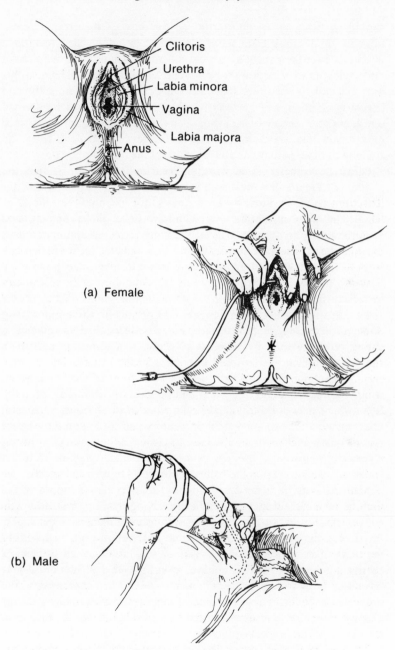

(a) Female

(b) Male

Figure 8.4　*Diagrams for teaching patients self-catheterisation.*

should be using an aseptic technique, because of the risk of cross-infection, and it must be explained to the patient why a clean technique is adequate for the patient's own use outside hospital. Most people will understand an explanation that everyone has a certain resistance to his own bacteria (germs), and as the bladder will be completely and regularly emptied, any bacteria which are introduced will be drained out again and so cannot take hold. The nurse (or doctor) must wear gloves and take extra precautions to protect the patient from the bacteria of other patients as well as those of the nurse or doctor.

Once the catheter is in position, women should be shown the position of the urethral meatus in a mirror, and locate by hand how far it is from an easily identifiable landmark, for example the clitoris or labia. The woman should then withdraw the catheter herself, and re-introduce it by parting the labia with the non-dominant hand, locating the meatus in a mirror. With a little practice most women can learn to self-catheterise by touch (indeed, some never manage to get a reasonable view in the mirror); this is an advantage, as the mirror can then be dispensed with.

Having successfully introduced the catheter two or three times lying down with the legs abducted, the patient is then asked to catheterise sitting on a lavatory, by touch if possible. If a mirror is needed, a shaving mirror may be adapted to hook over the front of the lavatory seat, or a suction pad attached to the seat or front of the bowl. Some women cannot manage this, and indeed there is a variety of positions which may suit individual preferences or disabilities. Squatting, standing with one foot on a stool or lavatory pan, sitting on the edge of a chair or wheelchair (with a U cut-out cushion if necessary), or using a posterior approach if the legs cannot be abducted, may all be found suitable, depending upon the patient's physical abilities and agility.

Male patients have far less difficulty than females in locating the urethral meatus, and may self-catheterise lying, sitting, or standing, as convenient. For the first few catheterisations most men use local anaesthetic (e.g. lignocaine gel) inserted into the urethra prior to inserting the catheter. Some women also prefer to use a little local anaesthetic or lubricant gel, either into the urethra or on the catheter. Single-use pre-lubricated or hydrophilic catheters are available as an alternative to the ordinary plastic catheters. These have been recommended as a means of preventing the recurrence of urethral strictures. However, they may also be used by patients practising intermittent catheterisation on a frequent and long-term basis. The manufacturers of these coated catheters suggest that they minimise the risk of potential complications.

Many people learn to self-catheterise competently in a single out-patient session or home visit. Others will be in hospital anyway, and some may benefit from a few days in hospital to perfect the technique under supervision. People with severe physical disabilities may take considerably longer to find a position and method that is reliable. Some women with limited movement in the hand and wrist may find a more rigid catheter easier to manipulate. Examples of these are the Scott semi-rigid pvc catheter or the metal Biscath. Alternatively, a nelaton with a handle may prove helpful, for example the Intex catheter as shown in Figure 8.3.

Frequency of catheterisation will vary with individual needs. Some people almost empty the bladder at micturition, and have a residual urine which slowly accumulates over a few days. Others are in complete retention and will need to catheterise five to six times a day. It should be done often enough to avoid incontinence wherever possible, as well as to ensure that the volume of residual urine obtained is always below 400ml. Once the technique is mastered, the patient may be sent away with an adequate supply of catheters and a simple instruction sheet and diagram (Table 8.1 or 8.2, overleaf), and Figure 8.4, page 185).

At home, each catheter is washed out after use under running water and dried (shaken and the outside wiped with a paper towel). It is then stored in a dry place until its next use, when it should again be held under a running tap prior to insertion. Many people use snap-sealing plastic bags to keep the catheter in a handbag or pocket between uses. Soaking the catheter in strong antiseptic solution is usually discouraged as unnecessary. It may also possibly be irritant to the sensitive urethral mucosa and has the potential to kill off normal flora, leaving the patient vulnerable to more harmful micro-organisms. Likewise, swabbing of the urethral meatus is not encouraged unless a discharge or vaginal infection is present. Each catheter is used for approximately one week and then thrown away (except in hospital, where a new catheter must be used each time to avoid cross-infection risks).

The importance of hand-washing is stressed to the patient. Women are instructed simply to wash their hands with soap and water. Then to part the labia and insert the catheter until urine flows. Once the flow ceases the catheter is withdrawn slowly, halting if the flow starts again. Men do exactly the same, some using lignocaine gel in addition when inserting the catheter as already mentioned.

Significant infection, when the patient is unwell, feverish and has

Table 8.1   Self-Catheterisation for Women (Patient Information Sheet)

1) Perform the catheterisation as often as your doctor or nurse has suggested. To start with, this should be every ..... hours.
2) Get your catheter, a mirror, and lubricant gel.
3) Wash your hands thoroughly with soap and water and rinse the catheter under the tap.
4) Position yourself in the most comfortable and convenient position. If you do not sit on the lavatory, you will need a jug or bowl for the urine.
5) Part the labia with one hand and, holding the catheter 2–3 inches from the tip, gently insert it into the bladder outlet until urine flows (see diagram).
6) When urine stops flowing, slowly withdraw the catheter. If the flow restarts, stop withdrawing until the bladder is empty. It is most important that the bladder is *completely* emptied at each catheterisation.
7) When the catheter is out, wash it under a running tap and shake it dry. Dry the outside with a clean paper towel or tissue and store it in a clean dry place (such as a resealable plastic bag) ready for the next use. If you are keeping a chart, record the urine volume obtained.
8) Use each catheter for one week (unless otherwise instructed) and then throw it away and use a new one. A supply of catheters is available from your chemist with a doctor's prescription.
9) You should drink 3–4 pints of liquid (any type) every twenty-four hours.

What should I do if . . .?

I see blood in the urine or on the catheter?
If this is a few specks, don't worry, if the bleeding persists or becomes heavy, contact the clinic.

The urine becomes smelly, cloudy, or if burning or a fever develop?
Bring urine specimen up to the clinic. You probably have a mild infection.

I cannot get the catheter in?
Don't keep trying, you will get sore. Abandon the attempt and try again later. If the difficulty persists and you are unable to pass urine yourself, seek help within twelve hours.

I miss and put the catheter in the vagina?
You will know because it will feel different and no urine will come out. Take the catheter out, wash it, and start again.

Clinic telephone No: .... (Hours ....)
In an emergency contact your own family doctor.

Table 8.2   Self-Catheterisation for Men (Patient Information Sheet)

1) Perform the catheterisation as often as your doctor or nurse has suggested. To start with this should be every ..... hours.
2) Get your catheter and lubricant gel.
3) Wash you hands thoroughly with soap and water and rinse the catheter under the tap.
4) Position yourself in the most comfortable and convenient position. If you do not sit on the lavatory, you will need a jug or bowl for the urine.
5) If you need to use anaesthetic gel, insert this into the tip of the penis, holding the penis slightly erect, then pinch gently to retain the gel. Wait four minutes for anaesthetic to take effect.
6) If you do not need anaesthetic gel, squeeze a small amount of lubricant gel along the catheter prior to insertion.
7) Holding the penis in a vertical position, gently insert the catheter until urine flows (see diagram). You may find that pretending to pass urine or coughing helps to overcome any resistance at the sphincter.
8) When urine stops flowing, slowly withdraw the catheter. If the flow re-starts, stop withdrawing until the bladder is empty. It is most important that the bladder is completely emptied at each catheterisation.
9) When the catheter is out, wash it under a running tap and shake it dry. Dry the outside with a clean paper towel or tissue and store it in a clean dry place (such as a resealable plastic bag) ready for the next use. If you are keeping a chart, record the urine volume obtained.
10) Use each catheter for one week (unless otherwise instructed) and then throw it away and use a new one. A supply of catheters is available from your chemist with a doctor's prescription.
11) You should drink 3–4 pints of liquid (any type) every twenty-four hours.

What should I do if . . .?

I see blood in the urine or on the catheter?
If this is a few specks don't worry. If the bleeding persists or becomes heavy, contact the clinic.

The urine becomes smelly, cloudy or if burning or a fever develop?
Bring a urine specimen up to the clinic. You probably have a mild infection.

I cannot get the catheter in?
Don't keep trying, you will get sore. Abandon the attempt and try again later. If the difficulty persists and you are unable to pass urine yourself, seek help within twelve hours.

Clinic telephone No: .... (Hours ....)
In an emergency contact your own family doctor.

pain, offensive urine or haematuria, is relatively uncommon. It will occur in one-quarter to one-third of patients at some time. It will usually respond to single-dose trimethoprim (400mg nocte), since most infections are *E. coli* from gut contamination. If there are recurrent episodes it may be advisable to give the patient a small supply of trimethoprim to take when needed. A urine specimen should be cultured if symptoms fail to respond.

Recurrent infection becomes a problem with a small minority of patients, and in this case the patient should be observed for any fault in technique. The volumes obtained should be measured to ensure that they are consistently below 400ml (infection results more often from catheterising too infrequently than from too frequently (Champion, 1976). Very occasionally it is necessary to advise changing the catheter more frequently. Only in rare cases does self-catheterisation have to be abandoned.

Asymptomatic bacteriuria is probably quite common in people self-catheterising (Lancet, 1979). Generally, unless the patient has vesico-ureteric reflux or is very young (under five years old), this does not matter and should be left untreated. Indeed, there is little point in obtaining routine urine samples. A sample is only indicated in the presence of symptoms. Treating asymptomatic infection predisposes to the development of more serious or resistant infection, and there is no benefit from eradicating a symptomless bacteriuria.

Where a patient has the dual problems of residual urine and hyperreflexic detrusor contractions, the aim of therapy should be to paralyse the bladder pharmacologically, for example using oxybutynin to abolish the contractions, and then to drain the bladder by intermittent catheterisation. This works well for many people with spina bifida, multiple sclerosis, or paraplegia.

The results from intermittent catheterisation are excellent. Up to 80% of patients with large-volume residual urine of neurogenic origin can regain continence. Wyndaele and Maes (1990) in a 12-year follow-up of 75 patients found chronic or recurrent infection in 42%, but the upper tract was well preserved and 92% were continent. Many people have avoided a permanent indwelling catheter, with all its attendant problems (see Chapter 9), or a urinary diversion by using ISC. Some people can gradually phase out catheterisation as normal voiding is re-established. Others must continue to catheterise indefinitely. The procedure is too new to be able to say with confidence what the long-term prospects are, but certainly at present they look very hopeful. Indeed, some people with ileal conduits are now being 'undiverted' back to using their own bladder with intermittent catheterisation. The technique is also being increasingly used with elderly patients with a voiding difficulty (see Chapter 11).

ACUTE AND CHRONIC MANAGEMENT OF A BLADDER AFTER SPINAL INJURY

It is crucial for the eventual rehabilitation of a paraplegic/tetraplegic patient and his or her bladder that good bladder management is started *immediately* after injury. The urological management of patients with spinal cord injuries is similar to that of patients with other types of neurogenic bladder dysfunction. It focuses on the prevention of upper renal tract complications, in addition to achieving successful relief of symptoms.

In the acute phase, immediately following injury, an indwelling catheter is often necessary. However, as soon as possible following stabilisation of the patient's condition, intermittent catheterisation is instituted during the early stages of recovery from spinal shock. During this period the problem is one of poorly sustained bladder contractions and erratic external sphincter behaviour, and the aim of intermittent catheterisation is to prevent over-distension of the detrusor muscle. Careful monitoring of residual urine volumes is essential.

Providing the patient has sufficient manual dexterity, he or she is taught how to self-catheterise. Where self-catheterisation is not possible, for example in the patient with limited dexterity or with a high spinal lesion, then assisted catheterisation should be considered. The technique can be successfully practised by a partner, relative or carer following a period of instruction, provided that this is acceptable to both parties. The presence of detrusor hyperreflexia may be controlled pharmacologically.

An individualised approach to the choice of treatment options is recommended for patients with spinal cord injuries (Fam and Yalla, 1988). In instances where self- or assisted intermittent catheterisation is not practical, then alternative forms of management must be considered to improve bladder emptying. Options may include bladder outlet surgery in male patients i.e. sphincterotomy together with condom drainage. This is often indicated in high tetraplegics where there is an increased risk of autonomic dysreflexia. Other indications for this type of surgery include vesico-ureteric reflux, hydronephrosis and pyelonephritis. The bladder may also be replaced by an ileal conduit or a continent diversion to allow urine drainage. An artificial sphincter may be useful in the management of lower motor neurone bladders to improve storage. In patients with a small capacity bladder, augmentation cystoplasty may be undertaken to increase bladder size.

REFERENCES AND FURTHER READING

Anderson, J. T. 1985. Disturbances of bladder and urethral function in Parkinson's disease. *International Urology Nephrology*, 17: 35–41.

Barrington, F. J. F., 1925. The effect of lesions in the hind and midbrain on micturition in the cat. *Quarterly Journal of Physiology*, 15: 82–102.

Barry, K., 1981. Neurogenic bladder incontinence: the consequences of mismanagement. *Rehabilitation Nursing*, 10: 12–13.

Betts, C. D., D'Mellow, M. T., Fowler, C. J., 1993. Urinary symptoms and the neurological features of bladder dysfunction in multiple sclerosis. *Journal of Neurology, Neurosurgery and Psychiatry*, 56: 245–50.

Blaivas, J. G., Barbalias, G. A., 1984. Detrusor-external sphincter dyssynergia in men with multiple sclerosis: an ominous urologic condition. *Journal of Urology*, 131: 91–4.

Champion, V. L., 1976. Clean technique for intermittent self-catheterisation. *Nursing Research*, 25, 1: 13–18.

de Groat, W. C., 1990. Central neural control of the lower urinary tract. In: Bock, G., Whelan, J., (eds). *Neurobiology of Incontinence*. Wiley, Chichester.

Eardley, I., Fowler, C. J., Nagendran, K., Kirby, R. S., and Rudge, P., 1991. The neurourology of tropical spastic paraparesis. *British Journal of Urology*, 68: 598–603.

Fam, B., Yalla, S. V., 1988. Vesico-urethral dysfunction in spinal cord injury and its management. *Seminars in Neurology*, 8, 2: 150–5.

Fay, J., 1978. Intermittent non-sterile catheterisation of children. *Nursing Mirror*, 146, 14: xiii–xv.

Guttmann, L., Frankel, A., 1966. The value of intermittent catheterization in the early management of traumatic paraplegia and tetraplegia. *Paraplegia*, 4: 63–84.

Hartman, M., 1978. Intermittent self-catheterisation. *Nursing*, 78, 11: 72–5.

Holland, N. J., Diesel-Levison, P., Schwedelson, E. S., 1981. Survey of neurogenic bladder in multiple sclerosis. *Journal of Neurosurgical Nursing*, 13, 6: 337–43.

Johnson, J. H., 1980. Rehabilitative aspects of neurologic bladder dysfunction. *Nursing Clinics of North America*, 15, 2: 293–307.

Kaye, K., Van Blerk, P. J. P., 1981. Urinary continence in children with neurogenic bladders. *British Journal of Urology*, 53: 241–5.

Khan, M. D., Starer, P., Singh, V. K., 1988. Neurologic basis of voiding disorders in patients with cerebrovascular accident. *Seminars in Neurology*, 8, 2: 156–8.

Kirby, R., Fowler, C. J., Gosling, J., Bannister, R., 1986. Urethrovesical dysfunction in progressive autonomic failure with multiple systems atrophy. *Journal of Neurology, Neurosurgery and Psychiatry*, 49: 554–62.

The Lancet, 1979. Clean intermittent catheterisation. *Lancet*, 2: 448–9.

Lapides, J., Diokno, A. C., Filber, S. J., Lowe, B. S., 1972. Clean intermittent self-catheterisation in the treatment of urinary tract disease. *Journal of Urology*, 107: 458–61.

Miller, H., Simpson, C. A., Yeats, W., 1965. Bladder dysfunction in multiple sclerosis. *British Medical Journal*, 1: 1265.

Pearman, J. W., 1976. Urological follow-up of 99 spinal-cord injured patients initially managed by intermittent catheterisation. *British Journal of Urology*, 48: 297–310.

Sotolongo, J. R., 1988. Voiding dysfunction in Parkinson's disease. *Seminars in Neurology*, 8, 2: 166–9.

Spiro, L. R., 1978. Bladder training for the incontinent patient. *Journal of Gerontological Nursing*, 4, 3: 28–35.

Wyndaele, J.-J., Maes, D., 1990. Clean intermittent self-catheterisation: a 12-year follow-up. *Journal of Urology*, 143: 906–8.

Chapter 9

Catheterisation

Brenda Roe, PhD, RN

*Senior Research Fellow, Health Services Research Unit,
Department of Public Health and Primary Care,
Oxford University*

The use of a hollow tube, or 'catheter', for urine drainage has a long history. The ancient Egyptians used gold catheters and the Greeks had bronze tubes for the relief of urinary obstruction (Cule, 1980). Reeds and rolled palm leaves were used for centuries by the Chinese. Modern technology has today resulted in a wide variety of catheters suitable for use in different situations. This chapter outlines how good catheter management can lead to the successful control of bladder function. Two categories of catheter are considered – the indwelling urethral (or Foley) catheter and the suprapubic catheter. (See Chapter 8 for intermittent catheter regimes.)

Overall, some 12% of patients in hospital have a catheter in situ at any one time (Crow et al., 1986). About 4% of people on community nursing caseloads have a long term indwelling catheter (Roe, 1989a).

INDWELLING URETHRAL (FOLEY) CATHETERS

It was not until the 1930s that Frederick Foley perfected a technique for the manufacture of a one-piece catheter and balloon, by the dipping and coagulation of latex on metal forms. Today the Foley catheter is the most commonly used of all urinary catheters. In its most usual form it has a double lumen shaft, one lumen for urine drainage, the other for inflation and deflation of the balloon, a rounded tip, and two drainage eyes proximal to the balloon (Figure 9.1).

There are many variations on this standard design, both in materials and construction. Table 9.1 (overleaf) summarises the most common variants in use. The size of a catheter is measured on the Charrière (ch) or French gauge (f.g.) – these are in fact identical and measure the external circumference of the catheters in millimetres, usually in graduations of 2mm. A 14 f.g. catheter therefore has an external circumference of 14mm.

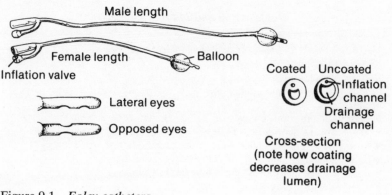

Figure 9.1   *Foley catheters.*

Indications for using an Indwelling Urethral Catheter

There are many situations in which an indwelling urethral catheter may be used. The most common indications are:

1) In the acute hospital setting, post-operative drainage, particularly after urological or gynaecological surgery, and during severe illness where accurate monitoring of urine output is needed.

2) Chronic or acute retention of urine, either short-term until the retention is treated, or long-term if treatment is impossible or unsuccessful.

3) The terminally ill patient may benefit from the use of a catheter if bladder management becomes a problem, either because of incontinence which is distressing, difficult to manage, or causing severe skin problems, or because micturition has become too frequent, too painful, or too difficult for the patient's comfort. A catheter may make the difference between relatives being able to cope at home, and a dying person needing hospital care.

4) Intractable urinary incontinence, at any age, in either sex and from any cause, may also be managed by an indwelling catheter. This, it must be stressed, should be very much a last resort, and a catheter should never be the first line of management for incontinence. But if, after full investigation and a trial of available treatments, the person remains so incontinent that the quality of his or her life is impaired and a normal lifestyle is impossible, a catheter may provide a very positive method of management. Patients who are too unwell or frail to undergo therapy for incontinence may also benefit.

Table 9.1   Types of Foley Catheter

MALE-LENGTH FOLEY CATHETER
Length: 40–45cm
Balloon sizes: 3ml (child), 5ml, 5–10ml, 30ml
Sizes: 8–30 f.g. in 2mm graduations
Material
- Plastic – short-term – 14 days
- Latex rubber – short-term – 14 days
- Siliconised – provides lubrication for insertion – short-term – 14 days
- Teflon-coated – medium term – 21 days
- Silicone elastomer-coated latex – long-term (> 21 days)
- 100% silicone – long-term (> 21 days)
- Hydrogel-coated – long-term (> 21 days)

FEMALE-LENGTH FOLEY CATHETER
Length: 20–25cm
Balloon sizes: 5–10ml, 10ml, 30ml
Sizes: 12–26 f.g.
Material
- Latex rubber – short-term – 14 days
- Teflon-coated – long-term – 21 days
- Silicone elastomer-coated latex – long-term (> 21 days)
- 100% silicone – long-term (> 21 days)
- Hydrogel-coated – long-term (> 21 days)

ROBERTS CATHETER
Length: 40cm
Balloon size: 10ml
Sizes: 12–24 f.g.
Material
- Teflon-coated – one eye below balloon for drainage.

DOUBLE BALLOON
Length: 40cm
Balloon sizes: 10ml, 30ml
Sizes: 16 f.g.
Material
- Latex rubber – double balloon for women – one each at internal and external meatus to prevent movement.

3-WAY CATHETER
Length: 40–45cm
Balloon sizes: 10ml, 30–50ml, 75–100ml
Sizes: 18–26 f.g.
Material
- Plastic or latex-rubber – some reinforced to prevent collapse with suction. For continuous irrigation.

Insertion of a catheter to control incontinence should only proceed after full discussion of the implications between doctor, patient, nurse and other relevant people (e.g. relatives). All parties to the decision must agree and accept the catheter. A catheter should never be inserted for the convenience of staff; it must always be a decision taken for the well-being of the patient. For some it may allow an independent life, free from the need for institutional care, or allow care by relatives who otherwise could not or would not cope with incontinence at home. For women who have no alternative to the absorbent pad, and for men who cannot use an appliance, a well-managed catheter can restore social continence and a full range of normal activities.

Selection of the Catheter

Once the decision to use an indwelling catheter has been made, the choice of catheter is crucial. It is not acceptable merely to use the first catheter that comes to hand from the store cupboard. Whoever is inserting the catheter should be aware of the range available and their different functions. Many hospital staff have been found to have poor knowledge and little training on catheter selection (Henry, 1992). Many catheters are badly stored, with little stock control. Mulhall (1992) found that two-thirds of hospital wards had some out-of-date catheters.

Size

The golden rule when selecting catheter size is to choose the smallest catheter that will drain adequately. For an adult this will normally be a 12, 14, or 16 f.g. Size 8 f.g. catheters are the smallest available for children, and for infants an infant feeding tube may be used. Sizes larger than 18 f.g. should never be used, except where heavy haematuria is anticipated (Wilson and Roe, 1986). It is all too common for patients presenting with pain and leakage of urine around the catheter to have a large catheter in situ (Kennedy et al., 1983a; Roe and Brocklehurst, 1987). The purpose of a catheter is not to occlude the urethra completely, like a cork in a bottle neck. The folds of the urethra normally close upon themselves (Pullen et al., 1982), and the smaller the catheter, the more easily the urethral folds can close around it.

Except at the sphincters, there should be adequate space around the catheter so that secretions from the paraurethral glands can drain. It has been suggested that if these glands are occluded, the secretions will accumulate and may become infected, which could then lead to an abscess or to stricture formation (Blandy, 1981) (Figure 9.2, overleaf).

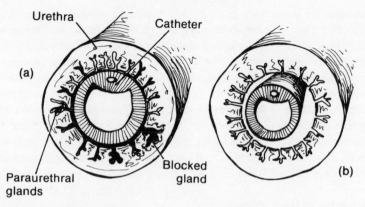

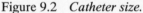

Figure 9.2 *Catheter size.*

A catheter which is too large will also risk causing a urethral pressure sore in men, either where it is gripped at the external sphincter or where it bends over the peno-scrotal junction (Blandy, 1981). This may be followed by sloughing granuloma and stricture formation (Figure 9.3).

Larger catheters do not necessarily have larger eyes in proportion, so will often block just as easily as smaller ones. Coated catheters have an especially small eye and lumen size in proportion to their f.g. size (Figure 9.1).

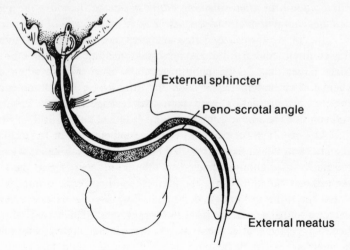

Figure 9.3 *Stricture sites.*

Balloon Size

Manufacturers indicate on their packaging of a catheter the maximum amount of fluid with which a balloon should be filled, 10ml or 30ml, according to the British Standard (BS1695). Very large balloons, 75ml and over, are intended specifically for controlling post-operative haematuria and should not be used for general purposes, although to date research has not established the benefits of larger balloons compared to smaller ones in controlling blood loss. A custom has grown up in the UK of using 30ml balloon catheters, filled with 30ml of water, as standard practice for routine drainage. Roe and Brocklehurst (1987) found that 58% (n=21) of community patients had catheters with 30ml balloons. This practice is not to be condoned and is the cause of many catheter-associated problems. In the USA the 10ml fill volume balloon is used routinely, and this practice is currently gaining acceptance in the UK. A larger balloon is not necessary to hold a catheter in place. The balloon is not designed to occlude the internal urethral meatus to prevent leakage – this is prevented by the bladder neck and sphincters gripping the catheter lumen – but merely to gently retain the catheter in the bladder to prevent it from falling out. Few catheters need more than 10ml of fluid for this purpose.

One major problem caused by using too large a balloon is the bypassing or leakage of urine around the catheter (Kennedy et al., 1983a). With all catheters, except the Roberts catheter, the drainage eyes are above the balloon. If a 10ml balloon is used this results in a small amount of residual urine, which is unable to escape, being left around the balloon. If the balloon has 30ml of water in it the residual urine volume is much larger, with a greater potential for infection (Figure 9.4, overleaf). It is thought that the larger balloon irritates the bladder and may provoke contractions, especially in an unstable bladder. Contractions will force the residual urine out around the catheter, and the larger the volume of residual urine, the greater the potential for leakage.

Thirty millilitres of water is heavy, especially when resting on the delicate and sensitive trigone of the bladder. This can lead to the patient experiencing discomfort or dragging, and repeated traction or pulling on the catheter may damage the bladder neck. It is sometimes stated that a large balloon is necessary to prevent confused patients from pulling the catheter out. This is not true, and it may be necessary to review whether a catheter is the most appropriate form of management for these patients. The weight and discomfort caused by a 30ml balloon in the bladder may indeed be the cause of the pulling.

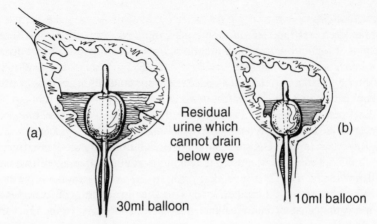

Figure 9.4   *Balloon size.*

Repeated traction upon a smaller balloon is less likely to damage the bladder neck. It is better to avoid the use of a catheter if a confused or uncooperative patient tends to pull at it.

Catheter Material
Until relatively recently, most catheters were made either from plastic (polyvinylchloride or polyurethane) or latex rubber. Plastic is soft at body temperature but rigid at lower temperatures and is often found by women to be uncomfortable, especially when sitting. Both plastic and latex rubber tend to develop cracks and encrustations (surface deposits) with prolonged use (after about two weeks). Plastic probably attracts less encrustation because its negative surface electrical charge discourages particle adhesion, although the clinical results of this are unproven. Both plastic and latex catheters are relatively cheap and suitable for short-term use, such as post-operative drainage. Some latex is not inert and problems have arisen with cytotoxicity, e.g. causing urethral strictures. All catheters must now conform to British Standard 1695 (1990).

Many attempts have been made to improve upon the latex catheter to provide a longer life, reduce encrustation and infection, and improve comfort. 'Siliconising' the surface of the latex catheter produces a lubricated surface, which is said to ease insertion and provide some lubrication. However the coating dissolves within hours of insertion, and as lubricant jelly is usually also used, insertion is seldom a problem. The extra cost of siliconised catheters is of debatable value.

Latex can be coated with Teflon, which is claimed to make the latex more inert and to give a smoother surface. This may reduce urethritis and is recommended by manufacturers for short- to medium-term use.

Many claims have been made for catheters coated or dipped in silicone elastomer – 'silicone-coated' – which should be distinguished from the 'siliconised' catheters described above. There does seem to be less encrustation with silicone-coated than with latex catheters in long-term use, and some reduction in tissue reaction (Blacklock, 1986). Manufacturers claim that they can be left safely in situ for three months without changing. It is possible that encrustation itself is not a major factor in catheter lifespan and many are changed for other reasons, especially leakage, long before encrustation has become a problem. It has yet to be determined whether the reduced lumen from the coating actually impairs drainage, encourages blockage, and shortens the catheter's life. Pure silicone catheters are not coated and the internal lumen tends to be proportionately larger.

Pure silicone and the more recent hydrogel-coated catheters are the most inert and least likely to encrust and are suitable for long-term use. Hydrogel seems to resist encrustation and biofilms (films of adherent bacteria), as well as being non-cytotoxic (Roe, 1993).

Catheter Design
For most purposes, a man will be catheterised with a male-length catheter and a woman with a female-length catheter with a 10ml balloon. There is no reason to use the longer catheters for most women, as their greater length makes them difficult to disguise under clothing and easier to pull accidentally. If a thigh drainage bag is used, they are also more likely to form a loop, which means that urine has to drain uphill into the bag. However, some women who are chairbound sometimes prefer to use the longer male-length. Whichever catheter is the most comfortable and convenient for the patient should be selected.

The Roberts catheter, which has one eye below the balloon, may be of use when leakage is a problem, e.g. with an unstable bladder. Urine which normally would not be able to drain may be squeezed out of the distal eye, rather than around the catheter by bladder contractions.

Most catheters have a semi-rigid rounded tip. Variations include the Tiemann tip, which is curved to aid insertion past an enlarged prostate, and a whistle tip which is open-ended to facilitate drainage of debris. Most catheters have two drainage eyes. These may be lateral (on the same side) or opposed (on opposite sides). The latter is possibly less likely to block (Figure 9.1).

The major design development this century since the introduction of the Foley is that of the conformable catheter. The conformable catheter has a section that conforms to the shape of the urethra (Figure 9.5). It allows partial filling of the bladder and intermittent emptying. By adopting the shape of the urethra, the catheter is intended to be more comfortable, less likely to encrust and to cause leakage of urine around the catheter (Brocklehurst et al., 1988). It is thought that the intermittent, rather than continuous, drainage which occurs with a conformable catheter may help to flush out the catheter periodically. At present the conformable catheter is only available for females but is currently being further developed for male patients.

Figure 9.5   *Conformable catheter.*

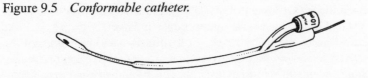

Insertion of an Indwelling Catheter
The decision to institute drainage by indwelling catheter is generally a medical one and should always be made by the responsible medical practitioner in conjunction with the patient, carer and nurse. The actual insertion should be done by a nurse or doctor who has received full instruction and who has had supervised practice in the technique, and is deemed competent. There is little obvious reason for the tradition that doctors or male nurses catheterise men, and female nurses catheterise women. So long as local chaperoning guidance is followed, any competent professional should be able to catheterise any patient.

The insertion of an indwelling catheter should always be performed using strict aseptic technique, whether in the home or in hospital (Bielski, 1980; Pritchard and David, 1988). In most situations, pre-packed catheter packs are available. The importance of selecting the right catheter has already been stressed. Ideally, the patient should have a bath prior to catheter insertion. If this is not possible, a thorough wash of the genital area with soap and water is essential.

For women, the key to successful catheter insertion lies in visualising the urethral meatus clearly. The patient should lie semi-recumbent with knees bent and abducted to either side as far as possible. An anglepoise light directed at the vulva can be very helpful. A cotton bud will help to locate the meatus if it is disguised among skin folds. Some women who find catheterisation painful may benefit from the use of local anaesthetic into the urethra. If the urethral opening is concealed, it may be easier to find with the patient in the left lateral position with her knees drawn up onto her chest, so that the anterior vaginal wall can be visualised from behind. Women with atrophic vaginitis may have a meatus which has 'migrated' up into the vagina.

In men, the foreskin should be retracted and the glans penis thoroughly cleaned. Local anaesthetic gel, e.g. lignocaine 1%, must be instilled into the penis using an applicator and then held in by gentle pressure, using the fingers for at least four minutes. The catheter is inserted while extending the penis vertically with gentle but firm lateral grasp. If resistance is met at the external sphincter, the patient is asked to relax and pretend to pass urine or to cough. The usual reason for encountering resistance at this point is insufficient anaesthesia. The catheter should never be forced in, but withdrawn and some more anaesthetic instilled, before re-inserting the catheter after a further four minutes. Catheter-introducers are dangerous in inexperienced hands and should only be used by a trained urologist. When the catheter still fails to pass, a smaller or softer one may be tried. If this fails, urological assistance should be sought. Once the catheter is in situ the foreskin must be replaced.

Most health authorities have their own detailed clinical procedures, guidelines and standards of care for catheterisation, and these should be consulted and followed. It is most important, because of product liability, to follow the manufacturer's printed instructions. Detailed written nursing records stating the type, size, volume of water in the balloon, batch number and date of insertion should always be kept.

Drainage Bags

Once a catheter has been inserted, it should immediately be aseptically connected to a sterile drainage bag. The type of bag will be selected according to the needs of the individual patient.

Most bags have a non-return valve at their inlet to prevent urine refluxing once it has entered the bag. Bags without this valve should not be connected directly to an indwelling catheter.

The patient who is bedbound or receiving continuous bladder irrigation will usually need a 2-litre capacity bag, which can be supported by a bed-hanger or floor-stand. These bags are also used for a short-term catheter and for overnight drainage with a long-term catheter.

Ambulant patients, especially those whose catheter is to be in for more than a few days, will need a smaller body-worn bag for use by day. It is not acceptable for a patient to carry around a 2-litre bag of urine like a handbag, in full view. The most usual body-worn bag is the leg bag (Ryan Wooley, 1987). This may have a capacity of 350ml, 500ml, 750ml or 1 litre, and is secured to the leg with straps which may be made from latex, fabric ties, elastic or foam rubber and Velcro. Leg-straps can cause problems if they are too tight (a full bag can be heavy), and some people develop a sensitivity to latex that can result in sores (Roe et al., 1988). The inlet may be short, for thigh-wearing, or longer to wear over the knee or on the calf, under trousers). The calf-bag is emptied by lifting up the bottom of the trousers. A thigh-bag can be emptied more easily if a small Velcro-fastened opening is made in the inner trouser seam.

Alternatively, a drainage bag may be suspended from a waist-belt, 'sporran' style (Figure 9.6). These bags hold up to one litre and have a side inlet to prevent kinking. As the weight is more evenly distributed, many patients find this more comfortable than leg-straps. Very obese patients may find that the waist-belt does not stay up easily, and immobile people must take care that the bag is below bladder level.

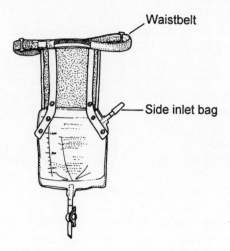

Figure 9.6 *Sporran with bag.*

Women find the sporran particularly useful under skirts, since there is no danger, as there is with a leg bag, of the bag sliding down and becoming visible.

Drainage bags, whether small or large, can be held in specially designed garments (pants, trousers or skirts) with an integral pocket for the bag (Figure 9.7). The plastic of the bag is not in contact with the skin, and even a 2-litre bag can be kept discreetly out of sight.

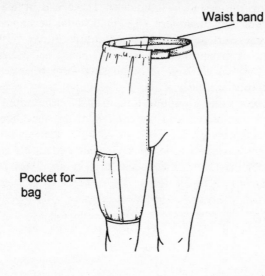

Waist band

Pocket for bag

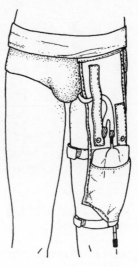

Figure 9.7   *Leg-bag garments.*

The selection of an outlet tap which the patient can manage easily and which does not cause the fingers to become wet with urine is important (Kennedy et al., 1983b; Glenister, 1987; Roe et al., 1988). Some people find a push-pull valve easy, others prefer a twist-and-pull type or a lever-action tap. Larger taps are often easier to manage, but may damage the leg. Taps are available which allow a night-drainage bag to be connected directly to the bottom of the smaller day bag without breaking the system (Figure 9.8). These can be used with cheaper non-drainable, single-use, bags in hospital or the home. If ordinary drainable bags are used in the home they may be washed out and re-used or disposed of, depending upon local policies and guidelines. In hospital all bags must be single-use because of the danger of cross-infection.

Some bags incorporate a quilting to spread the urine more evenly and allow the bag to conform to the contour of the leg. Others may have a fabric backing or an anti-kink device. Patients are very individual in their choice of drainage bag and need to be offered a range to find the best for their needs (Roe et al., 1988; Kohler-Ockmore, 1992).

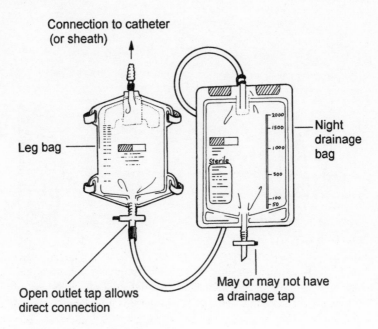

Figure 9.8 *Day-night link system.*

Valves and Straps

Opinion is divided on whether the catheter itself should be attached to the patient's leg. In some cases this could help to restrict traction on the catheter, in others it seems to increase it. Several catheter straps are available commercially.

The use of a catheter valve (Figure 9.9), in place of a drainage bag, is growing in popularity. This is said to maintain bladder capacity, reduce erosion and lessen catheter blockage by giving it a good flush out periodically. A valve also dispenses with the need to wear a bag, as the catheter can be emptied directly into a lavatory. This management is obviously not suitable for someone with a low-capacity unstable bladder, as leakage would occur between catheter releases. It is, however, a viable method for those who need a catheter because of voiding difficulties, and it deserves increased evaluation in future. It may also help to avoid some of the complications of long-term catheterisation, such as bladder shrinkage and erosion of the bladder wall (see below, page 216). Further research is needed on this (Roe, 1990).

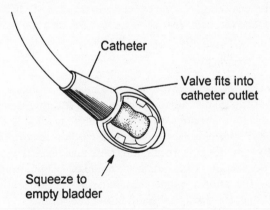

Catheter

Valve fits into catheter outlet

Squeeze to empty bladder

Figure 9.9   *Catheter valve.*

Infection and the Indwelling Catheter

The normal urinary tract has several defences against infection. Complete bladder emptying, the regular scouring action of micturition, and a competent sphincter mechanism all help to prevent bacterial invasion and to eradicate any micro-organisms promptly and completely. The introduction of an indwelling catheter into this normally sterile system provides three potential entry portals for infection: on the catheter itself during insertion, around the outside of the catheter via the urethra, and ascent up the lumen of the catheter. The first portal can be largely discounted if strict aseptic technique is used for insertion. The second is more of a problem in the short female urethra, but defences can be bolstered by ensuring that the catheter is small enough to allow free drainage of urethral secretions.

Ascending infection, via the catheter lumen, was the major source of infection in catheterised patients until the early 1960s. Prior to that, catheters were maintained on 'open drainage' with the end of the catheter open and draining into a non-sterile vessel. With this system, almost all catheterised bladders were infected within three to four days of insertion. Although this could be reduced, to some extent, by continuous antiseptic irrigation, infection rates remained high until the introduction of closed urinary drainage directly from the catheter into sterile sealed bags. This introduction of closed drainage has moved the point at which nearly all (95%) of catheterised bladders are infected, from twenty-four hours (Thornton and Andriole, 1970) to twelve days after catheter insertion (Garibaldi et al., 1974). This has been the biggest single advance in catheter care. It has meant that infection rates for catheters in situ for less than five days can be kept low in most situations, provided that the closed system is not interrupted, i.e. the catheter is never disconnected from the bag, and only opened when emptying.

However, as the duration of catheterisation continues an increasing proportion of patients with catheters will acquire a urinary tract infection, whatever precautions are taken, until nearly all are inevitably infected after two weeks. No method has yet been found which significantly reduces this rising infection rate, except the pragmatic approach of keeping the system scrupulously uninterrupted in the short term. Irrigation, routine washouts, systematic antibiotics and antimicrobals in the drainage bag all fail to alter this.

Most commonly the infecting micro-organisms are from the patients' own commensals, e.g. *E. coli*. However, almost any organism can invade the catheterised bladder, including more exotic bacteria, fungi and yeasts, which is why all attempts to prevent cross-infection are so important. Not all organisms are free floating, and they can adhere to the internal lumen of the catheter and drainage bag as part of a biofilm (Ramsay et al., 1989; Mulhall, 1991). Bacteria can also migrate upwards from the bag, past a non-return valve, in the form of biofilms (Mulhall, 1992). The development of biofilms and their interaction with catheter materials and bladder instillations form important lines of enquiry for current research. A decision to use a catheter for long-term bladder management must be made in the knowledge of the inevitability of infection.

Does this infection associated with catheters matter? One in ten patients admitted to an acute hospital will have an indwelling catheter at some point during their admission. Forty per cent of all nosocomial (hospital-acquired) infections are urinary tract infections, and 70% of these are associated with the use of an indwelling catheter. There is some evidence that those patients catheterised during admission are likely to have a longer stay in hospital, suffer more complications, and possibly have a higher incidence of fatal outcome to their hospital stay, than patients with similar illness but no catheter (Platt et al., 1982). The incidence of Gram-negative bacteraemias following catheterisation is low, but when it occurs it causes a 40% mortality. Those patients who are catheterised because they are acutely ill, or have had urinary tract surgery, are especially vulnerable to risks of serious complications.

If the catheter is likely to be in place short-term, it is certainly worth every effort to prevent or delay the onset of infection. Once the catheter is a permanent feature, infection has to be accepted. However, the importance of preventing any further contamination, in particular with drug-resistant organisms, is paramount. Therefore, the prevention of cross-infection and contamination is mandatory. Most of the evidence about the effects of infection from long-term catheters comes from patients with spinal injury. Many of these patients do suffer renal impairment; indeed, renal failure is the most common reason for death, apart from injury-related causes, and many are found to have scarred kidneys with pus on post-mortem examination (Warren et al., 1981).

Management of the Short-Term Indwelling Catheter

For the short-term catheter (intended duration up to 14 days) the primary aim of management is to prevent urinary tract infection. The first question must always be, 'Is this catheter really necessary?' Surprisingly often the answer is 'No'.

If the catheter is suggested because the patient has failed to pass urine, e.g. post-operatively, it may be possible to promote spontaneous voiding by ensuring that the patient is not in pain and has adequate privacy and comfort to pass urine, preferably on a lavatory or commode. Running taps, plenty of time and a hot cup of tea work well for many patients. If voiding is not achieved in the presence of a distended bladder or discomfort, an in-out catheter should usually be used in the first instance. Only after spontaneous voiding has failed to occur after several intermittent catheters should an indwelling catheter be considered.

In male patients who must have their urinary output closely monitored, but who are incontinent, a penile sheath is preferable to a catheter, provided that the bladder is emptying completely.

After much urological or gynaecological surgery, a suprapubic catheter is preferable to a urethral one because the catheter can be clamped while the patient tries to void, and simply unclamped if he fails (see page 221). This overcomes the problem of repeated catheter withdrawal and re-insertion in situations when some voiding problem is common. Some hospitals still use catheters routinely in certain situations, e.g. orthopaedic surgery, without consideration of individual needs and the risks involved.

If a urethral catheter is really necessary for short-term use, the duration of catheterisation must always be kept to an absolute minimum, preferably less than five days. A closed system between the catheter and bag must be maintained if at all possible. If a break is essential, e.g. to wash out a blocked catheter, then strict aseptic technique must be observed. If the need for irrigation is anticipated, for example after prostatectomy, it is best to insert a three-way irrigating catheter, remembering that the junction between irrigating fluid and catheter is another break in the system and must also be treated aseptically.

The drainage bag should be emptied when it is nearly full, but as infrequently as possible, using a 'no-touch' technique and a clean disposable urinal for each patient. Handwashing and the use of clean disposable gloves before and after any handling of the catheter or bag is very important and helps to prevent cross-infection. For the same reason, the bag should always be on a hanger and never allowed to touch the floor. Physically separating catheterised patients from each other in a ward may help to prevent cross-infection by acting as a reminder for nurses to wash their hands.

Drainage bags should not be changed routinely on short-term catheters. If the bag becomes clogged with debris, a new one can be substituted using aseptic non-touch technique; otherwise most bags will last up to seven days (DoH, 1991).

Meatal cleansing according to a person's daily hygiene, for both short-term and long-term catheterised patients, should involve careful washing of the genital area with soap and water. A bath or shower may also be taken using unscented soap and avoiding additives such as bubble bath. In men, the foreskin should be retracted, the glans penis cleaned and the foreskin replaced. The genital area should then be dried thoroughly with a clean soft towel. Talcum powder should be avoided as it can clog around the catheter and act as an irritant. Careful washing should also be encouraged after each bowel movement, and women must be instructed on correct perineal cleaning, i.e. using toilet paper from front to back, away from the catheter. Using antiseptic solutions for catheter care has no proven value and can lead to the development of resistant organisms (Stickler, 1991). Where the patient has any discharge of blood or mucus around the catheter, this should be carefully cleaned away using sterile cotton wool and water, if necessary.

Bladder washouts or instillations should not be used as a routine in short-term catheter management. They have no role in preventing infection and cause a break in the closed drainage system, which increases the opportunity for bacterial invasion. Likewise, systemic antibiotics have no place in the prevention of infection, and may indeed provoke the emergence of antibiotic-resistant strains. However, they should be used appropriately to treat infection in short-term catheterised patients, and the catheter should be removed.

Urine Specimens from Catheters

The drainage system does not need to be disconnected when taking a urine specimen from the catheter for microbiological examination, as most bags have a self-sealing sample port on the drainage tubing. The tubing may be clamped just below the port, and left for several minutes for urine to accumulate above the clamp. The sample port should be cleaned with 70% alcohol (e.g. an injection swab). The specimen is taken using a sterile needle and syringe, inserted via the sample port at an angle (to avoid going straight through the tubing and possibly injecting the nurse's fingers with infected urine). The urine should never be squirted into a specimen pot via the needle, since this can destroy any cells or casts present. The needle should always be removed first. Specimens should only be taken when (i) there are symptoms of urinary tract infection, (ii) treatment is intended and (iii) the catheter is to be removed completely or replaced with a new one if infection is found.

Urine specimens should never be taken from the drainage bag as this will be contaminated and will not reflect the state of the urine in the bladder. Wherever possible the specimen should be delivered to the laboratory for culture and sensitivity within one hour of sampling.

Long-Term Indwelling Catheter Management

As stated above, the use of a long-term catheter can be a very positive decision in patient care, but it must always be made bearing the risks of infection in mind. The likely benefits and costs should be considered for each patient individually. For younger patients with prolonged management by catheter, renal problems become a major cause of morbidity and mortality (Warren, et al., 1981). This is less relevant when a patient is very elderly or has a limited life expectancy. For younger patients, who may need a catheter for decades, every possible alternative should be seriously considered, such as a suprapubic catheter, intermittent catheterisation, an artificial sphincter, or urinary diversion via an ileal conduit.

The long-term catheter in a hospitalised patient should be managed in much the same way as the short-term catheter, but in the knowledge that an infected bladder is inevitable. Hospitals are prone to harbour multi-resistant organisms, and the aim must be to minimise cross-infection by strict adherence to the infection control policy.

The most important factor in successful home management is that the patient, or his relatives, should fully understand how to look after the catheter and drainage system. A fearful patient, afraid to touch the catheter, will be far less successful than the confident patient. To this end, ample time must always be given for the newly catheterised patient to discuss any worries, and careful instruction is vital. An information booklet is useful for reference (see Table 9.2 for an example, overleaf) and these are now widely available.

The patient must be shown and given supervised practice in caring for his catheter. This includes instruction on personal hygiene, changing day and night bags, how to empty the bag, how to wash bags out, if they wish to use this practice, and how to dispose of them. A leg bag may be worn during the daytime and a larger bag attached to it at night. After each change, the bag may be washed in warm soapy water (e.g. using washing-up liquid) and then hung up to dry thoroughly or be disposed of. The patient may be given the choice. Drainage bags have been successfully disinfected by researchers (Hashisaki et al., 1984), but to date we do not know whether patients who may be elderly and/or physically disabled can achieve the same successful outcomes. Each bag may be used for up to one week (DoH, 1991).

The patient is asked to drink plenty of fluid (at least two litres per day), to take reasonable exercise (to avoid debris accumulation) and to avoid constipation. Either a bath or shower may be taken, depending upon personal preference and circumstances.

CATHETER-ASSOCIATED PROBLEMS

Catheter Cramps

Most people experience abdominal cramps, often likened by women to menstrual pains, when a catheter is first inserted. A mild analgesic and simple reassurance that this is nothing to worry about will settle this within twenty-four hours for most patients. If cramps persist and are troublesome, the cause is usually an unstable bladder with contractions being experienced as discomfort. Sometimes a smaller catheter or a smaller balloon will stop this. Propantheline (15mg t.d.s.) or oxybutynin may also be an effective remedy. In some people the cramps are so severe that catheterisation is inappropriate, and another form of management has to be used.

Urethral Discomfort

Some urethral discomfort is common with an indwelling catheter, and this may have to be accepted. Silicone or silicone-coated catheters may be more comfortable than plastic or latex. The discomfort may be caused by too large a catheter mechanically distending the urethra, or occluding the paraurethral glands, leading to infection, urethritis, and an offensive discharge around the catheter. A smaller catheter should resolve this.

In post-menopausal women, discomfort may be caused by atrophic urethritis, and a course of oestrogen replacement therapy will relieve the discomfort (see Chapter 11).

Leaking Catheters

One of the most common reasons for catheter failure and premature change is leakage or bypassing. It is present in up to 40% of all patients with a catheter and is the reason for one-third of unplanned catheter changes (Kennedy and Brocklehurst, 1982; Kennedy et al., 1983a). This is particularly irksome if the catheter was instituted to control incontinence, as the patient is not only still wet but also has the additional problem of catheter care.

A leaking catheter is usually caused by too large a size catheter or by an unstable bladder. The bladder is irritated by the presence of the catheter and contracts uninhibitedly, squeezing urine out around the lumen of the catheter. Often using a smaller catheter decreases the irritation and thus the leakage. Also, with a smaller balloon there is less residual urine available to leak (see page 199). Anticholinergic medication may also help to dampen any unstable bladder contractions which

Table 9.2   Home Management of a Catheter

INSTRUCTIONS TO PATIENT

The catheter is a hollow tube which will drain your urine from the bladder into a bag. You will not need to pass water yourself. These simple instructions will help you to look after your catheter properly.

1) Wash the area around where the catheter enters your body thoroughly daily, or according to your personal hygiene needs. This should be done with unscented soap and warm water and the area dried thoroughly on a soft towel. When possible, a daily bath or shower may be taken. Avoid use of talcum powder in the area. Also wash the area thoroughly after a bowel motion.

2) Drink at least 4 pints (2 litres) of fluid in every 24 hours. This means about 1 cupful of liquid per hour when you are awake. The drinks do not have to be water – any other drink is just as good.

3) Wear the smaller drainage bag when you are up and connect the larger bag to the bottom of it at night. Always wash your hands thoroughly before and after changing the bags.

4) Each drainage bag will last about 1 week. After changing the large bag, wash it thoroughly in warm water with a mild detergent solution (e.g. washing-up liquid). A small funnel is useful to help fill the bag with fluid. Then hang it up to dry out thoroughly before next use. You may choose to dispose of your night bags rather than wash them through. The choice is yours. Generally a leg bag will last between 5 and 7 days, and should then be wrapped in newspaper and thrown away in the dustbin.

5) When possible take regular daily exercise.

6) Avoid constipation as this can prevent the catheter draining properly. If constipation is a problem, ask your nurse for advice.

7) Avoid bending or kinking the catheter tubing. Always keep the bag below bladder level to ensure good drainage.

Table 9.2 (continued)

Some Common Problems

1) Bladder spasms or cramps in the abdomen are common when you have a new catheter. They are nothing to worry about and usually pass off within a few days. If they persist, tell your nurse.

2) If no urine drains for several hours:
   - is the tubing bent or kinked?
   - is the bag below the bladder level? (It should be.)
   - is the bag connected the right way up?
   - have you been drinking enough?
   - are you constipated?
   - try moving or walking around, as this may dislodge a blockage.
   If 4 hours or longer pass and no urine has drained, call your nurse.

3) If your catheter leaks, this is not serious but should be reported to your nurse during office hours (9 a.m.–5 p.m.).

4) If the catheter falls out, call your nurse during office hours if you can pass urine. If you cannot pass urine yourself and your bladder becomes painful, seek immediate help from: ....

5) If you see blood in the urine do not worry, but report it at the nurse's next visit. If the bleeding is heavy, report it during office hours.

6) If your catheter is causing you problems during sexual intercourse, do not hesitate to discuss this with your nurse.

Your nurse is:

Address:

Telephone No. in office hours (9a.m.–5 p.m.):

Emergency No. for other times:

Please feel free to discuss any problems or queries you may have about your catheter with your nurse.

---

can contribute to the catheter leakage (propantheline is again useful here).

The catheter may also cause urine leakage because it is blocked. Flushing the catheter out with sterile water may unblock the catheter. Alternatively, it may be blocked because of kinked tubing or because the bag has been consistently above bladder level.

Some patients find a Roberts catheter helps to prevent leakage (see page 201).

Haematuria

Small amounts of blood in the urine of catheterised patients is common and of no importance. It is usually caused by trauma and infection. If haematuria becomes heavy and persistent, urological advice should be sought.

Infection

In the patient with a long-term catheter, infection is both inevitable and, in most cases, asymptomatic. It is futile to treat these infections as the urine is usually only cleared for a few days, if at all (Brocklehurst and Brocklehurst, 1978), and there is a danger of more pathogenic organisms invading the bladder, or of resistance developing. Prophylactic antibiotics or antimicrobal washouts have no place in long-term catheter management.

However, if the patient becomes ill the infection will have to be treated. Symptoms may include fever, rigors, loin pain, significant haematuria, and, in the elderly, the onset of sudden unexplained confusion. The catheter may have to be removed for treatment to be successful.

Various measures have been tried to acidify urine, and thus reduce infection, with as yet equivocal results. Cranberry juice may possibly help, as it is one of the few fruit juices not to be oxidised, and has been found to reduce both white and red blood cells in the urine (Rogers, 1991).

Erosion of the Bladder Wall

When a catheter is used for long-term continuous drainage, the bladder shrinks and collapses around it (Kritiansen et al., 1983). The tip of the catheter may therefore come into contact with the bladder wall and is thought to erode the bladder mucosa. There is some evidence that prolonged use of a catheter and the resultant negative pressures can cause pseudopolyps and mucosal irritation (Milles, 1965). Shrinkage of the bladder may be prevented by allowing partial filling and intermittent emptying, using a catheter valve and/or the conformable catheter (Roe, 1990).

Encrustation, Stones and Debris

Infection and secretions mean that most patients with a long-term catheter have some debris in their urine. This is a particular problem in immobile people, as debris accumulates and can eventually block the drainage eyes. Hence, patients are encouraged to be as mobile as possible. If the patient cannot move, regular passive changes of position are recommended.

All indwelling catheters become encrusted to some extent. The use of silicone or hydrogel-coated catheters may lessen this, but does not prevent encrustation. It can affect the lumen and eyes of the catheter by blocking them, and may make the balloon difficult to deflate. Some bacteria, notably proteus, produce the urea-splitting enzyme urease. When urease splits urea, it releases ammonia and free hydrogen ions. This process encourages the precipitation of salts from urine, classically the three phosphates of ammonium, calcium and magnesium, and causes encrustation of the catheter with resultant blockage. Some patients whose catheters encrust are prone to the development of bladder and kidney stones. In immobile patients, re-uptake of calcium from the bones may make more calcium available in the urine for stone formation.

Some patients seem more prone to debris, stones or encrustation than others. A few are inveterate catheter-blockers and for these people it is worth increasing their fluid intake, if tolerated. For habitual blockers, prophylactic washouts or instillations may prevent blockage (Brocklehurst and Brocklehurst, 1978). A variety of pre-packed sterile solutions are available, such as saline or weak citric acid, to acidify the urine (Kennedy, 1984; Roe, 1989b). To date, no research has been undertaken to ascertain the frequency with which intermittent bladder washouts should be given. Therefore, the frequency which suits the individual and maintains the patency of the catheter is the one recommended.

Some schools of thought question the use of bladder washouts due to the detrimental effects on the bladder urothelium (Elliot et al., 1989). Regular washouts have been shown to increase shedding of urothelial cells, with no significant reduction in crystal formation or encrustation (Kennedy et al., 1992). More research is required to establish the benefits or contraindications of bladder instillations. Often the patient or a relative can be taught to carry out intermittent bladder washouts. A further common clinical recommendation is for the patient to take large oral doses of vitamin C (as a tablet or in juice such as cranberry juice), in order to acidify the urine. This claim remains largely untested.

If a patient repeatedly blocks a catheter, there is no point carrying out excessive bladder instillations and the catheter should be changed more frequently. Alternatively, another form of management may have to be considered.

No Drainage

If a catheter has failed to drain any urine, or only minimal amounts, over a period of several hours, the cause should be investigated. Normally urine arrives in the bladder continuously, so it should drain continuously. Sometimes the explanation is that the drainage tube has inadvertently kinked. The bag may be overfull and will not admit further urine. A rectal examination may reveal that faecal impaction is interfering with catheter drainage.

The catheter may be blocked. It can be gently rolled between two fingers and encrustations may be felt. A bladder washout may unblock the lumen or eyes. Fifty millilitres of sterile water can be instilled and allowed to drain back. If nothing returns, further increments of 50ml can be added, up to a maximum of 200ml, unless of course the patient is already experiencing discomfort or an overdistended bladder. The water should not be removed by the suction of a syringe, because the walls of the catheter can collapse and occlude the lumen completely and the bladder mucosa may be sucked into the drainage eye. If a washout fails to unblock the catheter it should be removed and replaced. The removed catheter should be inspected for the site and type of blockage. If the second catheter fails to drain, the patient may be genuinely anuric. Provided that he is not dehydrated this is a sign of renal failure, and urgent medical attention must be obtained.

Sexual Activity

Sexual intercourse is possible for both men and women with a urethral catheter in situ. Men are usually advised to tape the catheter back along the shaft of the penis and wear a condom to keep it in place; women may tape the catheter to the inner aspect of the thigh to minimise movement. However, it is not a practice to be generally recommended, as the catheter may cause discomfort for both partners. Trauma to the urethra is inevitable, and repeated intercourse with a catheter in situ may cause eventual stricture formation. Intercourse will often also not be the pleasurable activity it should be. Urethral catheters are probably best avoided for a sexually active person, never forgetting that this includes older as well as the younger folk, and alternatives such as a suprapubic catheter should be considered.

If a urethral catheter is the management of choice, it may be feasible to teach the patient or partner to remove the catheter prior to intercourse and insert a new one afterwards. Women with a urethral catheter may find a lateral position or penetration from behind more comfortable for intercourse.

Since sexual activity is a difficult topic for many people to discuss, it will usually be up to the nurse to introduce it and encourage the discussion of problems. Roe and Brocklehurst (1987) have found that nurses do not volunteer information or advice on sexual matters to catheterised people.

CATHETER CHANGES

The interval between catheter changes should be determined by the individual patient's needs. Some people experience repeatedly blocked catheters and are best with a more frequent change to preempt problems. Others may be safely left for up to three months with no problems. A planned recatheterisation interval that avoids the occurrence of catheter problems, such as blockage and leakage, and which suits the individual client should be established and documented. It is a good idea to keep a supply of catheters and a catheter change kit in the patient's home, so that they are available when required. If possible, the patient or a carer should be taught how to catheterise themselves, so that they can be independent and less restricted by waiting for health service personnel.

Catheter Removal

To remove a Foley catheter, the water is drawn out of the balloon with a syringe via the inflation valve. The catheter can then be slowly pulled out. If encrustations are present, these can be very rough, and so care should be taken to be as gentle as possible.

The widespread practice of intermittent catheter clamping and release prior to catheter withdrawal, often called 'bladder training' and said to restore 'bladder tone', has no proven value for people who have had a long-term catheter. However there is some evidence to support its application in patients catheterised short-term (for less than six days, Roe, 1990). In most cases the bladder soon resumes normal filling and emptying, once the catheter is out, provided that fluid intake is adequate and the patient is allowed enough time, privacy and comfort in which to void. He should be warned that micturition may be uncomfortable at first and reassured that this is temporary.

If voiding has not been achieved within six hours of catheter removal, or if the bladder becomes distended or painful, an intermittent catheter will remove the residual urine and allow a further chance for normal function to return. When a catheter has been removed in the home, the nurse must always check later that day, and again the next day, to see that the patient has resumed normal voiding.

The Non-Deflating Balloon
Occasionally a catheter balloon will not deflate with a syringe. It is very important when inflating a balloon to use only sterile water and to be sure that no contaminants come into contact with the water, e.g. powder from sterile gloves. The inflation lumen is extremely narrow and easily blocked. If saline or other solutions are used, the solutes may precipitate out to block the lumen.

If the balloon will not deflate, it is not a good idea to attempt to burst it with extra water (it takes up to 100ml to burst a 10ml balloon, and up to 200ml to burst a 30ml one), as the trauma can damage the bladder mucosa and there is a high risk of leaving small particles of balloon in the bladder. These particles will almost always form the nucleus for stone formation. Nor should the balloon be dissolved, for example with ether. Chemicals can cause an acute chemical cystitis and there is again a risk of some particles of balloon remaining inside the bladder.

The fault may be in the valve or the inflation arm. If the water does not come out immediately, it should be left for up to twenty-four hours and attempts to deflate it repeated. If the balloon still will not deflate, the inflation channel must be blocked higher up. Unless the nurse is very experienced with this problem, this is the time for urological referral. The urologist might burst the balloon using a long stilette via the inflation lumen. Alternatively, the balloon can be punctured under local anaesthetic via the perineum in men, or the vagina in women, or with X-ray control via the abdominal route. With all these methods the catheter and balloon must be examined very carefully, and if there is any suspicion that they are incomplete, the particles must be removed at cystoscopy.

All cases of faulty catheters should be reported for investigation to the manufacturer and to the Department of Health, Medical Devices Agency (see Appendix 2).

CONCLUSIONS

The decision to catheterise must never be taken lightly and should always be made with both the benefits and risks in mind. One of the most important factors in the successful use of a catheter is good communication between all involved. Written records should always be kept of catheter size, type, changes, and problems. As with any other aspect of nursing care, planned management rather than ad hoc intervention will benefit the patient.

The more the patient is involved in the care of his catheter the better. If he handles it confidently and without fear, his independence will be greatly enhanced.

The catheter must always be there for a reason. Too often professional attention is focused on sorting out catheter problems rather than questioning, 'Why is it necessary?' If it causes more problems than it solves, take it out! There is still much to be learned about ideal catheter management. Much more research is needed before optimum management is available to all.

SUPRAPUBIC CATHETERS

A suprapubic catheter is a catheter inserted directly into the bladder via the anterior abdominal wall. It is always inserted by a medical practitioner in the first instance, either under general or local anaesthetic.

Indications
The suprapubic catheter is especially useful after pelvic or urological surgery, where the patient might have difficulty in resuming voiding. The catheter can be clamped for a trial of voiding. If unsuccessful, the catheter can merely be unclamped again, so avoiding repeated urethral catheterisations (Hilton and Stanton, 1980). The suprapubic catheter is likewise useful in acute retention, as voiding can be attempted without catheter removal.

A suprapubic catheter can be used for long-term drainage, especially in sexually active patients and those experiencing problems with urethral catheters. In some women the urethra may be closed surgically (Feneley, 1983).

The Catheters

There are several makes of suprapubic catheter. Sizes range from 6 f.g. to 16 f.g. Some are secured to the abdominal wall by a stitch or medical adhesive; others have a balloon for retaining the catheter (Figure 9.10). Foley catheters may also be inserted suprapubically and retained by inflating the balloon in the usual way.

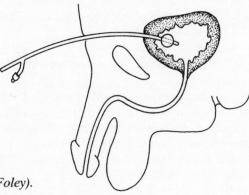

Figure 9.10
Suprapubic catheter (Foley).

Management

Suprapubic catheters are associated with lower infection rates than urethral catheters. This may be because the urethral defence mechanisms are left intact and the entry site is relatively easy to keep clean. The entry site should be inspected daily, and gently cleaned with mild soap and water. Some clinicians keep the entry site covered with a sterile dressing and some prefer to leave it uncovered. To date, no research has been undertaken to establish which practice should be adopted. Otherwise, management is the same as for urethral catheters: the same bags may be used and the same instructions given to patients. If the skin around the puncture site becomes infected, systemic antibiotics may be necessary.

Once the channel is established, the catheter can usually be easily changed by medical or nursing staff via the original channel, without further anaesthetic. When the suprapubic catheter is no longer needed, it can simply be removed. The opening in the abdominal and bladder wall normally closes spontaneously without complication.

REFERENCES AND FURTHER READING

Association for Continence Advice, 1991. *Recent Advances in Catheter Care* (proceedings of a study day). ACA, London.

Bielski, M., 1980. Preventing infection in the catheterised patient. *Nursing Clinics of North America*, 15, 4: 703–13.

Blandy, J. P., 1981. How to catheterise the bladder. *British Journal of Hospital Medicine*, 26: 58–60.

Blacklock, N.J., 1986. Catheters and urethral strictures. *British Journal of Urology*, 58: 475–8.

Brocklehurst, J. C., Brocklehurst, S., 1978. The management of indwelling catheters. *British Journal of Urology*, 50: 102–5.

Brocklehurst, J. C., Hickey, D. S., Davies, I., Kennedy A. P., Morris J. A., 1988. A new urethral catheter. *British Medical Journal*, 296: 1691–3.

Crow, R., Chapman, R., Roe, B., Wilson J., 1986. *Study of Patients with Indwelling Urethral Catheters and Related Nursing Practice*. Nursing Practice Research Unit, University of Surrey.

Crow, R., Mulhall, A., Chapman, R., 1988. Indwelling catheterisation and related nursing practice. *Journal of Advanced Nursing*, 13: 489–95.

Cule, J., 1980. Forerunners of Foley. *Nursing Mirror*, 150, 5: i-vi.

Department of Health. 1991. *Drug Tariff*. Department of Health, London.

Elliot, T. S. J., Gopal Rao, G., Rigby, R. C., Woodhouse, K. 1989. Bladder irrigation or irritation? *British Journal of Urology*, 64, 4: 391–4.

Feneley, R. C. L., 1983. The management of female incontinence by suprapubic catheterisation, with or without urethral closure. *British Journal of Urology*, 55: 203–7.

Ferrie, B. G., Glen, E. S., Hunter, B., 1979. Long-term catheter drainage. *British Medical Journal*, 2: 1046–7.

Flynn, J. T., Blandy, J. P., 1980. Urethral catheterisation. *British Medical Journal*, 281: 928–30.

Garibaldi, R. A., Burke, J. P., Dickman, M. L., Smith, C.B., 1974. Factors predisposing to bacteriuria during indwelling urethral catheterisation. *New England Journal of Medicine*, 291, 5: 215–19.

Glenister, H., 1987. The passage of infection. *Nursing Times*, 3, 22: 68–73.

Hashisaki, P., Swenson, J., Mooney, B., Epstein, B., Bowcutt, C., 1984. Decontamination of urinary bags for rehabilitation patients. *Archives of Physical Medicine and Rehabilitation*, 65: 474–6.

Henry, M., 1992. Catheter confusion. *Nursing Times*, 88, 42: 65–72.

Hilton, P., Stanton, S. L., 1980. Suprapubic catheterisation. *British Medical Journal*, 281: 1261–3.

Kennedy, A. P., Brocklehurst, J. C., Robinson, J. M., Faragher, E. B., 1992. Assessment of the use of bladder washouts/instillations in patients with long-term indwelling catheters. *British Journal of Urology*, 70: 610–15.

Kennedy A. P. 1984. A trial of a new bladder washout system. *Nursing Times*, 80, 46: 48–51.

Kennedy, A. P., Brocklehurst, J. C., 1982. The nursing management of patients with long-term indwelling catheters. *Journal of Advanced Nursing*, 7: 411–17.

Kennedy, A. P., Brocklehurst, J. C., Lye, M. D. W., 1983a. Factors related to the problems of long-term catheterisation. *Journal of Advanced Nursing*, 8: 207–12.

Kennedy, A. P., Brocklehurst, J. C., Faragher E. B., 1983b. A comparison of 10 urinary drainage bags. *Nursing Times*, Aug 17: 56–60.

Kohler-Ockmore, J., 1992. Urinary drainage leg bags. *Community Outlook*, Nov: 29–33.

Kritiansen, P., Pompeius, R., Wadstrom, L.B., 1983. Long-term urethral catheter drainage and bladder capacity. *Neurology and Urodynamics*, 2: 135–43.

Milles, G. 1965. Catheter-induced haemorrhagic pseudopolyps of the urinary bladder. *Journal of the American Medical Association*, 193, 13 Sept: 968–9.

Mulhall, A., 1992a. Catheter tips. *Nursing Times*, 88, 13: 80–2.

Mulhall, A., 1992b. The bladder model: clinical implications. *Nursing Standard* 7, 5: 25–7.

Mulhall, A., 1991. Biofilms and urethral catheter infections. *Nursing Standard*, 5, 18: 26–8.

Platt, R., Polk, B. F., Murdock, B., Rosner, B., 1982. Mortality associated with nosocomial urinary tract infection. *New England Journal of Medicine*, 307, 11: 637–42.

Pritchard, A. P., David, J. A., 1988. *The Royal Marsden Manual of Clinical Nursing Procedures*, 2nd edn. Harper and Row, London.

Pullen, B. R., Phillips, J., Hickey, D. S., 1982. Urethral lumen cross-sectional shape, radiological determination and relationship to function. *British Journal of Urology*: 399–407.

Ramsay, J. W. A., Garnham A. J., Mulhall, A. B., Crow, R. A., Bryan, J. M., Eardley, I., Vale, J. A., Whitfield, H. N., 1989. Biofilms, bacteria and bladder catheters. *British Journal of Urology*, 64: 395–8.

Roe, B. H., 1989a. Catheters in the community. *Nursing Times*, 85, 36: 43–4.

Roe, B. H., 1989b. Use of bladder washouts: a study of nurses' recommendations. *Journal of Advanced Nursing*, 14: 494–500.

Roe, B. H., 1990. Do we need to clamp catheters? *Nursing Times*, 86, 43: 66–7.

Roe, B. H., 1992. Use of indwelling catheters. In: Roe, B. H., (ed) *Clinical Nursing Practice*. Prentice Hall, Hemel Hempstead.

Roe, B. H., 1993. Catheter-associated urinary tract infections: a review. *Journal of Clinical Nursing*, 2, 4: 197–204.

Roe, B. H., Brocklehurst, J. C., 1987. Study of patients with indwelling catheters. *Journal of Advanced Nursing*, 12: 713–18.

Roe, B. H., Reid, F. J., Brocklehurst, J. C., 1988. Comparison of four urine drainage systems. *Journal of Advanced Nursing*, 13: 374–82.

Rogers, J., 1991. Pass the cranberry juice. *Nursing Times*, 87, 48: 36–7.

Ryan Wooley, B., 1987. Aids for the management of incontinence. King's Fund, London.

Stickler, D. J., 1991. The role of antiseptics in the management of patients undergoing short-term indwelling bladder catheterisation. *Journal of Hospital Infection*, 16: 89–108.

Thornton, G. F., Andriole, V. T., 1970. Bacteriuria during indwelling catheter drainage: Effect of a closed sterile drainage system. *Journal of the American Medical Association*, 214: 339–42.

Warren, J. W., Muncie, H. L. J., Bergquist, E. J., Hoopes, J. M., 1981. Sequelae and management of urinary infection in the patient requiring chronic catheterisation. *Journal of Urology*, 125: 1–8.

Wilson, J., Roe, B., 1986. Nursing management of patients with an indwelling urethral catheter. In: Tierney, A. J., (ed), *Clinical Nursing Practice*. Churchill Livingstone, Edinburgh and London.

Chapter 10

Faecal Incontinence

Lesley Irvine, RGN, HEd Cert
Continence Adviser, Swansea NHS Trust

Incontinence of faeces is the most embarrassing, socially unacceptable and demoralising of symptoms. Whether in the home or in hospital, coping with chronic faecal incontinence is an almost unbearable burden, distasteful for both the sufferers and carers, and is frequently associated with social stigma.

As with urinary incontinence, faecal incontinence is a symptom and must have a cause. Since accurate diagnosis of the underlying problem leads to a substantial cure-rate, persistent uncontrolled faecal incontinence should with good management be rare. In practice this is not always the case, and chronic faecal incontinence may be thought of as the poor relation of chronic urinary incontinence. Nurses are in a key position to change society's attitude to this demoralising problem. Chronic faecal incontinence is significantly less prevalent than chronic urinary incontinence, although the two may coexist.

About one adult in two hundred living in the community suffers regular faecal incontinence. Table 1.3 (page 7) gives a detailed breakdown of the best overall figures yet available (Thomas et al., 1984). More recent studies have suggested an even higher prevalence. Talley et al. (1982) found that 7% of people over 65 years living at home had weekly faecal incontinence or wore pads. It tends to be a significantly under-reported symptom which many elderly or disabled people, and those with ano-rectal and colonic disorders, accept and disguise because of shame and embarrassment without seeking medical help (Leigh and Turnberg, 1982). The vast majority of people with faecal incontinence receive no professional help (Table 1.4). In addition, the public and nursing perception is that little can be done to help.

By far the highest prevalence of faecal incontinence occurs in elderly people in long-stay institutional care. The commonest cause in the elderly is constipation, with faecal impaction and spurious diarrhoea – often the result of decreased mobility and inadequate fibre and fluid intake. Many surveys of patients in hospital wards for elderly people have reported faecal incontinence in up to half of all patients, and certainly a prevalence of 10%–20% is common. Amongst the elderly mentally infirm in hospital, over two-thirds may be faecally incontinent (Rands and Malone-Lee, 1990). On general hospital wards, 2%–3% of patients are likely to be incontinent of faeces (Egan et al., 1983). This may be acute short-term, or long-term chronic incontinence. The high rate in hospitals adds enormously to the burden of nursing or caring for long-stay patients, as well as to the unpleasantness associated with the job.

In the majority of cases it is a reversible or avoidable situation. It is important for health service managers to know what proportion of their health service funds are spent on managing chronic incontinence. If incontinence was dealt with more efficiently, the resources freed up could be channelled to other priority areas.

PHYSIOLOGY OF NORMAL BOWEL FUNCTION

The main functions of the colon include dehydration and storage of waste products from the ileum to form faeces. Folds in the mucous membrane result in a greater surface area for the removal of water, electrolytes and some metabolites. Mucous secretion adds potassium to the waste matter and patients with chronic diarrhoea may become significantly potassium depleted; this is of particular importance in the elderly, who are especially vulnerable to potassium depletion. The more the colon contracts, the greater the absorption of fluids. Thus reduced colonic contractility is associated with looseness of bowel action and increased contact contractility with constipation. About 600ml of fluid are received per day by the colon from the small intestine and this is eventually reduced to 150–200ml of faecal matter.

Movement of waste matter along the colon is controlled by the intrinsic nerve plexus in the bowel wall. This may be stimulated by physical and neurological activity, by emotion or mental stress, or by eating, all of which cause the release of complex gut hormones. Both eating and the sight or smell of appetising food cause the caecum to empty into the colon, the 'gastro-colic response', mediated hormonally. This often stimulates a 'mass movement' of faeces through the colon, provoking defaecation reflexes. The mass movement is coordinated by local reflexes. Sleep greatly reduces colonic activity.

Normal habit varies greatly between individuals from as frequently as two motions per day to once every 2–3 days (Connell et al., 1965). However, it should be remembered that what has become 'normal' on a highly refined Western diet is often far from optimal, as the high incidence of bowel disorders in the West testifies. Normally one good-volume, formed, but soft and easily passed stool per day, without excessive urgency, flatus, or abdominal discomfort, is probably the best objective for most people to aim at. Variations of this frequency of bowel action are seldom cause for concern unless the criteria above also fail to be met.

THE NORMAL MECHANISM OF FAECAL CONTINENCE

To understand faecal incontinence it is necessary to understand the mechanisms that enable one to be continent. We maintain faecal continence by the delicate coordination and balance of the neurological and muscular activity of the colon, rectum and anus.

This is dependent on several factors (Irving and Catchpole, 1992):

1) An effective barrier to outflow provided by the internal and external anal sphincters.
2) A capacious, passively distensible and evacuable reservoir, i.e. the normal rectum.
3) Intact anal sensation.
4) Bulky and firm (but not hard) faeces.

When faeces enter the rectum there is an immediate sensation of rectal fullness and impending defaecation. The sensory nerve endings responsible for this are probably located in the muscle around the rectum rather than in the rectal wall itself. When the rectum is distended by about 150ml of faeces, the internal anal sphincter, which is a smooth-muscle (autonomic) sphincter, relaxes completely, allowing faeces to pass into the anal canal. The external sphincter however, which is striated muscle, is under both autonomic and voluntary control (Figure 10.1). If defaecation is not convenient, the external sphincter is contracted, leading to the full defaecation reflex being inhibited from continuing to completion. The external sphincter maintains a continuous tonic contraction, even at rest, and this can be greatly augmented for short periods by voluntary contraction. If the defaecation reflex is voluntarily inhibited, the stool will be returned to the rectum until a more convenient time for voiding. The anal canal is lined with very sensitive epithelium, which can distinguish accurately

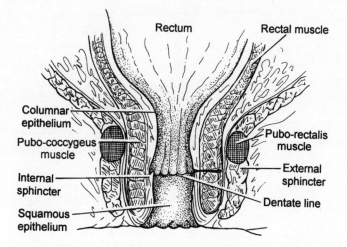

Figure 10.1 *Coronal section through pelvic floor.*

between gas, fluid and solid matter entering the anal canal, even during sleep. This is important, as flatus can be passed without faecal incontinence occurring, and even fluid diarrhoea can be retained by most people for a short time.

If the defaecation reflex is not inhibited, i.e. if it is convenient to defaecate, the external sphincter will relax completely and, with minimal abdominal effort, rectal contractions will expel the stool, aided by gravity.

The muscular supports of the pelvic floor, especially the pubo-rectalis muscle, help to maintain a double right-angle between the anus and the rectum which acts as a flap valve (Figure 10.2, overleaf). This is thought to aid continence during physical activity. If abdominal pressure is raised, the pressure merely closes the valve more effectively. The importance of the part played by the acute ano-rectal angle acting as a closure valve has been questioned by recent research (Orrom et al., 1991). It may help in preventing stress incontinence of faeces, but is probably secondary to the integrity of the sphincter muscle and pelvic floor muscle strength. There is a reflex contraction of the pelvic floor in immediate response to effort.

Normally the anus seems to have a cyclic (15 per minute) pattern of contraction, which may assist continence and anal cleanliness by retrograde propulsion of faecal matter before the need to

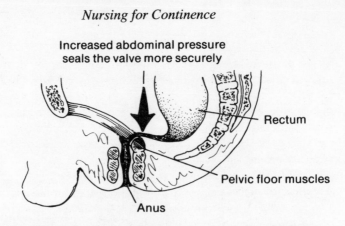

Figure 10.2 *Anatomical arrangement at ano-rectal junction. The arrangement at the ano-rectal junction results in the formation of a flap valve. The anterior wall of the lower rectum impinges upon the closed anal canal, and any increase in abdominal pressure appears to seal the valve more securely.*

defaecate. The soft vascular submucosal tissue above the dentate line (Figure 10.1) also aids the occlusion of the canal (Irving and Catchpole, 1992). It is chronic enlargement of the venous plexuses in this tissue, usually due to chronic repetitive straining to defaecate, that produces the troublesome problem of internal haemorrhoids (piles).

FAECAL INCONTINENCE

Incontinence of faeces is the involuntary passage of faeces and/or flatus, at an inappropriate time and in an inappropriate place.

Minor Incontinence
Occasional soiling of underwear, incontinence of flatus, or both can be the result of anal disorders such as skin tags, or prolapsing haemorrhoids. Poor local hygiene can result (Henry, 1988).

Deficiency of the internal anal sphincter and rectal prolapse can lead to incontinence of flatus and increasing risk during episodes of diarrhoea.

Usually minor problems are dealt with by treatment and reassurance by the GP, coupled with haemorroidectomy and excision of skin tags by minor surgery. Manual stretching of the dentate line as a treatment for internal haemorrhoids may lead to chronic minor faecal soiling.

Major Incontinence

This is the involuntary passage of solid faeces, or of diarrhoea. It causes great distress, anxiety, loss of self respect and social isolation. It may be caused by trauma to the pelvic floor, the sphincter or the anal canal, e.g. as a result of childbirth. Neurological disorders such as stroke, multiple sclerosis and dementia, where faecal impaction and/or loss of cortical control may be the cause, can lead to involuntary passage of faeces.

Broadly, the causes of faecal incontinence can be divided into three categories: those indicating underlying intrinsic disorders of the colon, rectum, anal canal and anus; disorders of the autonomic and voluntary nervous system; and those resulting from faecal impaction.

ASSESSMENT OF FAECAL INCONTINENCE

Nursing assessment, which is very dependent on the experience and motivation of the nurse, should include a careful history of the problem, with consideration of the patient's likely reluctance to discuss it due to embarrassment, in as much privacy as possible. Diet, mobility, fluid intake, the environment and reactions to it should all be closely observed and their relevance determined. Table 10.1 (overleaf) shows an assessment of defaecation/faecal incontinence checklist which the nurse might find helpful. The nurse must ask key questions to ascertain which particular syndrome is being dealt with, to determine the type and cause of a faecal incontinence, and to enable realistic planning of treatment. For example, is the condition related to ulcerative colitis and diarrhoea, or to constipation, or is it incontinence secondary to childbirth?

Whatever further investigations may be indicated, the history plays a key role in diagnosis and determining treatment. Ideally, assessment should be a dual medical and nursing one. A high input of clinical awareness and motivation of both disciplines is necessary to help treat the problem.

Table 10.2 (page 234) lists investigations that might be undertaken to confirm the diagnosis as to the cause of faecal incontinence. Investigations and examinations range from digital examination, proctoscopy, rigid and flexible sigmoidoscopy to endo-anal ultrasound and electromyography (EMG). The latter two are becoming increasingly useful tools in investigations of the rectum and anus. Barium enema studies are useful if malignancy or diverticular disease are suspected.

Table 10.1   Assessment of Defaecation/Faecal Incontinence Checklist

---

NAME: ASSESSMENT DATE:

Problem as perceived by patient/carer:

Has patient a known systemic disorder – if so, state:

Past usual frequency of bowel action: Range:

Present usual frequency of bowel action:

Usual time of day:

Any associated habits/events:

Does patient complain of constipation?

If so, what is understood by this?

Does patient get sensation of the need to defaecate/pass urine?

Can patient control this sensation?

Average time taken for bowel action:

Does patient have to strain?

Is defaecation associated with pain? If so, where and duration:

Any bleeding?   Fresh or altered blood: Mixed or separate:

Mucus:

Problematic flatus: Continent of flatus:

Scybala: Ribbon stools:

Usual consistency of faeces: Do faeces float?
                                       Do faeces flush?

Usual amount of faeces:

Does patient experience urgency?   How much warning time?

Diet: Any food taken for bowels?
       Any food avoided for bowels?
       Average daily fluid intake: Type:

Laxative use: Present:
              Past history of use:

What other drugs taken?

History of perianal problems: (particularly obstetric)

Faecal incontinence?

If yes: Nature of soiling:
          Sensation of incontinence:
          Frequency of incontinence:

Obvious evidence of faecal soiling:

Incontinent of flatus:

Table 10.1   (continued)

Result of rectal examination:
Any recent change in bowel habits?
Urinary urgency/urge or stress urinary incontinence?
Toilet facilities:
> Problems with using lavatory:
> If bedpan/commode used, reaction to this:
> Aids needed?

Ability to cleanse after defaecation:
Mobility impaired?
Attitude   – Patient
> – Carers

Are any bowel problems anticipated with current illness/condition?
Can the patient always obey defaecation urge when it occurs?
If not, why not?

Assessment summary:

Planned action:

Review date:

Table 10.2   Investigations for Constipation/Faecal Incontinence

History and clinical examination

Digital anal examination – function of sphincter muscles
                           – impacted faeces in rectum
                           – abnormalities

Proctoscopy   – to examine rectum

Plain X-ray   – impaction in large bowel

Endoscopic examination of rectosigmoid and anal canal – for any abnormalities, inflammatory or neoplastic changes

Endo-anal ultrasound   – integrity of anal sphincter

MRI scan   – integrity of anal sphincter

Defaecating proctogram – perianal descent
                           – ano-rectal angle
                           – rectal prolapse
                           – rectocele
                           – adequacy of rectal emptying

Ano-rectal manometry   – function of sphincteric muscles
                           – measures pressure within anal canal, resting & squeezing, and perception thresholds for distending stimuli
                           – air distension – pressure should fall with volume rise (ano-rectal inhibition reflex)

(2/3 of patients with idiopathic faecal incontinence have reduced anal resting pressure)

Balloon expulsion studies– determine efficiency of faecal expulsion.

Electromyography   – registers muscular activity at rest, during voluntary contraction and during straining. 'Anal mapping' of response in different part of anal canal

Pudendal nerve latency   – efficiency of pudendal nerve responses

Saline infusion test   – for continence to liquids

Colonic transit studies   – records time taken for faecal matter to pass through the colon. Radio-opaque markers – normally 80% are passed by day 5.

Whilst ano-rectal manometry remains a useful tool, the key diagnostic weapon nowadays is endo-anal ultrasound. This involves insertion of a small probe into the lower bowel and evaluating directly on the X-ray screen the integrity of function of, particularly, the anal sphincter (Law et al., 1991; Kamm, 1995). MRI scanning can also be used to evaluate the sphincter.

UNDERLYING INTRINSIC DISORDERS OF THE BOWEL

These will be principally in the large bowel, but may have their aetiology in the small bowel.

Diarrhoea

Severe diarrhoea, particularly if fulminant (i.e. developing suddenly or explosively) increases the likelihood of the person becoming faecally incontinent. Table 10.3 lists the more common disorders which can cause diarrhoea and faecal incontinence. The cause must be determined by investigation. Faecal incontinence tends to be a common, but seldom reported and seldom asked about, accompaniment to many of these disorders (Leigh and Turnberg, 1982). In addition, any fluid and electrolyte loss will need correcting as part of the management regimen.

Those with impaired mobility, diminished sensation or awareness, or an already impaired sphincter mechanism are more likely to experience incontinence as a result of diarrhoea than otherwise healthy individuals. Lower-bowel carcinoma is the commonest malignancy of old age, but any recent persistent change in bowel habit should be investigated in all age groups. Treatment for incontinence from these causes will obviously involve treating or controlling the underlying disease process.

Table 10.3   Common Causes of Diarrhoea

Ulcerative colitis – blood, mucus and diarrhoea

Crohn's disease/regional ileitis – blood, mucus and diarrhoea

Diverticular disease – diarrhoea or constipation

Villous adenoma of the rectum

Carcinoma of the rectum (may also present as constipation and/or rectal bleeding – dark blood mixed with the faeces)

Infection – acute or chronic (may be associated with disease contracted abroad, e.g. dysentery – bloody diarrhoea)

Irritable bowel syndrome – very variable bowel behaviour

Radiotherapy-induced, causing damage to bowel wall

Drug-induced (e.g. broad-spectrum antibiotics, laxative abuse, iron, which should be discontinued if possible)

Muscle-Ring Deficiency Impairing Anal Function

The muscles of the pelvic floor support the anal sphincter. A rise in abdominal pressure tends to force the rectal contents down and out. Any weakness will cause a tendency to faecal stress incontinence. Figure 10.3 shows that with muscle weakness the flap-valve formed by the ano-rectal angle is lost. Surgical treatment to restore the flap valve seems to result in better anal sphincter muscle function and better anal sensation, despite doubt as to relevance of the ano-rectal angle itself.

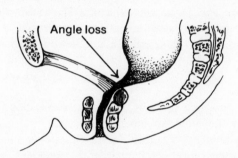

Figure 10.3   *Flap valve lost with muscle weakness. With muscle weakness the flap valve formed by the ano-rectal angle is lost. Surgery to correct this appears to result in better anal sphincter muscle function and improved anal sensation.*

Sphincter damage may be the result of congenital abnormalities, e.g. spina bifida or of later trauma, e.g. obstetric, epidural, or after anal surgery. Sultan et al. (1993 a & b) have found that 10% of women develop new bowel symptoms following their first vaginal delivery, and one-third sustain structural damage to one or both sphincters. Forceps delivery is associated with an 80% incidence of structural sphincter damage. A lifetime's habit of straining at stool may also be implicated in pelvic floor muscle weakness, which, if mild, may respond to pelvic floor exercises. These should be taught very much as exercises for urinary stress incontinence (see Chapter 6), but concentrating on the posterior rather than anterior portion of the pelvic floor.

Rectal tone should be assessed on digital examination using the index finger. The patient is instructed to squeeze, which brings into use the perineal muscles. Treatment is by encouraging regular contractions of the posterior portion of the pelvic floor, graded to the individual's abilities, which should then be practised up to ten times daily for at least three months, with an increasing number and length of contractions as muscle strength increases. The patient must also be advised firmly to desist from all straining during defaecation.

The physiotherapist may use electrotherapy to assist or augment pelvic floor exercise. All the same methods apply as for urinary stress incontinence (see Chapter 6). Weighted cones have also been reported for use rectally (Fox et al., 1991).

As a guideline for the need for surgery, most people with muscle weakness severe enough to cause incontinence of solid stool require surgical repair to restore continence. Table 10.4 lists the operations most used for faecal incontinence.

Table 10.4   Surgical Procedures

Idiopathic Faecal Incontinence – for poorly functioning anal sphincter, canal and pelvic floor

Post-anal repair

Sphincteroplasty (anterior sphincter plication and levatorplasty)

Total pelvic floor repair

Gracilis muscle transposition + implanted electrical stimulator (not fully evaluated to date) – for loss of substantial part of external sphincter in patients with motor denervation (Baeten et al., 1991)

Continent Stoma   –the appendix is re-implanted into the caecum in a non-refluxing manner, with the other end brought onto the abdomen as a channel which can be catheterised. Antegrade washouts produce colonic emptying (Malone et al., 1990).

Rectal Prolapse

Abdominal rectopexy –with colonic resection if slow colonic transit time
                    –often followed by residual problem of constipation and incomplete evacuation

Perineal rectopexy/puborectoplasty

Delormes operation   –sometimes poor results for continence.

Constipation

Total or sub-total colectomy with ileorectal anastamosis
    for slow transit constipation

Colectomy with pelvic floor retraining
    for slow transit constipation and pelvic floor dysfunction

Colostomy for intractable constipation/faecal incontinence

There is evidence that chronic straining at defaecation, or a prolonged second stage of labour, may not only cause direct muscle damage but may also damage the nerve supply of the pelvic floor by prolonged stretching of the nerve fibres (Parks, 1980; Snooks et al., 1984), although more recent work has cast some doubt on this as the major mechanism of obstetric damage (Kamm, 1994). This may be exacerbated if the normal mechanism of limiting pushing in the second stage is blocked by epidural anaesthesia. If the straining has also induced rectal prolapse, which may also occur in children with cystic fibrosis, this should be corrected first. Some, but not all, cases of rectal prolapse with faecal incontinence may in addition require a post-anal repair, strengthening the weakened or damaged anal sphincter.

Fistula

A fistula is an abnormal passage connecting the cavity of one organ with another or with the surface of the body. A recto-vaginal fistula is usually caused by obstetric trauma and is mostly seen in developing countries. It may occasionally arise from bowel disease (e.g. Crohn's disease) or following pelvic radiotherapy for bowel, bladder or reproductive organ neoplasms. Excision and surgical repair of the fistula is needed.

NEUROGENIC DISORDERS

The medulla and higher cortical centres of the brain have a role in coordinating and controlling the defaecation reflex. It is therefore likely that any neurological disorder which impairs the ability to appreciate or inhibit impending defaecation will result in a tendency to incontinence, similar in causation to the uninhibited or unstable bladder. For example, the paraplegic person, either with a traumatic lesion, acute or chronic myelitis, or secondary to carcinoma (often prostatic), may lose all direct sensation of and voluntary control over bowel activity. Neurological disorders such as multiple sclerosis, diabetic neuropathy, cerebrovascular disease and dementia may affect sensation, or inhibition, or a combination of both. Incontinence occurring in the demented person will sometimes be because of physical inability to inhibit defaecation. With others it is because the awareness that behaviour is inappropriate has been lost.

The Paraplegic or Tetraplegic Patient

Often the patient receives only indirect indications of when the rectum is full and defaecation imminent. Various autonomic indicators, such as tachycardia, sweating or flushing, are often present and it is important for each individual, and where appropriate carers, to learn to become sensitive to his or her own internal indicators if continence is to be achieved. If the lesion is above the cauda equina it is usually possible to stimulate a defaecation reflex voluntarily, once the period of spinal shock is past. This is only useful if the rectum is full, so each person must learn to diagnose a full rectum correctly and then act upon it before an involuntary reflex causes incontinence. For many, the reflex can be initiated by dilating the anus, either with a finger or an anal dilator. Some people with paraplegia experience the same autonomic indications when the bladder is full.

Cauda Equina Lesions

Where the defaecation reflex is disturbed because of damage to sacral S_2–S_3 nerve roots, defaecation is often extremely difficult to manage, and total uncontrollable incontinence is common. The sphincters, devoid of nerve supply, are usually lax and patulous (gaping open), and allow faeces entering the rectum to pass straight out. Until recently it has been thought that if a person with neurogenic faecal incontinence fails to achieve adequate voluntary control, the problem is best managed by artificially inducing constipation, and then planning controlled bowel evacuations. Now it is recommended that keeping the bowel empty may be more beneficial, and attention to adequate dietary fibre, fluids, mobility and a regime of laxative medication to promote regular emptying of the bowel should lead to a more normal lifestyle, and prevent the toxic effects of 'planned' constipation – chronic malaise or confusion.

CONSTIPATION

Severe constipation with impaction of faeces is the most common cause of faecal incontinence, and it certainly predominates as a cause among older people and those living in institutional care. Chronic constipation leads to impaction when the fluid content of the faeces is progressively absorbed by the colon, leaving hard, rounded rocks, or scybala, in the bowel. This hard matter promotes mucus production and bacterial activity, which causes a foul-smelling brown fluid to accumulate. If the rectum is overdistended for any length of time, the internal and external anal sphincters become completely inhibited and relaxed, giving a patulous sphincter which freely allows passing of this material as 'spurious diarrhoea'. The patient's symptom will usually be of a leakage of fluid stool without any awareness or control. Obviously, if the diagnosis of the true cause of this is missed and the patient wrongly treated for diarrhoea with a constipating agent, the condition will be aggravated. Some of the scybala may also be passed from time to time by gravity or pressure from the formation of more faeces above.

Many patients with impaction will have hard faeces in the rectum, and this can easily be detected by a digital rectal examination (which is mandatory in assessment). But for some, the impaction is higher up and cannot be detected by digital examination, which may persuade the examiner that constipation is not the problem. Alternatively, the rectum may be filled with soft putty-like faeces (Barrett, 1993). Continuous faecal soiling in the presence of a loaded rectum suggests faecal impaction, whatever the consistency of the stool.

The Causes of Constipation

Constipation, the underlying cause of faecal impaction with consequent faecal incontinence, has many possible causes (Table 10.5).

'Constipation' means different things to different people, and is a difficult term to define. Many people will claim to be constipated if they do not pass a daily bowel motion. If the motion is of a soft consistency and easy to pass without undue effort or straining, this is not true constipation. 'Constipation' refers to motions which are hard and difficult to pass, usually also at irregular or infrequent time intervals. As well as causing incontinence, impaction can lead to intestinal obstruction, to mental disturbances (including apathy and possibly agitation or confusion), to rectal bleeding, and to urinary retention, with possible overflow incontinence.

Simple Constipation

Simple constipation, i.e. that with no underlying bowel pathology, is often self-induced. It may be caused by lack of regular exercise, or low food or fluid intake (low fluid intake often being caused by fear of urinary incontinence), or by poor diet, especially one low in fibre or residue. In older people this may be for financial or social reasons or because of dental problems, or a painful mouth and gums. Some older people require dietary fibre in a form that does not need chewing, e.g.

Table 10.5   Common Causes of Constipation

CAUSE	EXAMPLES OF CAUSES
Simple constipation	Low-residue diet Dehydration Environmental factors – e.g. toilets – inadequate provision and siting – dirty and smelly, lack of privacy, lack of toilet paper, cold, etc. Attitudes of patients' carers and society in general
Motility disorders	Irritable bowel syndrome Idiopathic megacolon (Hirschsprung's disease) Spina bifida
Psychiatric disorders	Depression Confusion Anorexia nervosa
Local pathology	Anal fissure, Haemorrhoids Diverticular disease Large bowel obstruction
General pathology	Endocrine disorders (e.g. hypothyroidism, diabetes mellitus) Cachexia from carcinomatosis
Iatrogenic	Drug-induced, Immobility Poor nursing management

shredded wheat. Physical activity is an important stimulus to colonic activity, and mass bowel movements are rare in very immobile people. Diminished awareness may lead to ignoring the call to stool.

The environment may be important in causing constipation. Some lavatory pedestals are too high to allow the feet to rest comfortably on the floor, so additional help from the abdominal muscles cannot be employed during defaecation. This may be especially important in older people, whose muscle tone may already be decreased. Lavatories which are cold, uncomfortable or inconveniently situated may encourage the ignoring of rectal sensations, as well as making it more probable that inadequate time will be allowed for a completed bowel action. Privacy is also important for complete defaecation, and where privacy is lacking defaecation may be delayed or only partial. This may be true of a child at school, inhibited by the older children having a secret cigarette in the lavatory, or by no locks on vandalised doors. It may be the person who shares accommodation and fears that others are waiting, or may be conscious of the odour. Or it may be the patient in hospital who can hear the nurse hovering outside the door and waits until next time in the hope of less haste and greater privacy. Many people have the ability to delay defaecation almost indefinitely, and impaction may result.

Motility Disorders

The normal transit time of food through the gastrointestinal tract has been measured by radio-opaque markers, and is between three and seven days from mouth to anus for most people. Disorders such as irritable bowel syndrome or diverticular disease, itself probably caused by the constipating effect of Western low-residue, low-fibre, high-carbohydrate diet, can lead to constipation, sometimes alternating with diarrhoea. Some people have an idiopathic slow transit time due to a megacolon which is dilated and redundant. It is likely that transit time increases with advancing age. Slow transit time – eight to fifteen days is not uncommon – allows increased water absorption and encourages the formation of impaction. In older people this may lead to the 'terminal reservoir syndrome', where a hugely distended lower colon is never completely emptied.

Psychiatric Disorder

Depression, confusion and dementia can predispose an individual to constipation. Conversely, constipation may be the underlying cause of confusion. Anorexia nervosa, self-purgation and some of the psychoses, e.g. schizophrenia, may underlie apparent constipation.

Secondary to Local or General Pathology

A large-bowel carcinoma may present as constipation or rectal bleeding. Haemorrhoids, anal stricture, or any painful ano-rectal disorder will tend to cause inhibition of defaecation and thus constipation. Endocrine disorders, notably hypothyroidism or diabetes mellitus, with neurological complications may be the underlying pathology.

Since haemorrhoids occur very frequently, and since their management may be an intrinsic part of dealing with bowel problems, the regimes in current use for treatment of this avoidable condition are summarised in Table 10.6.

Table 10.6   Treatment for Internal Haemorrhoids

Suppositories ⎱
High-residue diet ⎰ early stages

Injection 5% phenol ⎱ effective when there is minimal prolapse
Infra-red coagulation ⎰ of haemorrhoids

Rubber band ligation ⎱ for moderate-sized prolapsing haemorrhoids
Cryosurgery ⎰

Dilation – for tight overactive internal and sphincter. If sphincter is weak, perineal descent or chronic diarrhoea may be present.

Haemorrhoidectomy by ligation and removal at surgery for large severely prolapsing haemorrhoids.

Iatrogenic

Constipation may be induced. Analgesics, especially opiates, anticholinergics, and anti-parkinsonian drugs are among the many having this effect. It is worth noting that people over 65 years comprise 20% of the population and that they receive 50% of all prescribed drugs (Macphee and Brodie, 1992). Alternatively, constipation may develop because of a period of enforced immobility, for instance post-operatively. It may also be induced by poor nursing management – for instance, requiring a patient to defaecate perched on a bedpan in bed, a most unnatural act, both because of the inappropriate position adopted and the lack of privacy. The straining and effort, not to mention stress, involved in attempting defaecation on a bedpan are often considerably greater than the effort of getting up to use the commode or lavatory. In cardiac patients, and post-operative patients, straining at stool is a known precursor of cardiac arrest and sudden death, often associated with major pulmonary embolism. Young women in particular may have anismus, a failure of the puborectalis muscle and external sphincter to relax on straining, resulting in chronic intractable constipation.

Constipation in Elderly People

An older person may have a combination of many of the above mentioned problems causing constipation. Wilkins (1968) has described a vicious circle of constipation in elderly people (Figure 10.4, overleaf). Factors may combine to maintain constipation.

Many elderly people are obsessed with their bowels, often from a lifetime's habit of weekly purgation and persistent beliefs that a bowel which is not completely cleared regularly can become 'toxic'. Older

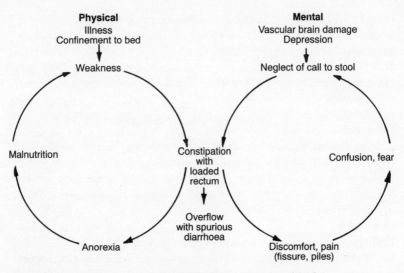

Figure 10.4 *Vicious circles of constipation in the elderly.*
(Wilkins, 1968)

people often attribute any feeling of malaise or ill health to infrequent bowel actions. Many are chronic laxative abusers (Connell et al., 1965; Sekas, 1987). This practice in itself may cause problems and eventually damage colonic activity, leading to nerve impairment and a 'cathartic' colon. There is no real evidence that healthy, active old people are more likely to be constipated than younger people. Prophylactic laxative-taking is best avoided, unless constipation is a known problem which cannot be resolved by other means. Because of some atrophy of bowel mucosa and muscle, transit times do rise somewhat with age. Elderly patients should be reassured that some decrease in frequency of defaecation is normal with age, and taught not to equate this with 'constipation' unless motions also become hard and difficult to pass.

Elderly people who live in institutional care often suffer from persistent faecal incontinence. Whilst this is often secondary to faecal impaction, simply disimpacting the bowel does not always solve the problem. Rands and Malone-Lee (1990) found that intensive treatment over a two-month period reduced impaction, but not incontinence. There was also very poor staff compliance with prescribed regimes. It seems that the causes and treatment of faecal incontinence in long-stay care are complex and multifactorial, and insufficient research has been done as yet to make definitive recommendations on treatment.

Investigation of Constipation and Faecal Impaction

Given the large number of possible causes outlined above, constipation with faecal impaction and incontinence should always be investigated and the underlying causes remedied, where possible. A rectal digital examination will reveal most impactions, although occasionally only soft faeces are present and the rectum may even be empty. A plain abdominal X-ray will reveal higher impaction if this is suspected. Many causes are quite easily treated, such as changing a drug regime, treating hypothyroidism or haemorrhoids, or acquiring a new set of dentures so that solid food containing more fibre can be chewed.

Further investigation will depend on the clinical picture. Reference to Table 10.1 for an assessment checklist and Table 10.2 for possible investigations may be helpful.

Treatment of Incontinence Caused by Impaction

The first necessity is to clear the faecal impaction. A manual evacuation of the faeces will rarely be necessary and should only ever be performed by a nurse who has been properly trained in the procedure. More usually a course of disposable enemas daily (phosphate if the faeces are soft and dioctyl if hard), for seven to ten days, or until no further return is obtained, is the best method of clearing impaction. A single enema is seldom sufficient, even if an apparently good result is obtained, because impaction is often extensive and the first enema merely clears the lowest portion of the bowel. Many patients' fear of enemas stems from the days of large volume soap-and-water enemas, which were both extremely uncomfortable and usually messy. These should no longer be used. The modern low-volume (100–150ml) disposable phosphate enema causes minimal discomfort and, if administered with careful prior explanation and due attention to privacy and dignity, does not generally cause much distress. The newer 'micro' (5–10ml) enemas are even more acceptable.

If faecal incontinence persists once the bowel has been totally cleared, and a plain abdominal X-ray may be helpful to confirm this, it can usually be assumed to be neurogenic in origin rather than caused by impaction.

Once the impaction is cleared, every effort must be made to prevent recurrence. Attention to diet, fluid intake, mobility, lavatory facilities and drug regimes may be sufficient. Some patients will additionally need to use agents to keep their bowels regular. There is a huge variety of laxatives available. They can be divided into four categories:

bulking agents, stool softeners, chemical laxatives, and per rectum evacuants.

Laxatives (Table 10.7)

Bulking laxatives work by being hydrophilic, i.e. attracting water into the stool. Usually faeces are 60–70% water, and a mere 10% increase in water content softens the stool considerably. Natural unprocessed bran is probably the most satisfactory bulking agent, but proprietary brands, such as Isogel, are available. Bran, because it is mixed with food and chewed, is less likely to form a bolus, especially if taken with adequate fluids, and therefore has a low risk of leading to intestinal obstruction. Fibre may also be taken as high fibre cereals. Bulking agents eaten as granules carry a slight risk of adhering together as a bolus.

It must be remembered that bulking agents will take several days to reach the colon. Impaction should be cleared before initiating this treatment. If not, the additional bulk will merely accumulate above the impaction and add to the amount of faeces which needs to be cleared. Bulking agents will increase the water content and size of stool, and decrease gut transit time, thereby increasing frequency of defaecation. They should be used with care for patients with diminished rectal sensation, those who ignore the call to stool and those with known terminal reservoir syndrome. Side effects include worsening of abdominal distension and wind. If fluid intake is inadequate, increased bran intake will exacerbate the impaction of faeces. The gradual introduction of bulking agents will tend to minimise problems.

Stool softeners are oral laxatives intended to alter stool consistency. Once the commonest softener was liquid paraffin. The use of liquid paraffin should have been discontinued as so many harmful effects have been noted. These include interference with digestion, binding of fat-soluble vitamins, possible deposits in lungs from inhalation leading to lipoid pneumonia, paraffinomas (deposits in the tissues), and faecal incontinence. Likewise, castor oil should not be in general use. It works by stimulating the small bowel to massive activity, leading to complete bowel clearance within two hours in most people. Currently Picolax seems to be the laxative of choice for one-off clearances (e.g. prior to X-ray examinations). The water, electrolyte and nutrient loss involved in the use of castor oil make it unsuitable for repeated use, especially with older people.

Chemical, or irritant, laxatives work by stimulating colonic peristalsis. The most commonly used are senna (e.g. Senokot) and

Table 10.7   Commonly-Used Laxatives

CATEGORY	NOTES/CONTRAINDICATIONS	EXAMPLES
Bulking agents	Introduce gradually, only after impaction cleared. Avoid if patient has loss of rectal sensation or terminal reservoir syndrome. (Ensure sufficient fluid intake).	Natural bran Fybogel Isogel Normacol
Stool softeners	(See text): avoid general use of castor oil	Castor oil Dioctyl (osmotic also)
Irritant/chemical	Use minimal effective dose	Senna Bisacodyl
Bulking and stimulating agent	Flatus/distension may be a problem	Manevac
Osmotic laxatives	Flatus may be a problem	Milk of magnesia Lactulose Dioctyl (softener also)
Rectally-administered	Some patients may need assistance or find use unpleasant	Suppositories (e.g. glycerine, bisacodyl) Enemas (e.g. phosphate, micro enemas)

bisacodyl (as Dulco-Lax). As they are selective to the colon, they do not upset the whole gut and have a minimal effect on fluid and electrolyte balance and gut flora. For prolonged administration, the smallest effective dose should always be used.

Osmotic laxatives, for example the sugar lactulose, attract water and so soften the stool. Some patients find it causes a bloated feeling and excessive flatus.

Of the rectally-administered laxatives, the disposable small volume enemas are probably the most convenient, but their use usually necessitates help. For lesser problems, glycerine or bisacodyl suppositories may be found effective and can be used independently by many people.

Often the best regime for each individual will only be found by trial. It is most important to prevent a recurrence of impaction, as incontinence will otherwise usually return. When dealing with patients in a home or hospital this will often involve close observation of each person's bowel habits. The traditional nursing practice of merely asking each patient if the bowels have been opened and marking 'yes' or 'no' on the TPR chart or in the nursing notes is insufficient, and fails to provide an adequate duty of care. Great vigilance is needed to avert the preventable condition of incontinence caused by impaction. The patient must be asked in more detail about the motions – their consistency, amount, ease of passage, and about any feelings of discomfort, bloating or incomplete evacuation.

The nurse must respect the patient's dignity and be sensitive to likely embarrassment, and choose an opportunity of asking such questions in private. Questions asked in front of visitors or other patients are less likely to be fully answered and spontaneous comments may be discouraged. If the patient cannot be relied upon for an accurate account, it is the nurse's responsibility to observe the stool and note its characteristics herself. The difficult passage of one small hard pellet per day, which all too often is recorded as 'bowels open' and assumed to be evidence that all is well, is usually the exact opposite – a pointer to impending impaction. Where this is suspected, the nurse may need to perform a rectal examination with a lubricated index finger to ensure that impaction is not developing. The momentary discomfort caused by a digital rectal examination is minimal compared to the distress and inconvenience resulting from faecal impaction and incontinence.

Meticulous observation, coupled with optimism and a belief that impaction is avoidable, can greatly reduce the prevalence of faecal incontinence in our caring institutions. The paradox is that although the message is simple, the results are often poor, perhaps because of the sometimes helpless and hopeless attitude of the carers and their patients.

SURGERY FOR FAECAL INCONTINENCE AND CONSTIPATION

There have been many recent advances in the surgical management of faecal incontinence, rectal prolapse and constipation. The techniques now in common use are listed in Table 10.4. This is clearly a very specialised field (Madoff et al., 1992; Keighley, 1991) and the success rate remains variable.

Most patients feel that there is an improvement in the degree of continence. Keighley reports to date that total pelvic floor repair appears to achieve the best results for idiopathic faecal incontinence. However, for some patients a feeling of incomplete evacuation – accompanied by some residual motion at the entrance to an incompletely closed anus, or small involuntary leakages – can persist for some time. Advice should be given on dietary and laxative management to produce a regular complete, formed stool. The treatment should be tailored to the individual's symptoms and needs, and may include the use of suppositories in conjunction with optimising the gastro-colic reflex. Frequently loperamide is useful for controlling post-operative diarrhoea.

Surgery for constipation should only be undertaken if constipation cannot be cured medically. The patient should be followed up and offered advice and counselling where appropriate. Detailed descriptions of surgical options are given in Henry and Swash (1992) and Kamm and Lennard-Jones (1994).

PREVENTION OF FAECAL INCONTINENCE

Much faecal incontinence can be prevented. Alterations to lifelong dietary habits could prevent many disorders, such as diverticular disease and possibly carcinoma, which may later cause incontinence. Regular laxative use or abuse should be avoided, as it may cause colonic and nerve damage. Avoidance of straining at stool could help to preserve pelvic floor integrity, as will better obstetric care, with a shortened second stage of labour. Internal anal sphincter dysfunction is an important factor in faecal incontinence in the elderly. Public education about fluid intake, the importance of establishing a regular bowel habit, suitable diet and avoiding laxatives and straining, could in future prevent many problems. Nonetheless it remains an uphill struggle to change long-ingrained behaviour and habits.

Abdominal massage has been reported as beneficial in controlling constipation, both for women with chronic constipation (Fox et al., 1991), and for people with cerebral palsy (Emly, 1993). It seems that prolonged firm massage (15–30 minutes) can promote colonic mass movements and stimulate voluntary evacuation, often thirty minutes later.

For those who come under the nurse's care, greater thought should go into the need for privacy, comfort and adequate time for defaecation. The importance of diet, fluids, exercise, a correct toilet height and relevant drug regimes must be stressed. Nurses who create an environment geared to the promotion of continence, who have an attitude that this is a preventable or reversible condition, and who are prepared to make strenuous efforts to closely monitor the bowel function of all their patients, will do much to prevent the misery of faecal incontinence.

FAECAL INCONTINENCE IN CHILDREN

The majority of children are continent of faeces by the age of four years, but 1% are still having problems at seven years. As with bladder control, more boys than girls are incontinent, suggesting that developmental factors may be relevant, as boys mature more slowly. Knowledge of normal developmental milestones is of considerable importance in this age group.

Faecal incontinence or soiling in childhood, sometimes referred to as 'encopresis', has, like nocturnal enuresis, long been regarded as evidence of psychiatric or psychological disorder in the child. Psychological factors are certainly important, but it is not true that most faecally incontinent children are disturbed (Morgan, 1981). The effects on the child of this condition should not be underestimated. Other children can be very cruel to anyone who is different, especially with a problem which makes the incontinent child appear dirty and babyish to his peers.

It is not difficult to see how the incontinence arises in many cases. The child often has fastidious, over-anxious parents with unrealistic expectations of potty-training, who are frequently not prepared to be convinced by nurses or doctors about modifying their own attitudes to the problem. The child is punished for soiling, so tends to inhibit defaecation, both in the pants and in the pot. Often, when attempting potty-training, the child is repeatedly sat on the pot in the absence of a full rectum and simply cannot perform. The situation becomes fraught with anxiety, and bowel movements become associated with unpleasantness in the child's mind. Parents reinforce this by telling threatening stories of what will happen if there is no result. He therefore retains faeces and becomes constipated. Defaecation is then also difficult and painful.

The tension created while on the potty or lavatory is often relieved later when out playing. 'Respite defaecation' occurs when the child relaxes – a formed stool is passed into the pants. This may seem like deliberate naughtiness to the parent who has just spent time encouraging its passage in the correct place.

Once this pattern is established, the child may even become impacted and suffer spurious diarrhoea. Tension at home, or lack of privacy or bullying at school, can both lead to deliberate retention. The child is made to feel guilty about his incontinence, although he has no control over it, and may try to conceal it by hiding the faeces or clothing. This may be misinterpreted as deliberate dirty habits – in fact it is rare that a child uses deliberate smearing or soiling as a weapon against parents.

The incontinent child and his parents should be assessed for their attitude to the problem. A history of difficult defaecation since birth might indicate Hirschsprung's disease. An abdominal examination may suggest impaction. Inspection of the perineum may show a skin tag suggestive of an anal fissure. Rarely, a congenital abnormality of the rectum or anus may be present. A rectal examination may prove traumatic for the child, and should probably only be done by a doctor when it is clearly indicated and in the presence of a parent or guardian. An abdominal X-ray can confirm suspected constipation.

Buchanan (1992) advocates a 'whole child' approach to soiling, including a package of treatment to meet the child's physical, psychological and social needs. The focus is on empowering the child to take responsibility for his own bowels, and educating him on how to do so.

The majority of children can be treated by disimpaction of the bowel, clear explanation and reassurance, and the use by parents of simple rewards for appropriate defaecation. Parents should be encouraged to make toileting more relaxed and less threatening for the younger child by keeping him company in the lavatory, and reading a story or singing a song. Punishment for soiling should never be used, as this merely aggravates the anxiety over defaecation. Neither should clean pants be rewarded, as this might reinforce retention of faeces. Regular laxatives and sensitive counselling and support will remedy most problems. A star chart can be helpful as it is rewarding to the child and monitors progress. A home visit is often useful (Keating, 1990). Older children can be involved in the charting of their dietary fibre or laxative intake and also of the result.

Sometimes advice will include practical measures, such as the use of a footstool to support dangling legs to aid defaecation, or a lower lock that the child can reach to ensure privacy, or getting him up ten minutes earlier so that he has time to empty the bowel before school. Adequate fluid, fibre and exercise are all important (but not necessarily easy to achieve if the child is not motivated to cooperate). If the child is incontinent at school, he will need an emergency clean-up kit (e.g. wipes, clean pants, bag for soiled pants). Teachers must be aware of the problem, and encouraged by the family and health professionals to be constructively sympathetic.

If the child does prove to be disturbed, as a few do, then psychotherapy or child guidance may be indicated.

The child with learning difficulties may be in exactly the same position as other children – retaining faeces because of the unfavourable response they produce in others. Conversely, incontinence may produce much commotion and attention and so become rewarding. Behaviour modification programmes of appropriate prompt rewards and gradually withdrawn prompts will cure many children of incontinence (see Chapter 14). If the incontinence has a neurogenic basis, e.g. some children with spina bifida, careful monitoring of the bowel habit and action will enable the implementation of planned defaecation, with up to one half becoming continent (King et al., 1994).

The health visitor has an important role in educating parents to avoid many problems of faecal incontinence arising in children. Clear practical advice on potty-training, and support for those experiencing problems, will often prevent incontinence at an early stage.

FAECAL INCONTINENCE IN DEMENTED PEOPLE

Advanced dementia or confusional states may result in faecal incontinence caused by the loss of social awareness of appropriate behaviour. The person who has no insight that defaecation should only be in clearly defined receptacles has no reason to voluntarily delay defaecation, so the stool is usually passed as soon as it enters the anal canal. Sometimes the knowledge that certain receptacles are designated for the purpose is retained but the ability to identify them is lost, and the demented person may use a totally inappropriate receptacle, such as a waste-paper bin or a sink, in which to pass faeces. Others remember to remove clothing and to sit or squat, but will do so wherever they happen to be at the time. Some lose all apparent awareness and pass the stool into their underpants or the bed. Some demented people lose all appropriate toilet behaviour, but retain an appreciation that something is wrong and become agitated or start wandering, apparently aimlessly, just prior to being incontinent.

It must never be assumed that dementia alone is sufficient reason to explain faecal incontinence, without investigation and exclusion of other causes. Continence is deeply ingrained in most of us, and it is often one of the last social skills to be lost. The demented person may be incontinent because of diarrhoea from any cause; because the same neurological damage which has caused dementia has also affected the ability to voluntarily control the defaecation reflex; or, most commonly of all, because of faecal impaction. The majority of demented people are not faecally incontinent. Unless the dementia is profound, incontinence is most often found to have other causes.

Where the patient gives any impending signs of defaecation (for example, restlessness is a very common symptom of full bladder or bowel), there will usually be enough time to prevent incontinence by appropriate toileting. This is dependent on all those looking after that person knowing exactly what signs to look for and what they mean. Spotting this characteristic behaviour for each person is a vital part of the nursing assessment of faecal incontinence in each individual.

It may be possible to retrain the demented person towards more socially acceptable habits. It is often possible to establish a routine of defaecation, for example, half an hour after a hot meal or drink. Principles of reality orientation and behaviour modification (see Chapters 11 and 14) are equally applicable to faecal as to urinary incontinence. Rewarding continent behaviour may restore continence in many demented people.

Education and training in the prevention, treatment and management of faecal incontinence and constipation should be available and undertaken by all nurses in order to alleviate the misery these symptoms cause.

Where there are combined lower urinary tract and faecal disorders, a unified approach to diagnosis and optimum management should be sought from the specialist consultants, continence adviser and the multidisciplinary team (Mathers and Swash, 1988).

INTRACTABLE FAECAL INCONTINENCE

For a few unfortunate people, faecal incontinence proves resistant to treatment. These people will need support and counselling, as well as practical advice.

Protection

Protection will be needed to preserve the sufferer's dignity and protect the environment. Many of the garments used for urinary incontinence are suitable (see Chapter 15). Specifically, those with a disposable pad worn directly next to the perineum are most suitable. If faecal incontinence alone is present, a high absorbency is usually not needed and relatively thin pads may be used. If large formed stools are passed, some people find a shaped pad most successful at containing the stool until it can be disposed of. Marsupial pants and washable underpads are not suitable for faecal incontinence.

Smell

The odour of faeces is a particularly difficult problem. Obviously, prompt action to dispose of the faeces and scrupulous personal hygiene (with regular baths or showers if possible) is the best management, but even this will not always prevent smell. Proprietary deodorants, obtainable from pharmacists, may help if used on a pad, clothing, or in the air. Each patient may find that certain foods aggravate smell and are best avoided. Smell is one of the intractable problems associated with faecal incontinence.

Anal Plug

A promising development is an anal plug to control faecal incontinence. It is made from polyurethane sponge, which is compressed by a water-soluble coating for easy insertion. Once in place, the coating dissolves and the plug expands to its full size (Mortensen et al., 1991).

REFERENCES AND FURTHER READING

Association for Continence Advice, 1991. Faecal soiling in childhood. *Proceedings of a Study Day*. ACA, London.

Baeten, C. G. M., Konsten, J., Spaans, F., 1991. Dynamic graciloplasty for treatment of faecal incontinence. *Lancet*, 338, 8776: 1163–5.

Barrett, J. A., 1993. *Faecal Incontinence and Related Problems in the Older Adult*. Edward Arnold, London.

Blackwell, C., Williams, A., 1989. *Encopresis*. Enuresis Resource and Information Centre, Bristol.

Buchanan, A., Clayden, G., 1992. *Children Who Soil*. John Wiley, Chichester.

Cavara, K., Prentice, A., Wellings, C., 1991. *Caring for the Person with Faecal Incontinence*. Ausmed Publications, Melbourne, Australia.

Clayden, G. S., 1989. Constipation in childhood. *British Medical Journal*, 299: 1116–17.

Clayden, G. S. and Agnarsson, U., 1991. *Constipation in Childhood*. Oxford University Press, Oxford.

Connell, A. M., Hilton, C., Irvine, G., Lennard-Jones, J. E., Misiewicz, J. J., 1965. Variation of bowel habit in two population samples. *British Medical Journal*, ii: 1095–9.

Egan, M. Plymat, K., Thomas, T., Meade, T., 1983. Incontinence in patients in two district general hospitals. *Nursing Times*, 79, 5: 22–4.

Emly, M., 1993. Abdominal massage. *Nursing Times*, 89, 3: 34–6.

Fox, J., Sylvestre, L., Freeman, J. B., 1991. Rectal incontinence: A team approach. *Physiotherapy*, 77, 10: 665–72.

Hancock, B. D., 1992. Haemorrhoids: ABC of colorectal diseases. *British Medical Journal*, 304: 1042–4.

Henry, M. M., 1988. Faecal incontinence and rectal prolapse. *Surgical Clinics of North America*, 68, 6: 1249–54.

Henry, M. M., Swash, M. (eds), 1992. *Coloproctology and the Pelvic Floor* (2nd edn). Butterworth Heinemann, London.

Irving, M. H., Catchpole B., 1992. Anatomy and physiology of the colon, rectum and anus. ABC of colorectal diseases. *British Medical Journal*, 304: 1106–8.

Kamm, M. A., 1994. Obstetric damage and faecal incontinence. *Lancet*, 344: 730–3.

Kamm, M. A., 1995. Functional disorders of the colon and anorectum. *Current Opinion in Gastroenterology*, 11: 9–15.

Kamm, M. A., Lennard-Jones, J. E. (eds), 1994. *Constipation*. Wrightson Biomedical Publishing, Petersfield, UK.

Keating, P., 1990. Constipation. *Community Outlook*, December: 4–10.

Keighley, M. R. B., 1991. Results of surgery in idiopathic faecal incontinence. *South African Journal of Surgery*, 29, 3: 87–93.

King, J. C., Currie, D. M., Wright, E., 1994. Bowel training in spina bifida: importance of education, patient compliance, age and anal reflexes. *Archives of Physical Medicine and Rehabilitation*, 75: 243–7.

Law, P. J., Kamm, M. A., Bartram, C. I., 1991. Anal endosonography in the investigation of faecal incontinence. *British Journal of Surgery*, 78: 312–4.

Leigh, R. J., Turnberg, L. A., 1982. Faecal incontinence; the unvoiced symptom. *Lancet*, 1: 1349–51.

Macphee, J. A., Brodie, M. J., 1992. Drugs in the Elderly. *Medicine International*, 101: 4258–63.

Madoff, R. D., Graham Williams, J., Caushaj, P. F., 1992. Faecal incontinence. *New England Journal of Medicine*: 1002–7.

Malone, P. S., Ransley, P. G., Kiely, E. M., 1990. Preliminary report: the antegrade continence enema. *Lancet*, 336, 8725: 1217.

Mathers, S., Swash, M., 1988. Faecal incontinence. *International Disability Studies*, 10: 164–8.

Miner, P. B., Donnelly, T. C., Read, N. W., 1990. Investigation of mode of action of biofeedback in treatment of faecal incontinence. *Digestive Diseases and Science*, Vol. 35, No. 10.

Morgan, R., 1984. Behavioural treatments with children. Chapter 8: *Faecal Soiling*. William Heinemann Medical Books, London.

Morgan, R., 1981. *Childhood Incontinence*. William Heinemann Medical Books, London.

Mortensen, N., Smilgin Humphreys, M., 1991. The anal continence plug: a disposable device for patients with anorectal incontinence. *Lancet*, 338, 8762: 295–7.

Orrom, W. J., Miller, R., Cornes, H., Duthie, G., McC., Mortensen, N. J., Bartolo, D. C. C., 1991. Comparison of anterior sphincteroplasty and post-anal repair in the treatment of idiopathic faecal incontinence. *Diseases of the Colon and Rectum*, 34, 4: 305–10.

Parks, A. G., 1980. Faecal incontinence. In: Mandelstam, D., (ed), *Incontinence and its Management*. Croom Helm, Beckenham.

Rands, G., Malone-Lee, J., 1990. Urinary and faecal incontinence in long-stay wards for the elderly mentally ill; prevalence and difficulties in management. *Health Trends*, 22, 4: 161–3.

Sekas, G., 1987. The use and abuse of laxatives. *Practical Gastroenterology*: 33–9.

Snooks, S. J., Swash, M., Setchell, M., Henry, M. M., 1984. Injury to innervation of pelvic floor sphincter musculature in childbirth. *Lancet*, ii: 546–50.

Sultan, A. H., Kamm, M. A., Hudson, C. N., Bartram, C. I., 1993a. Anal sphincter disruption during vaginal delivery. *New England Journal of Medicine*, 329: 1905–11.

Sultan, A. H., Kamm, M. A., Bartram, C. I., Hudson, C. N., 1993b. Anal sphincter trauma during instrumental delivery. *International Journal of Gynaecology and Obstetrics*, 43: 263–70.

Talley, N. J., O'Keefe, E. A., Zinsmeister, A. R., Melton, J. L., 1992. Prevalence of gastrointestinal symptoms in the elderly: a population-based study. *Gastroenterology*, 102: 895–901.

Thomas, T. M., Egan, M., Walgrove, A., Meade, T. W., 1984. The prevalence of faecal and double incontinence. *Community Medicine*, 6, 3: 216–20.

Wilkins, E. G., 1968. Vicious circles of constipation in the elderly. *Postgraduate Medical Journal*, 44: 728.

Books for Patients

Chiarelli, P., Markham, S., 1992. *Let's Get Things Moving – Overcoming Constipation*. Gore and Osment, NSW, Australia.

Nicol, R., 1989. *Coping Successfully With Your Irritable Bowel*. Sheldon Press, London.

Schuster, M. M., Wehmueller, J., 1994. *Keeping Control: Understanding and Overcoming Faecal Incontinence*. Johns Hopkins University Press, Baltimore and London.

Chapter 11

Continence in Older People

Jean Swaffield, MSc, RGN, RSCN, DN, DNT, FETC, PWT
Senior Lecturer, Department of Nursing & Midwifery, Glasgow University

Although prevalence studies have shown that incontinence becomes more common with increasing age, they do not show that incontinence is an inevitable part of ageing. Unfortunately, the myth that there is nothing that can be done for incontinence in old age has been responsible for formulating much of society's view on the subject. Consequently, in the recent past, senior citizens have not always received a fair assessment of their problems and were often treated by palliative measures rather than thorough investigation. More positive approaches are now in evidence.

Devoting a separate chapter to elderly people does not imply that older adults should be investigated and assessed any differently from younger people. However, this chapter highlights certain age-related problems that may affect the elderly person's continence status, as well as bringing to the attention of the reader the current changes in health policies which may have a profound effect on care and assessment at home, or in residential and nursing homes.

Surveys of incontinence in elderly people in Britain have provided widely differing prevalence rates. This is due to lack of standardised terminology and differences in sampling methods. About 14–20% of people over 65 living in a community setting have some degree of incontinence, while it is found to be within the range of 25–50% among those living in institutions (Mohide, 1992). Of these elderly people, women are more likely to be incontinent than men; frail elderly women, over 85, being the most affected.

For many people, incontinence in old age may not be a new or even recent problem. Some have hidden or secretly managed the problem for a long time and are only confronted with facing up to incontinence when they require nursing, medical treatment or admission to hospital for some other disorder. It may also come to light when 'significant others' are no longer available to help. Many learn to cope in their own way, but for others it causes a serious disruption to social integration. They may be uncomfortable and ashamed. Carers may have found caring for incontinent relatives and friends a burden, which has precipitated admission to institutions and nursing homes. Sanford (1975) showed that faecal incontinence, persistent disturbance at night and incontinence in an opposite-sexed parent, were least tolerated and could lead to requests for institutional care or social service help.

However, many relatives do look after severely incontinent people in the community with great devotion, and tolerate a considerable workload and disruption to their household and family life.

Britain is experiencing an unprecedented increase in the numbers of individuals surviving to old age. The over-85 age group is increasing most rapidly (OPCS, 1987). This is occurring at a time when there has been a rationalisation of hospital beds and a major change of government policy in the care of elderly people and the use of hospital facilities. There has been a move to reduce long-term hospital beds and a shift to the use of private residential and nursing homes for those receiving social security payments for care. At the same time, general practitioners have been made responsible for screening people over 75 years and for the assessment of their social and health care needs. From 1993, the responsibility for assessing the care needs of elderly people passed to local authorities (via social services staff) rather than community nurses, although joint protocols may be used (National Health Service and Community Care Act, 1990).

Without careful planning, integration of policies, staff training and a willingness to use team approaches, the assessment, care and treatment of incontinent elderly people might be jeopardised.

It is important that older people are enabled to live high-quality independent lives in the community. To achieve this, there is a need to identify and effectively assess and treat people suffering bladder and bowel dysfunction and to introduce strategies to prevent incontinence.

A change of attitude towards ageing needs to be fostered, and a positive approach to the promotion of continence among health educators is one of the hallmarks of good health provision. The identification of and support for carers must be a cornerstone of good community care services; continence services should be widely available and clearly advertised. Practical help and advice should be actively disseminated to those who may be too embarrassed or ashamed to seek help. A recognition of this need is stated in the English DoH report 'An agenda for action on continence services' (1991), and the need to advertise and audit services was clearly identified in the report 'Community continence services' (Rooker, 1992).

OLDER PEOPLES' ATTITUDE TO INCONTINENCE

While there appears to be an increasingly more open discussion of topics that were considered unsuitable for general conversation two decades ago, those who are very elderly may still hold views that belong to a previous era. Mention of bodily functions may cause embarrassment and highlight an ignorance of the way the body functions. The use of the individual's own words to describe micturition and defaecation may be the starting point for further discussion on the subject. For many people, incontinence may still retain the 19th century usage of 'wanting in self restraint, especially in regard to sexual appetite', and they fear being labelled in this way.

Passing urine and faeces is considered a private act. On admission to hospital or in other establishments it is important to respect the value of privacy, even when patients may require assistance for these basic needs. Curtains can hide them from sight, but do not disguise the sound, smell and knowledge of what is going on behind the curtain. This may cause a failure to relax and lead to constipation or incomplete bladder emptying and discomfort where a commode must be used.

It is important to offer a hand-bowl after using a commode, and maintain the patients' normal hygiene. If these normalities are ignored, patients may be reluctant to use the commode before meal times because they cannot cleanse themselves.

Many people have always feared catching diseases from public toilets and will not therefore sit on hospital toilets. Attention to cleanliness and comfort in all toilets, and the proper cleaning of commodes and bedpans, are very important to people in communal living accommodation. Nurses should ensure that toilets are kept to a high standard of hygiene.

For disabled people who live at home, the social interactions between family and friends may need to be considered before commodes are introduced to the bedroom or living room. The consequence of inadequate discussion can lead to a reduction of visitors to the home, or embarrassment and inhibition by the patient in using the commode in case of being interrupted.

When nurses are using the nursing process, or are involved in primary nursing care, the ability to understand the wishes and values of the patient are more easily recognised and acknowledged. In the case of patients in nursing homes it is important that carers are familiar with patients' needs and are aware of their individual preferences for personal hygiene. Care staff will only be able to achieve this if they work with small groups of patients and avoid toileting patients from across the whole population of residents.

THE PHYSIOLOGICAL EFFECTS OF AGEING ON CONTINENCE

The Ageing Kidney

There is a considerable reduction in glomerular filtration rate (GFR) with advancing age. On average, a 60-year-old kidney is half as efficient as a 30-year-old one and the number of glomeruli halves between 30–70 years. The whole organ shrinks – the cortex more than the medulla. Renal flow, GFR and creatinine clearance all fall, while glomerular and tubular basement membranes all thicken.

The control of blood chemistry declines and older people are less able to produce a concentration of urine in response to dehydration, dispose of a fluid or acid load, and conserve sodium (Na^+) or potassium (K^+). Drugs will tend to accumulate in the body, increasing the likelihood of toxic effects.

The ageing kidney is also less efficient in converting vitamin D into its active form. This makes osteomalacia more likely, and vitamin D given for treatment less effective (Roberts, 1989).

The kidney receives a smaller proportion of cardiac output by day, although this may return to normal at night when the demands of other organs are lessened. This may explain why many elderly people have a disturbed diurnal rhythm of urine production compared with young adults, who produce most urine by day and relatively little when asleep. Older people often produce urine at the same rate day and night, or even produce more at night. This is more pronounced in confused and demented people, possibly due to their generally disturbed circadian rhythms (Armstrong-Esther and Hawkins, 1982). It is also found in patients with heart diseases, where the heart and kidneys function best when the body is at rest and the demands of other organs lessened.

Urinary Tract Infection

Infection in the bladder or kidneys is common in old age. This may be due to failure to empty the bladder properly, to bladder neck obstruction or to problems with neurological control resulting in contractions of the detrusor muscle being uncoordinated, with the relaxation of the urethral sphincter. The ageing immune system may also be generally less efficient.

261

Significant bacteriuria is present in 20% of women over sixty-five and men over seventy-five living at home (Brocklehurst et al., 1968). In hospital this rises to 30%–40% of long-stay inpatients. The criteria for diagnosis of a significant urinary tract infection (UTI) is commonly recognised as more than 10^5 colony-forming units per millilitre. The vast majority of infections are asymptomatic and probably harmless; opinions differ as to the use of antibiotics, which may prevent the problem turning into a kidney infection, but once antibiotics are stopped the bacteriuria often reappears. Resource implications are an issue in general practice (Brumfitt and Hamilton-Miller, 1987). Failure of therapy or reinfection are common, so if one or two courses of antibiotic fail to clear the infection it should be left alone (Brocklehurst, 1977), or other reasons explored for stasis of urine or infection.

Most UTI's in old age are confined to the bladder. The clinical picture may include mental confusion, incontinence and dysuria and urgency. Extra fluids will reduce the reproduction rate of bacteria and wash them out of the bladder, but may dilute the effect of any antibiotics taken. Where pyelonephritis is suspected, and this is more common in men with prostatic obstruction, the clinical picture may include, in the acute attack, fever, loin pain, frequency and dysuria. Chronic cases may be asymptomatic until signs of renal failure are apparent and the patient shows signs of tiredness, anorexia, confusion, nausea and vomiting. Treatment by antibiotics and treatment of the predisposing causes will be required (e.g. removal of prostatic obstruction).

Most UTI's are low-grade and chronic, often associated with voiding difficulties and residual urine. The commonest form of bladder neck obstruction in men is benign prostatic hyperplasia (BPH), and in women the underactive bladder or constipation are the most common cause of residual urine. One of the commonest neurological conditions causing stasis of urine and possible infection is multiple sclerosis.

It has not been proven that urinary tract infection causes incontinence, nor indeed vice versa. An acute cystitis may precipitate incontinence in someone at risk, and should therefore be treated. A chronic infection is unlikely to be the cause of incontinence.

Age Changes in the Bladder
The incidence of multiple bladder dysfunction increases with age. There is an increased tendency for the bladder to be trabeculated (have fibrous bands) and the detrusor muscle to become unstable, and there is

loss of supporting elastic tissue. Fibrosis becomes more common, possibly as a consequence of chronic infection and distension, and may result in bladder neck stenosis and voiding difficulties.

The urethral mucosa may prolapse down through the external urethral meatus, and this can form an ulcerating carbuncle. The significance of this is unknown, but it tends to be associated with incontinence. If painful or bleeding, it can be treated with vaginal oestrogens (see below).

As elastic tissue and muscle weaken, stress incontinence becomes more common in women (see Chapter 6). With atrophy of all pelvic organs, the urethral meatus may recede along the vaginal wall, out of sight. This causes great difficulty if a catheter is to be inserted, and the woman may have to be catheterised in a lateral position, from behind, with flexed knees.

Mixed pathologies should always be considered when assessing an older incontinent person. It is far more likely than with younger patients that there will be more than one bladder abnormality, such as an unstable detrusor *and* stress incontinence, or a voiding problem with unstable contractions. This means that an initial decision must often be made as to which is the dominant problem, in order to treat that one first. Sometimes more than one therapy can be used at the same time, for instance where bladder training for an unstable bladder is combined with pelvic floor exercises for stress incontinence. Other combinations may be treated one at a time; for example, where there is an unstable bladder and outflow obstruction the instability, if dominant, should be treated first, because if outflow resistance is lowered first the incontinence is likely to worsen.

Hormone Changes
The urethra and trigone in the female are formed embryologically from the same hormone-dependent tissue as the vagina. When fully oestrogenised, the surface of the urethral wall is very soft and convoluted, forming many folds which interdigitate to form an efficient watertight seal (Figure 11.1, overleaf).

Oestrogen levels decrease following the menopause. In many women this loss does not produce any problem, however the walls of the urethra may become a lot less soft and the folds less pronounced so that closure is less efficient (Figure 11.2). Coupled with decreased mucus production, which lowers surface tension, the result is that both stress incontinence and leakage during uninhibited detrusor contractions are more likely to arise.

(a) Side view   (b) Cross-section

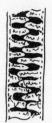
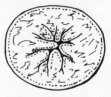

Figure 11.1   *Well-oestrogened urethra (note interdigitating folds giving efficent closure).*

(a) Side view   (b) Cross-section

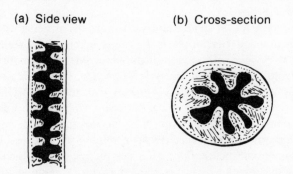

Figure 11.2   *Oestrogen-deficient urethra.*

With increasing age a larger area of the urethra and trigone become oestrogen-sensitive. Lack of oestrogen may cause a urethritis and trigonitis. The patient will suffer symptoms similar to cystitis – dysuria, frequency and often urgency. This will be associated with a vaginitis ('atrophic' or 'senile' vaginitis), which can be detected easily by looking at the vulva which will appear red, inflamed, and often dry. There may be secondary infection. Much of the perineal discomfort commonly attributed to the effects of incontinence in elderly women is probably in fact a symptom of atrophic vaginitis. Considerable excoriation, and even adhesions, may develop. If the diagnosis is in doubt a histological smear will confirm it.

Oestrogen replacement therapy will remedy these conditions. Ideally this should be a very low dose. A combined oestrogen and progestogen will avoid problems of endometrial stimulation if the patient has a uterus. Oestrogen is available as a pessary or cream for local application, but some older women find the vaginal applicators difficult or uncomfortable to use, and doses may be loaded into the applicators inaccurately. Oral preparations and slow-release patches are available for those who cannot manage a vaginal dose. (Considerable dexterity is necessary for vaginal application and some women find it distasteful or impossible, particularly the nulliparous.) Oral oestrogens may carry a higher risk of side effects. Oestrogens should not be used for women with a history of thrombo-embolic disease or malignancy of the reproductive system. On a low dose the therapy can be given continuously or via a '3-month on, 3-month off' basis. Withdrawal bleeding is rare. Patients should be warned that with pessaries or cream used at night they may get a white discharge on rising in the morning. They should be advised that this is of no importance, as the active hormone will have already been absorbed.

It is established that oestrogen can produce a subjective improvement in a patient's symptoms and well-being; however, objective measurements have not substantiated a decrease in urine loss (Fantl et al., 1994).

The Prostate
Benign prostatic hyperplasia (BPH) is discussed in Chapter 7. The incidence of prostatic malignancy increases in old age and is present in 30% of men over seventy, rising to 80% over ninety. Most of these malignancies are latent and do not affect life expectancy. However, the possibility of an obstructive tumour should be considered in men who experience an altered micturition pattern, especially difficulty in passing urine.

As with younger patients considering transurethral resection of the prostate, counselling on the effects of any post-operative impotence and retrograde ejaculation should be given. It should not be assumed that older patients are uninterested in sexual intercourse and their own sexuality.

Surgery is now a possibility for more elderly patients previously considered unfit for surgery, because of the advent of new techniques in anaesthesia and simpler procedures for some conditions.

The Ageing Bowel and Constipation
This topic is dealt with in Chapter 10.

Neurological Conditions

Ageing and neurological disease make bladder dysfunction more common in old age. Predominant is an unstable detrusor, with a very high proportion of all old people having some degree of instability. Parkinson's disease, cerebrovascular accidents and multiple sclerosis are three diseases that frequently affect an older person's continence.

Neurogenic voiding difficulties can occur in all the complex combinations described in Chapter 8. It is also likely that with the increased incidence of autonomic neuropathy associated with ageing, the number of both men and women with functional (non-anatomic) obstruction from detrusor-sphincter dyssynergia increases. The urethral sphincter does not relax completely during micturition or else closes too soon, resulting in incomplete emptying and residual urine, which may lead to retention of urine with overflow incontinence and possibly also to an increased risk of urinary tract infection.

Bladder sensation can change with age. Instead of perceiving the sensation of bladder filling at about half of capacity, as young people do, many older people first feel the desire to void at, or very near to, bladder capacity. To the active and mobile old person this can represent a considerable problem, as they will have to stop whatever they are doing and find a toilet. To an immobile person, or to someone with an unstable detrusor or painful arthritis, this can result in incontinence; there is not enough time between sensation and the actual release of urine to reach a toilet.

Diabetes

Over the age of seventy, 30% of women and 20% of men have diabetes. However mild a form of the disease is present, it can have a profound effect upon the bladder, particularly leading to damage to peripheral nerves and an underactive bladder (see Chapter 8). Many of the underactive bladders seen in old age are directly related to diabetic neuropathy.

Undiagnosed diabetes may present as polyuria and polydipsia: vulval irritation with reddened swollen labia and possibly a candida albicans infection; or with overflow incontinence. Screening for diabetes should be routine among elderly people with urinary symptoms. If a urine test detects sugar, a glucose tolerance test is usually then performed to confirm the diagnosis.

Mental Impairment

Most people become mentally less flexible and adaptable, to some extent, as they age. Many react with confusion and even aggression to circumstances which have suddenly or unexpectedly altered. Some suffer accelerated age changes, resulting in dementia. The specific problems and management of the mentally impaired elderly incontinent person are dealt with later in this chapter.

Disability

Multiple pathology is common in old age. Many elderly people with bladder or bowel problems also have other disorders to contend with, many of which will affect the ability to be continent. Neurological disorders not only directly influence bladder function but also often impair ability to cope with it. A parkinsonian tremor or a hemiparesis may make independent toileting slow, or even impossible. Heart or lung disease may make the patient so slow or breathless that the lavatory cannot be reached in time. Arthritis may limit mobility and dexterity. Depression is common in old age and may lead to apathy, self-neglect and incontinence. Alcoholism may likewise be overlooked as a reason for gradual deterioration in mental and physical state, with concomitant incontinence. Treatment of these disorders may result in a consequent improvement in continence.

IATROGENIC FACTORS

With more complex treatments, hospital organisation and pharmacological treatments, these may in fact cause more problems than they cure. Increasingly, iatrogenesis is being recognised as an issue in continence promotion (Donaldson, 1983; Miller, 1985).

Drugs

Multiple drug usage is common among elderly people. Many drugs have side effects on bladder function that can contribute to incontinence (see Table 2.2, pages 26–7), (Keister, 1989). Stopping unnecessary prescriptions, lowering the dose of a diuretic, or using a less rapid-acting one, decreasing sedation or changing to an alternative medication for a particular disorder, may improve or cure the problem. Drugs with anticholinergic properties must be carefully monitored in those with normal or underactive bladder function, as their introduction may cause retention of urine.

Fluids

The habit of restricting fluids to control incontinence can reach dangerous proportions in some old people, who may drink almost nothing. Many already have a precarious metabolic stability, and severe fluid and electrolyte imbalance may result. Dehydration, malaise, constipation and confusion can follow.

Older people often find drinking large quantities of fluid difficult, as it makes them feel bloated. When encouraging people to drink reasonably (ideally more than one litre per twenty-four hours), it is important to find out what they like and when they prefer to drink. Many who find water or squash unpalatable can drink the same volume of strong tea or stout with little problem (providing, of course, that the preferred drink does not aggravate the bladder).

Institutional Organisation

Many research studies have shown that the organisation of care in an institution can affect the independence of the patient (Goffman, 1961). Task orientation and a lack of individualised patient care prevents self attainment or development (Miller, 1985; Robertson, 1986; Swaffield, 1988). If patients are not seen as individuals, it is unlikely that the individual needs of the patient with incontinence will be diagnosed correctly or that care will be planned individually as a consequence. In routine approaches to toileting, the patient fits into a regime which may not suit their own pattern of daily defaecation and micturition, and which in fact leads to incontinence. The introduction of the nursing process and primary nursing care offer possible solutions to individual toileting needs. The use of audit for long-term care wards and homes for elderly people, such as that produced by the Royal College of Physicians (1992), offers scope for individual and functional evaluation of the continence services offered. This can then lead to improvements in the standards of continence care.

THE SOCIOLOGY OF INCONTINENCE

Attitudes

In our society there appear to be two conflicting norms regarding incontinence and elderly people. On the one hand older people are expected to be continent, yet the myths are maintained that past a certain age or with certain diseases, incontinence is inevitable. The consequence of this affects opportunity for treatment, as very often patients and their carers fail to seek continence. It is important therefore to educate the public concerning what can be achieved through accurate assessment. This will ensure that more people know that help is available. Services should be presented in such a way that people are not embarrassed or lose dignity, but are welcomed and involved in positive health promotion (Armstrong, 1980).

Health promotion focused towards continence among old people involves creating an environment in which an optimal level of functioning, including bladder and bowel control or management, is achievable.

Triggers

In examining the reasons for consulting a doctor, medical sociologists have demonstrated that unless there is an acute painful condition, most people go to a doctor for a social reason or because an event has triggered the decision to consult (Zola, 1973; Scambler, 1986). Professionals have therefore to use opportunistic patient contacts to raise the issue of continence.

Opportunity

In the assessment of people over 75 years the practice nurse, district nurse and health visitor have the opportunity to discuss continence. They will be able to refer on, as necessary, according to protocols set up before such programmes of assessments are commenced.

In discussions on joint protocols to be established by social care and health care agencies, it is important that those responsible for assessing the needs of elderly people are fully educated in the need for an assessment of the causes of incontinence, and that they have a positive attitude towards treatment rather than assuming the negative approach of assessing just for incontinence products.

Wherever patients are assessed for health, in well women clinics or in other consultations, opportunities to discuss continence problems will be presented (Swaffield, 1986).

Independence

For most elderly people the greater the functional independence allowed by the environment, the greater is their potential for continence. However, many are reticent in asking for personal physical help even though they have urgency; while there may not always be someone immediately available when needed to help, they may object to the loss of privacy when help is offered. This in turn may prevent turning to the services of doctors and nurses for treatment. There is a need when educating relatives to ensure that they encourage maximum independence for the patient.

Beds should be at the correct height for the individual to be able to get out of easily at home, and nurses should make sure that adjustable height beds are returned to patient-friendly heights after use in hospital. At home it helps if the mattress is neither too soft nor sags in the middle, as this can make rising difficult. Chairs should also be of the correct height, not too soft or deep, and have armrests at an appropriate height to aid leverage.

A good walking aid, whether stick, tripod or frame, can greatly improve mobility, speed, and confidence in visiting the toilet independently. Clothes should be attractive and easy to adjust, and any incontinence product should be able to be easily removed and replaced by the wearer.

OTHER IMPORTANT ENVIRONMENTAL CONSIDERATIONS

Toilet Facilities
In Western societies privacy is considered important for toilet purposes, with segregation of the sexes. Toilets should have a door which is easy to open and lock. The seat must be the correct height for easy sitting and rising. (See Chapter 13 for modifications which can be made and alternative urinals and commodes for those who cannot get to the toilet.)

Distance
An older person, especially one with impaired mobility, generally needs to have fast access to the toilet. Because many feel sensation only at or near capacity, urgency is often considerable. Once urgency is felt it may not be possible to rush. The Scottish Home and Health Department have estimated that 30–40 feet is the optimum distance between the starting point and the toilet for an elderly person. This means situating toilets near day areas in homes, hospitals and day centres, and may involve structural alterations in the patient's own home. The route also needs to be unobstructed and without stairs if mobility is limited.

Identification of Toilet Facilities

In unfamiliar surroundings, being able to identify the correct toilet quickly and easily is important. Clear signposts in public places as well as in hospitals and homes, and clear labels on doors are required. It is easy to misunderstand a Ladies or Gents symbol such as Edwardian hats and bonnets, and this may make people who have made such a mistake nervous to venture out for fear of repeating the incident. Clear and large labelling, colour-coded doors and unambiguous well-lit signs at an appropriate height (remembering that many older people have a diminishing height) are all aids to achieving independence. Where memory is a problem, some units have found that following a coloured line on the floor to a toilet door of the same colour, is helpful.

EMOTIONAL AND PSYCHOLOGICAL FACTORS

As with younger patients, psychological factors are important with elderly people, although a direct causative role is unproven. The onset of incontinence may be observed following a stressful significant event such as bereavement or admission to hospital. Occasionally, incontinence is perceived by others as deliberate, conscious and attention-seeking behaviour. This cannot simply be assumed – the behaviour must be investigated. If someone feels the need to gain the attention of others in this drastic manner, it should alert professionals to the need for further investigation of that individual's needs. A manipulative person, if successful in gaining attention by being incontinent, will repeat the process, and a behavioural assessment is indicated to ascertain how it might be possible to redirect the need for attention.

TREATMENTS

General Considerations

Identification of patients who require assessment and treatment for incontinence will remain a problem of hidden need until services are effectively advertised. Most Health Authorities and Boards have continence services and urodynamic clinics. A number of drop-in clinics are being established.

A good nursing assessment (see Chapter 3) will reveal many problems which can be remedied, but for those who do not respond to nursing measures a full urodynamic assessment is indicated. Few old people find this unduly distressing or uncomfortable if conducted in a private and relaxed atmosphere.

The full range of treatments are applicable to the elderly incontinent person: the options should be explained and the decision made jointly with the patient, and sometimes with the carer, as to how the treatment should proceed. Some people are reluctant to undergo invasive treatment such as surgery, and prefer reliable containment. Drug therapy should be used with care in older people, as many are more sensitive to side effects than younger people. Provided treatments are introduced cautiously and gradually, and evaluated, all standard preparations may be used. For example, great care is needed with anticholinergic drugs, which are contradicted in the presence of glaucoma. Time spent teaching the patient will increase understanding and compliance with prescribed regimes. With improvements in surgical techniques and varying approaches to anaesthesia, surgery is increasingly feasible for all those who need it.

Intermittent Catheterisation
(A fuller discussion of the techniques involved is given in Chapter 8.)

Voiding problems and a large volume of post-micturition residual urine become increasingly common with advancing age. Where surgical or pharmacological treatments are inappropriate or unsuccessful, the use of intermittent catheterisation should be considered. Many elderly people retain sufficient dexterity to catheterise themselves, although the urethral meatus may be more difficult for a woman to find if it has migrated back along the vaginal wall. If the patient cannot manage, a spouse or relative may be willing to learn the procedure, although it should never be presumed that both parties will feel comfortable with this. Otherwise, nursing help must be employed. Whether in hospital or community, if removing the residual urine will keep the patient continent, every effort should be made to ensure that this is done. Older people often require intermittent catheterisation far less frequently than younger people with voiding problems (see Chapter 8), as often the residual urine accumulates gradually. Once per day, or even on alternate days, is sometimes enough to restore continence. With a proportion of patients, bladder function will return over a period of weeks, so that catheterisation can be discontinued as residual volumes drop.

Instituting an intermittent catheterisation regime on a ward or in the community often involves a considerable readjustment of nursing routines (and attitudes). Once the idea has been accepted and the appropriate equipment ordered (such as adequate numbers of catheter packs and a good anglepoise light), it soon becomes routine. Nurses become acquainted with any anatomical idiosyncrasies of the patient, and each catheterisation only takes a few minutes, especially if timing is planned to fit in with the individual patient's daily routine (e.g. before getting up in the morning, so that undressing and dressing are unnecessary). It must be emphasised that when a nurse performs a catheterisation this should always be done aseptically, because of the risks of cross-infection. If the patient or a relative is doing it at home, a clean technique is perfectly acceptable (see Chapter 8).

ELDERLY PEOPLE WITH MENTAL INFIRMITIES

Only one in four people are likely to become mentally infirm in extreme old age. For those who do, there is a great spectrum of impairment, from slight memory loss and coarsening of personality traits to severe confusion and dementia. If impairment is severe, the individual may need institutional care. However, the majority of elderly mentally infirm people are cared for by relatives in their own homes.

Incontinence is seldom an inevitable feature of memory loss or dementia. Many people with dementia are not incontinent, as continence is so deeply ingrained in most people's socialisation that it is often one of the last social skills to be lost. Often, other causes of incontinence are overlooked and left untreated. The individual may be faecally impacted, have a urinary infection, or be immobile (King, 1979; 1980). Also, lower urinary tract dysfunction or a concomitant illness such as diabetes can be the precipitating factor. Depression, the most common affective disorder in older adults, often mimics dementia.

Elderly mentally infirm people depend on familiar surroundings for their level of functioning. Many of those living in their own homes, with familiar people and objects, can maintain a relatively normal lifestyle, even with quite advanced mental impairment. Sometimes incontinence results from disorientation, especially in changed surroundings. It is difficult for those with dementia to learn new things, and they may never become accustomed to a strange environment, even after prolonged residence. In a hospital or a home, clear signs and good lighting coupled with verbal reminders may help to promote continence. Patients should if possible be allowed to use the toilet with which they are familiar. A commode should not be introduced unless absolutely necessary, as to a disorientated person this may resemble an armchair, and may be counterproductive if its function is not understood.

Many older people do not like being asked if they wish to use the toilet and may deny their need, if not asked discreetly. A nurse asking publicly and in a loud voice will often be met with a refusal, or denial, even hostility.

It is important to expect continence. Too often demented people are expected to be incontinent and not given the opportunity or encouragement to be dry. In institutions, the routine may be geared to everyone being incontinent, with regular washing and changing routines. Indeed, it can be easier for staff, in the short term, to have a monotonous regular routine rather than positively promoting continence through rehabilitation and retraining, (Wells, 1975). If the nursing process is applied to each patient, realistic continence goals may be set for each individual.

Behavioural Assessment

An individual behavioural assessment can help to determine why incontinence is occurring. Some units have a clinical psychologist or clinical nurse specialist attached who can liaise with colleagues in the community. These health care professionals can make a valuable contribution to a team assessment of an elderly demented person who is incontinent.

If an individual cannot communicate his needs verbally, observation for any typical behaviour occurring prior to micturition or defaecation, e.g. getting up, wandering, pulling at clothes, or other verbal or non-verbal cues, should be established. If such cues are discovered and all carers made aware of them, needs can be responded to appropriately. By discovering the patient's past and present life history, what sort of person the patient was and what were his or her major past interests, activities and pet hates, it may be possible to deduce that incontinence is a symptom of apathy, protest or despair at a currently unacceptable life situation. If someone who has always been a solitary and shy person is expected to become accustomed to living, sleeping, dressing and eating with twenty-five other people, neither known nor naturally liked, it is not difficult to see why a formerly fastidious personality might crumble under the strain. Many people do become incontinent for the first time upon admission to residential accommodation, or soon thereafter, and this may be related to loss of independence, personal responsibility, and a sense of self-worth. It may also happen when being obliged to sell a home and move in with a son or daughter or other relative.

Some people seem to employ the defence mechanism of regression under such circumstances – becoming passive, dependent and often incontinent (Swaffield, 1988). By regressing to an infantile state they may be able to avoid facing the reality of their unacceptable situation. Occasionally incontinence can be interpreted as an expression of anger, as one of the few weapons available to the individual to use against carers. Incontinence may occur in the presence of one particular carer, or during a certain disliked activity or event – for example while being dressed or when pop music is on the radio, but not during preferred activities such as occupational therapy or watching certain TV programmes. It is often observed that patients who are seemingly 'hopelessly' incontinent on a ward may be dry for a whole day on a coach trip or other special occasion or outing.

Conversely, continence may also be due to the extra care given by particular nurses. Cheater (1987) showed in her study of nurses' attitudes to incontinence that continence in some patients only occurred when certain nurses were on duty.

The consequences of incontinence are also important to the behavioural assessment. In some circumstances incontinence may become rewarding, since it gains attention and creates a fuss. This is especially true in a socially impoverished situation such as an understaffed institution. The individual may get very little attention when dry or going to the lavatory independently – the staff are busy giving care to those who really need it. If incontinent, however, the individual will usually gain attention, often promptly. A member of staff will come, talk, touch, and usually smile. The patient may be taken to the bathroom for a wash or to be changed. Even if the staff member is angry or hostile, this may be better than no communication at all. The continent person may have nobody to talk to him between breakfast and lunch. The incontinent person gains physical and social contact every time incontinence occurs.

Great care must be taken not to attribute incontinence automatically to deliberate attention-seeking. It is seldom a conscious choice, especially for the confused person. However, it is important to be alert to staff practices which unwittingly reinforce the very behaviour that is least wanted. The same may be true of patients in the community. The incontinent person may benefit from considerably increased attention (e.g. the district nurse, the supplies officer delivering pads, the home care assistant to wash the sheets and give a bath, may all start to visit), whereas before becoming incontinent very few people visited. Again, it should not be interpreted as the patient's conscious choice to be incontinent, but there is certainly little incentive to try to remain dry.

In advanced dementia all social realisation of the desirability of continence may be lost. The individual may become completely uninhibited and, with no reason to try to hang on, will pass urine and faeces as and when he or she needs to. If the concept of a right and wrong place becomes meaningless, then clothes, bed, floor or furniture may be used indiscriminately. Urine and faeces are no longer seen as dirty or unpleasant, and may be played with or smeared when discovered. This will often seem particularly unacceptable behaviour to relatives or staff. Sometimes the recognition of what a lavatory is meant for is lost, so that even when taken to one, it is not used appropriately. The patient may sit on the toilet and do nothing, then be incontinent soon afterwards, or the restless person may refuse to sit at all. Alternatively, the distinction between a lavatory and other receptacles is lost, so that urine or faeces are passed into wastepaper bins, buckets, or any other receptacle which is to hand.

Most people have a lifetime of conditioned reflexes to pass urine while seated with no clothing over a toilet, in privacy and with the sensation of a full bladder. This familiarity needs to be utilised in helping people with dementia. It is all too easy to upset these conditioned reflexes by offering confusing stimuli (Newman, 1962). The individual may be repeatedly taken to the toilet when the bladder is not full, if no one has found out the most likely times that the toilet will be needed. Demented people who are being looked after often lead very regular lives, with meals and drinks served at routine times of the day. Each person's bladder and bowel will react differently to this – no two people are likely to have identical patterns of elimination, but the pattern for each individual is likely to be similar each day. An accurate chart will reveal any such pattern. If a confused person is repeatedly taken to the toilet and does not need to use it, the conceptual recognition of the purpose of the toilet will be destroyed. Likewise, a lack of privacy may militate against the use of the toilet.

It is not appropriate to sit those who are incontinent on an underpad with a bare bottom. Not only does this mean a lack of dignity for the patient but also gives a message that it is alright to pass urine or faeces there. This can lead to paradoxical micturition patterns – the individual does not pass urine if taken to the toilet but is incontinent as soon as he is relaxed, quiet and comfortable again in a chair or bed. This can be most frustrating and annoying for the carers, who often feel that the behaviour is deliberate. It must be understood that the individual is seldom trying to be awkward, but is merely responding to the confusing mixed stimuli provided by the carer.

It is common for those with dementia to deny the existence of their own incontinence. Sometimes they are well aware of the problem but are too ashamed to admit it to others. This can lead to attempting to hide the evidence – concealing soiled clothes or pads in a cupboard, or putting a clean sheet over a soiled one. Often the situation can become most unpleasant before anyone realises what is happening. If confronted, the person may become hostile and abusive or try to blame someone else (or the cat). Sometimes the person may be denying the situation even to himself, and be so distressed by his incontinence that he genuinely does not consciously know that it is happening. Often, in advanced dementia, the individual will be as oblivious of incontinence as he seems to be of his surroundings.

Nursing Interventions

Reality Orientation

It is very important to maintain a reality-orientated environment for confused elderly people, in order to keep as many conditioned responses to normal cues operative as possible. It has often been noted in hospitals that if patients are dressed in their own clothes (including appropriate underwear), and have their own possessions around them with plenty of stimulation and activities, incontinence is much less frequent. Information must be repeated frequently if it is to be retained. Staff should use the patient's own name often, in the form which the patient prefers (whether first name or surname or a lifelong nickname). Frequent use of diminutive endearments ('dearie', 'love') do little to keep the individual in touch. Conversation should include repeated use of reality cues – about time, place, weather, family or events.

Clear, easily-read clocks, calendars and signposts at an appropriate height can all help failing memories. Most institutions are attempting to move away from the large, featureless day area where everyone sits around on plastic chairs in a large circle (making any eye contact or communication difficult), with the endless drone of a TV set which no one is watching. Even within the constraints of staff and resource shortages, many small alterations can be made towards individualising care. Covering a hospital locker with photos and reminders of family, friends and former home, or having a large mirror with the person's name clearly written above his reflection, may help to remind the patient who he is. While recent memory may be poor, longer-term memories may be intact, and old records, picture books or conversations about the war often bring pleasure and recognition. People who are seemingly very confused may still be able to perform a lifetime's repetitive activity – a housewife may help with bedmaking, even if the result is slow and somewhat untidy. Art, drama and occupational therapy should all be used to the full where available. Many long-stay settings now have pets (such as a cat or budgie), outings, and frequent voluntary visitors. By keeping people as stimulated and occupied and as motivated as possible, and by using carefully planned repeated information for teaching, it is possible to maximise the level of functioning of confused people. This is of course desirable in its own right. As an added bonus, continence is often greatly improved.

Behaviour Modification

Behaviour modification techniques may be used to help confused elderly people to be continent, in much the same way as for people with learning difficulties (see Chapter 14). By reinforcing the desired behaviour (i.e. continence, and passing urine or faeces in the correct place) and extinguishing the undesired behaviour (i.e. incontinence), it is often possible to use the theories of operant conditioning to promote continence (Burgio, 1986).

The aim is to reverse the attention pattern outlined above – to give attention, praise and physical contact for continence, and to withdraw these when incontinence occurs. To be effective, everyone who comes into contact with the patient must understand and carry out the procedure, so that consistency is maintained. Every time someone approaches the individual and he is continent, he should be rewarded (by a smile, praise, a hug – an appropriate reinforcer should be chosen for each patient). If using the lavatory correctly, or he indicates the need to go appropriately, the reinforcement should be given as promptly as possible. When incontinence occurs it must of course be dealt with, but this should be done with a minimal amount of fuss and attention – no smiles, no conversation, and minimal physical contact. Punishment is not warranted. This procedure can be used for day incontinence (Grosicki, 1968), or night incontinence (Hartie and Black, 1975; Barker, 1979), and will, if used consistently over a sufficiently long period, often several months, restore continence for some individuals. It is often possible to teach relatives to use such a programme at home if they are highly motivated.

Advanced Dementia

In the advanced stages of dementia all these attempts to achieve continence might fail. It is important that carers (whether relatives or staff) are not made to feel guilty or inadequate because of such failures. For some people incontinence does become inevitable, even with the best available care and treatment. At present we have to accept this. Regular toileting, if the individual will use the toilet, may 'catch' some of the incontinence in the daytime, especially if it is timed to coincide with the most likely times as revealed by an incontinence chart. There seems little point in repeated awakenings at night as the patient will often become more confused if tired, and will usually benefit more from a good night's sleep than from repeated toileting, unless obviously awake and agitated.

Probably the most important aspect of care is to provide high-quality incontinence pads, in ample quantities, and of a type which are as easy as possible to use. A good pad will protect the skin, protect the environment and clothing, minimise odour, and maintain the dignity of the individual. (The selection and use of continence products is discussed in detail in Chapter 15.) Wherever the demented person is being cared for, it should be possible to relieve many of the most unacceptable aspects of incontinence, and enable him to spend his last years in relative comfort.

INCONTINENCE IN TERMINAL ILLNESS

Many people become incontinent, often doubly, in the final stages of a terminal illness. This can be a tremendous burden on carers and cause psychological suffering to the patient. Incontinence of urine may occur because of any of the causes outlined elsewhere in this book. The most likely causes include neurological disease and cerebral clouding, the effects of which may often be exacerbated by immobility and loss of independence. It can also be the result of constipation. Faecal incontinence can often be prevented by good bowel management – to prevent constipation and impaction or to regulate the neurogenic bowel (see Chapter 10).

Vigorous investigation will seldom be desirable for a terminally ill person, but some incontinence can be reversed by judicious use of drugs for an unstable detrusor, the use of hand-held urinals, and by alerting carers to the need for individual but regular toileting regimes. If incontinence persists, a good quality pad or appliance may contain it.

If leakage is heavy, or movement to a urinal or commode becomes painful and difficult, an indwelling catheter should be seen as a positive alternative. If the patient accepts a catheter, long-term risks can be discounted and it may enable a dying person to spend the last days at home. Relatives can be reassured that if they sleep or go out, the patient will not be lying in a pool of urine or needing assistance. Catheter education given to relatives will be an essential teaching role for the nurse discharging a patient home or when supervising care.

A bladder or bowel fistula as part of a terminal illness can prove tremendously distressing, and is one of the most difficult problems to deal with. A faecal collector, a wound drainage collector or stoma equipment may be adapted to prevent digestion of the skin by enzymes. Failing that, a highly absorbent pad in an adult size or an adult diaper may be effective in management.

Uncontrolled incontinence makes the development of a pressure sore more likely, and in the emaciated person this risk is increased. For women, a catheter should prevent this occurring and thereby avoid extra pain and distress. Men may find a penile sheath is as effective as a catheter, as long as the carer is sure that the bladder is emptying completely.

CONCLUSION

Throughout this chapter the need for a good knowledge base of the causes of incontinence in older people has been advocated. Nurses and carers have a responsibility for changing the myth that age inevitably brings incontinence. The need to see each elderly patient as an individual and as having individual bladder and bowel habits has been presented as crucial to the diagnosis of the cause of incontinence. The progress of treatment of those with a contributing disease, in dementia and during a terminal illness has been highlighted. Throughout the changes in the Health Service and the differing environments of care following the implementation of the NHS and Community Care Act in 1993, it is essential that protocols are jointly arranged so that positive care is given to elderly incontinent people, rather than an acceptance of incontinence (Swaffield, 1994). The multidisciplinary team must also evaluate the outcome of the care given, through a systematic review of cases (Swaffield, 1995). Careful assessment of individual needs for products to manage intractable incontinence is needed when the other treatment and management options have been exhausted or are inappropriate.

REFERENCES AND FURTHER READING

Armstrong, D., 1980. *An Outline of Sociology as Applied to Medicine.* John Wright, Bristol.

Armstrong-Esther, C. A., Hawkins, L. H., 1982. Day for night. Circadian rhythms in the elderly. *Nursing Times* 78, 30: 1263–5.

Barker, P., 1979. Nocturnal enuresis; an experimental study involving two behavioural approaches. *International Journal of Nursing Studies*, 16: 319–27.

Brocklehurst, J. C., Dillane, J. B., Griffiths, L., Fry, J., 1968. The prevalence and symptomatology of urinary infection in an aged population. *Gerontologica Clinica*, 10: 242–53.

Brocklehurst, J. C., 1977. The causes and management of incontinence in the elderly. *Nursing Mirror*, 144: 15.

Brocklehurst, J. C., 1978. The genitourinary system. In: Brocklehurst, J. C. (ed), *Textbook of Geriatric Medicine and Gerontology* (2nd edn). Churchill Livingstone, Edinburgh and London.

Brumfitt, W., Hamilton-Miller, J. M. T., 1987. The appropriate use of diagnostic services. Investigations of urinary infections in general practice – are we wasting facilities? *Health Bulletin* 45, 1: 5–10.

Burgio, K., 1986. Behavioural geriatrics: application of operant procedures to the control of urinary incontinence. *Behavioural Therapy*, 9: 67.

Cheater, F., 1987. Incontinence: a nursing perspective. *Nursing Times*, 18, 83: 46.

Department of Health, 1991. An agenda for action on continence services. Department of Health, London.

Donaldson, L. J., 1983. Survival and functional capacity. *Journal of Epidemiology and Community Health*, 37: 176–9.

Fantl, J. A., Cardozo, L., McClish, D. K., 1994. Estrogen therapy in the management of urinary incontinence in postmenopausal women: a meta-analysis. *Obstetrics and Gynaecology*, 83, 1: 12–18.

Goffman, E., 1961. *Asylums*. Doubleday Anchor, New York.

Grosicki, J. P., 1968. Effect of operant conditioning on modification of incontinence in neuropsychiatric geriatric patients. *Nursing Research*, 17: 304–11.

Hartie, A., Black, D., 1975. A dry bed is the objective. *Nursing Times*, 71: 1874–6.

Keister, K. J., 1989. Medication of elderly institutionalised incontinent females. *Journal of Advanced Nursing*, 14, 11: 980–5.

King, M. R., 1979. A study of incontinence in a psychiatric hospital. *Nursing Times*, 75, 26: 1133–5.

King, M. R., 1980. Treatment of incontinence. *Nursing Times*, 76, 23: 1006–10.

Miller, A., 1985. Nurse patient dependency – is it iatrogenic? *Journal of Advanced Nursing*, 10: 63–9.

Mohide, A., 1992. The prevalence of urinary incontinence. In: Roe, B. H., (ed), *Clinical Nursing Practice*. Prentice Hall, London.

NHS and Community Care Act, 1990. HM Government, Westminster.

Newman, J. L., 1962. Old folks in wet beds. *British Medical Journal*, 1: 1824–7.

OPCS, 1987. *Registrar General's 1987 Estimates*. HMSO, London.

Roberts, A., 1989. The ageing urinary system. Systems of life 169, Senior systems; 34. *Nursing Times*, 85, 10: 59–62.

Robertson, I., 1986. Learned helplessness. *Nursing Times*, 82, 51: 28–30.

Rooker, J., 1992. *Community Continence Services*. Labour Party, London.

Royal College of Physicians of London, 1992. *The CARE Scheme. Clinical Audit of Longterm Care of Elderly People*. RCP, London.

Sanford, J. R., 1975. Tolerance of debility in elderly dependents by supporters at home: its significance for hospital practice. *British Medical Journal*, 3: 471–3.

Scambler, G., 1986. Illness behaviour. In: Patrick, D. L., Scambler, G., (eds), *Sociology as Applied to Medicine*. Balliere Tindall, England.

Swaffield, J., 1986. Avoiding incontinence – health education and preventive care. *Nursing*, 10: 6–7.

Swaffield, J., 1988. Motivating for continence. *Nursing Times*, 84, 43: 56–9.

Swaffield, J., 1994. The management and development of continence services within the framework of the NHS and Community Care Act 1990. *Journal of Clinical Nursing*, 3: 119–24.

Swaffield, J., 1995. Quality audit – a review of the literature concerning delivery of continence care. *Journal of Clinical Nursing* (in press).

Wells, T., 1975. Promoting urinary continence in the elderly in hospital. *Nursing Times*, 71, 48: 1908–9.

Zola, I, 1973. Pathways to the doctor: from person to patient. *Social Science and Medicine*, 7: 677–89.

Chapter 12

Continence in the Community

Mary Dolman, BSc, RGN, ET
Continence Adviser, East Berkshire Community Health NHS Trust

The majority of incontinent people live in their own homes, but others will be in residential or extended-care units or nursing homes, and some will be in a community hospital for long- or short-term respite care. Increasingly the emphasis is for care within the community, with a decrease in long-term hospital care. This chapter discusses continence care and services available for people in the various community settings. Much of what has been written in the rest of this book applies equally to people in the community, no matter which community setting they are in, so this chapter should not be read in isolation.

COMMUNITY ISSUES

Prevention

Nurses need a sound knowledge of bladder and bowel control before it is possible to educate and communicate effectively with the members of the community at large.

Prevention can start with school nurses educating all pupils about good bladder and bowel care as part of the healthy lifestyle message, as well as teaching senior girls about the function of the pelvic floor muscles. Physical education teachers may also get involved, and incorporate pelvic floor exercise within a general fitness programme. Midwives should emphasise the need for pelvic floor exercises to pregnant women; post-natally, the general practitioner, health visitor or practice nurse have an ideal opportunity at the six-week check-up to ask questions about bladder or bowel control. Table 12.1 (overleaf) summarises simple potential health education messages for the community.

Home Care

Most incontinent people live in their own homes and cope with their incontinence, often remarkably well, managing to control the problem

Table 12.1   Health Education for Continence Promotion

Avoid constipation. Eat a balanced diet.
Adequate fluid intake, approximately 3 pints (1.5 litres) daily.
Effective pelvic floor exercise programme for women for LIFE.
Allow normal bladder function: fill, store and empty completely.
Recognise the role of oestrogen.
Do not become overweight.
Limit medications wherever possible.
Keep a healthy mind and body.
Encourage people to talk about elimination concerns.
General fitness and exercise benefits pelvic floor tone.
Treat chronic cough, give up smoking?
Avoid voluntary frequency ('just-in-case' micturition).
Don't ignore signals from a full bladder or bowel indefinitely.

---

so that it creates only minimal disruption to their lives. At best, there may be just a little extra laundry or more items for disposal. But where incontinence is very heavy, or poorly managed, it can become such a burden that it dominates home life, eventually leading to a breakdown of the ability to live independently or to be maintained at home by carers. Success in managing incontinence at home will often depend upon who is available and their willingness to help, what washing and disposal facilities there are, and which services can be mobilised to assist.

Self-Care

The taboo on talking about elimination problems is at last lifting. People now have the opportunity to look after their own bladder and bowel problems by talking to knowledgeable nurses in the community and following their advice. Many measures can be taken towards self-care, but people need information to enable them to make informed choices. And even with good information, people may fail to comply with health care advice.

A poor diet may be due to the lack of motivation to prepare meals, especially for people living alone, and the high cost of fresh food. Others do not have the knowledge to select a 'balanced' diet with adequate fibre content. The effort of shopping or cooking may deter from proper self-care. Nutritional advice, arrangements for shopping or the provision of meals-on-wheels could overcome some problems. Liaison with the community dietitian may also be helpful.

Personal hygiene may be a problem, often due to apathy. The patient may need encouragement to re-establish personal hygiene to avoid skin and odour problems. Personal assistance may be needed.

Care Givers in the Home

Most care givers in the home are family members, close relatives, or partially-trained home carers, and as such have often not been adequately prepared for promoting continence or managing incontinence. It has been estimated that there are over six million informal carers in the UK. Given the strong intrusion of urinary or faecal incontinence into everyday life, it seems remarkable that people do not always seek advice or help earlier or more frequently.

Someone who is not completely self-sufficient in toileting is dependent on others. The availability of help at the required time will often determine whether or not incontinence occurs. An individual's toileting pattern can be recorded on a weekly chart. This will identify the times a carer needs to prompt or assist that person to the toilet. If, however, the incontinent person lives alone, or with an elderly, frail spouse, effective management must be planned by the visiting community nurse.

When incontinence occurs, the longer the time lapse between wetting and changing, the greater the likelihood of discomfort, skin problems and odour. Many district nurses will realise the need for frequent visits to the individual for toileting or changing appliances and can arrange for home carers (either health or social services) to do this. Planning a regime within available staffing levels is often very difficult (even unrealistic in some cases), but it is necessary to try to organise the team, particularly to meet the needs of a disabled person living alone.

The help that is available may be unacceptable, either to the patient or to the carer. Many people are embarrassed for a partner or offspring to aid with toileting, especially to assist in the more intimate tasks of cleansing and washing. They may be ashamed of wet or soiled clothing and prefer not to seek or accept help, even when needed. A partner may be willing to assist in all the activities of daily living except elimination. It should not be assumed that because a relative is willing to care, they will also be at ease with all the tasks that this entails. A daughter who will readily feed, wash and dress a parent may draw the line at cleaning up excreta. A carer who will tolerate much inconvenience and hard work may not tolerate the continual problems of incontinence, and it is at this stage that respite care is essential.

Certain treatments for incontinence may be impossible to implement when no one is available to help. Bladder training can be particularly difficult. It is no use working out ideal toileting times for someone who is dependent and alone. No amount of medication or training can postpone micturition indefinitely. For the forgetful, an alarm clock may be useful, but it has to be reset for the next time. People who are forgetful about visiting the toilet will also forget to reset the alarm. The hard-of-hearing may benefit from a vibrating or flashing light mechanism, but this is body-worn and only operates once urine has started to flow. This system is not successful for all frail elderly people, but should be kept in mind as a possible method of management.

Where a family is caring for a very incontinent person in the home, their role must be recognised and supported. Too often those who appear to be coping well are left alone, when really they could benefit from more help, both as support and practical measures. Where the official support is stretched to its limits there are voluntary organisations which may be able to help. Such organisations as the Multiple Sclerosis Society, Association for Spina Bifida and Hydrocephalus, the Red Cross, the Women's Royal Voluntary Service and Age Concern may provide practical help as well as support and advice. Appendix 2 gives addresses of voluntary organisations. Most have a telephone service which can offer advice and information leaflets on the varied aspects of incontinence and its management.

Incontinent people and their assistants need to know what help is available and how to access it. Most health authorities have a continence adviser who acts as a resource person and he or she will have the knowledge to point people in the right direction.

Respite Care
Respite care enables the individual to be admitted into a twenty-four hour care facility in order to give the principal carers at home a 'break'. Respite care facilities are available in most communities, either in a community hospital or residential or nursing home. Carers often feel guilty about the planned separation, and good communication skills are needed by the nurse to emphasise the psychological benefits for all concerned. The district nurse is usually the key person to arrange respite care and it can be planned at frequent intervals, e.g. two weeks in every six, for a heavily dependent individual.

ASSESSMENT AT HOME

The emphasis should always be on ways to keep people continent, and the assessment will highlight the action which can be taken by the nurse to promote continence. Community nurses should be trained by the continence adviser to do a continence assessment (see Chapter 3). Table 12.2 suggests some factors specific to a home assessment. The assessment should not be merely a requisition for pads or appliances. Community nurses can ask for advice from the continence adviser on treatment or investigations rather than just ordering incontinence pads. Most continence advisers will do a joint home visit with a community nurse when necessary. This assists the nurse in learning. Decisions should be a team effort wherever possible and this may include advice and assessment from the general practitioner, community physiotherapist or occupational therapist.

Table 12.2   Factors to Consider in Home Assessment

Double/single bed: patient sleeps alone or with spouse.
Bed protection: mattress covers, draw sheets.
Washing machine: would reusable bed/chair pads be appropriate?
Upstairs/downstairs toilet: distance to toilet.
Commode required: can it be unobtrusive? Who will clean/empty it?
Toilet adaptations: raised seat, grab rails, toilet frame.
Carpet protection: non-slip plastic covering.
Disposal of incontinence pads.
Community laundry service.
Odour control.
Who else lives with the client or visits regularly?
Ventilation.
Standards of hygiene.
Availability of home carers/nurses.
Voluntary organisations: meals on wheels, taxi services, WRVS.
Pad delivery services.

Nearly all health authorities now have a community policy and assessment form which community nurses complete to order incontinence pads for an individual at home. Very often the policy states the minimum/maximum daily pad allowance for an individual because of budget restrictions. Although this is not totally satisfactory, it does give a measure of control on the budget. The total needs may not be met by the health authority – a 'help towards' the need is all most budgets will allow.

When an individual requires incontinence pads, the assessment form is usually sent to the continence adviser or nurse manager for authorisation to supply the patient. The patient is informed of the collection times from the issuing point, usually a health centre. In some communities a pad delivery service operates. Reassessments should be made at four- or six-monthly intervals for the supply to be continued and to make adjustments to the requirements, if necessary.

The community continence service should have a computerised database which stores patient records and information, products used, stock control and costings (e.g. Thompson, 1990). The assessment forms received from community nurses should be put directly into the computer. The information (such as monthly and annual expenditure, caseload per carer) enables the continence adviser to monitor assessments so that advice and support can be offered to the community nurse if problems become apparent. A computerised service is essential to produce information for managers and predict future trends and costs.

THE HOME ENVIRONMENT

Where large quantities of pads are used in the home, disposal can be a problem. There are no fully biodegradable plastics available. Although some companies claim that their products are biodegradable, the plastic is in fact mixed with starch, which enables the polymers to break down into very small pieces that cannot be seen by the human eye, but which nevertheless remain in the soil.

Most people simply wrap used pads or appliances in newspaper or a polythene bag and put them in the dustbin, but this may contravene public health regulations in some areas. Refuse collectors in many districts are not obliged to collect rubbish which is known to contain incontinence pads. In practice, most turn a blind eye – provided that a sealed bin-liner is used. However, it makes good and practical sense to ask the local authority for their guidance on the procedure they would want to be followed in their area.

Some health authorities issue disposal sacks with their deliveries of incontinence pads. These may be heavy-duty plastic bags or waxed paper sacks. The environmental health department may offer a soiled pads collection service on a weekly basis. Indeed, some specify that all incontinence items should be collected by this service rather than by the domestic refuse service.

Disposal is even more of a problem for incontinent people who venture out of the home. Few male public toilets have any disposal facilities, and even female toilets with sanitary-towel incinerators or bins seldom have a suitable receptacle for larger pads. Going to work, visiting friends and relatives – indeed any social situation – can present a problem for disposal of used products, and most people simply have to wrap up the used items and take them home.

There has been a move towards the increased use of reusable items. This method of management may not be suitable for many people, and assessment will determine which facilities are available. Many people do not have a washing machine, spin drier or tumble drier. Some do not have a decent-sized sink, hot water, or a garden for drying reusable pads. There may be no laundry service, and in some cases the home is literally taken over by the volume of soiled or drying linen. If only one sink is available, it is unhygienic to have to wash soiled laundry in the same place as food and crockery. Arthritic hands cannot wring linen effectively, and frail people may not be able to wash efficiently to remove traces of soiling. The costs and problems of washing reusable products may outweigh the cost of disposable items.

There is often a shared responsibility between health and social services to provide a laundry service, but the demand for the service may be greater than the capacity. Unless the service is very efficient and reliable, the incontinent person is at risk of being left without linen when a delivery is delayed. Collections and deliveries may only be on a weekly basis and soiled linen can become most unpleasant within that time. There is an urgent need to provide an efficient laundry service if care in the community is to work. Thought also has to be given on how to avoid users of the service being stigmatised, for example by having to leave distinctive bags on the doorstep, and ensuring that people have sufficient linen to enable them to wait for deliveries. Some authorities operate a linen loan service.

A few people can take advantage of launderette facilities at a day centre and some local authorities will provide washing machines via the social services. People in receipt of benefits may be entitled to claim a single payment to meet extra costs incurred because of incontinence. Certain charitable organisations offer a one-off payment to replace such items as a bed, chair or clothing.

Appendix 2 gives the Department of Social Security Freephone number to call for details of benefits available.

COMMUNITY SERVICES

Most health authorities where a continence adviser is employed offer regular community continence clinics, and these are often available for all age groups and both sexes. The advantage of the clinic is that the specialist nurse will usually take self-referrals, so an embarrassed patient does not have to go to the doctor first. Continence clinics should be advertised in prominent locations, e.g. surgery waiting areas, the library notice board and local papers, with a named person and telephone number to contact. Eye-catching posters can help to inform the general public of how common bladder and bowel problems are, and also that advice and treatment are available.

The district nurse and general practitioner and health visitor are the key people to mobilise services for disabled and elderly people, school nurses and community medical officers for school-age children, and health visitors for children under five years. These key people should know how to liaise with specialist areas for the particular need of the patient/client. For example, a child with behavioural disturbance and enuresis may well be referred to a clinical psychologist.

Team work – knowing when to refer and to whom – is the essence of a community team member. There is a growing number of services available to help keep an individual in their own homes. Perhaps the fastest growing is the community psychiatric nursing service, with expertise on clients with psychiatric disorders and dementias.

Nursing terminally ill people at home can be made easier by support from teams of Marie Curie nurses and Macmillan nurses. Their role is slightly different. Macmillan nurses counsel and visit the home on a regular basis for short periods. Marie Curie nurses can sit with the patient day and/or night and perform nursing care. It is usually possible to arrange an emergency provision of incontinence products for terminally ill patients.

The community team includes social workers who advise on grants for home adaptations and financial assistance. The community physiotherapist may be asked to improve mobility or teach correct lifting techniques. The occupational therapist can assess self-care skills and improve these with instruction or aids. The chiropodist or optician may help a person to remain independent, by assessing walking and vision. Home care assistants can clean a home, organise washing, shopping, bathe an individual or prepare food, and these services and their availability often determine whether or not a person can remain at home.

Luncheon clubs, day centres, or good-neighbour schemes can provide social contact or practical help to an individual. Having a caring environment often preserves an individual's continence, or brings the problem out in the open so that help and treatment can be given.

It is the responsibility of community 'key workers' to devise individually-tailored packages of care to enable people with care needs to remain in their own homes for as long as is feasible.

Community Hospital Care

Within any community hospital unit there will generally be a day centre, rehabilitation wards and facilities for respite and long-stay care, including for elderly or mentally ill people. These facilities are increasing throughout the country because of the increasing elderly population. The goals for continence will be the same in any of these areas, and some standards for care are given below.

When a patient is in hospital for rehabilitation, the success or failure of the rehabilitation programme will often be determined by whether the incontinence can be brought under control, either by cure or appropriate containment. All members of the rehabilitation team must be involved in trying to restore the individual to continence: the nurse in planning bladder training and creating a positive environment, possibly involving reality orientation or behaviour modification (see Chapter 11); the physiotherapist by mobilising the patient; the occupational therapist by enhancing independence in daily living activities, improving dexterity and assessing for the most appropriate aids; the social worker addresses social and financial problems and the doctor prescribes any necessary medication or specialised investigations. Continence is everyone's responsibility and hence standards of care must be interdisciplinary. Because continence often requires an interdisciplinary assessment to set goals and plan an individual's care, the team must develop and agree the same standards and have the same aims, objectives and measurable outcomes for clinical audit. (See Table 12.3, overleaf, for an example of a mission statement, aims and objectives.)

Individual Assessment

The importance of individual interdisciplinary assessment of a patient in a rehabilitation or long-stay ward cannot be over-emphasised. Many studies have found that multiple problems are usually contributing to incontinence for each person, but that each will have a unique

*Table 12.3   Community Hospital – Interdisciplinary
Continence Service*

MISSION STATEMENT

All elderly persons have the right to be continent. They are entitled to a complete interdisciplinary assessment to establish the cause of the urinary/faecal incontinence. Investigations and interventions will be initiated to enable the elderly person to achieve continence. Where continence is unachievable, the individual will be managed in the most appropriate way to preserve dignity and quality of life.

AIM

Nurses, physiotherapists, occupational therapists, social workers, liaison visitors to the elderly and the medical staff will be involved in assessing each individual's physical, psychological and social ability to remain continent.

OBJECTIVES

1) To rehabilitate the elderly person to self-care wherever possible.
2) To determine the amount of supervision/help required for toileting.
3) To enable the incontinent elderly person to manage continence with the correct appliances or aids according to individual need.
4) All members of the interdisciplinary team will have knowledge and skills in promoting continence and managing incontinence.

(Dolman, 1993)

combination of factors needing attention (Lepine et al., 1979; King, 1979, 1980). Untreated medical conditions, drug side effects, constipation, urinary tract infection, immobility, depression, disorientation and a whole variety of other problems may be implicated (see Chapters 2 and 3 for the causes and assessment of incontinence). Until it has been discovered why each person is incontinent, any attempt at remedy is unlikely to be effective. Although such individual assessment is initially time-consuming, the long-term benefits include the patient's dignity as well as satisfaction for the nurses.

Standards

It would be difficult for any member of the interdisciplinary team to work in isolation on a common problem such as incontinence, and all members of the team need to set standards from which to work. This prevents overlap of work and the team is able to work to the same set of goals. A measurable outcome will be easy to audit and the quality of care can be determined.

The three examples in Table 12.4 have been extracted from standards in the author's Community NHS Trust (Dolman, 1993). There are ten standards applicable to the rehabilitation and long-stay wards, and there is also a section for the day hospital. This unit has introduced clinical audit for the interdisciplinary team for care of the elderly.

Table 12.4   Example of Standards for the Interdisciplinary Team

---

CARING FOR ELDERLY PEOPLE. REHABILITATION/LONG-STAY WARDS

Standard 1

Patients who have urinary or faecal incontinence twice or more a month will commence a continence chart (frequency/volume chart) for one week.

STRUCTURE

A continence chart will be used as part of the assessment for one week.

PROCESS

1) All members of the interdisciplinary team involved with the patient will record on the continence chart
2) The following data will be recorded:

TU = toilet used
TNU = toilet not used
D = dry
W = wet
BO = bowels open
FI = faecally incontinent

OUTCOME

1) The frequency of incontinence will be determined.
2) Further investigations may be indicated so that the type of incontinence can be diagnosed.

---

continued overleaf

Table 12.4   (continued)

Standard 2
The interdisciplinary team will assess the patient for the contributory factors to incontinence.

STRUCTURE
The Barthel Index will be used to assess the contributory factors to incontinence (Mahoney, 1965).

PROCESS
Team members will record the scores as follows:

BOWELS   2 = continent, self-administers suppositories or laxatives
              1 = accidents less than one a week, aid with enema from someone else
              0 = any worse grade of incontinence

BLADDER   2 = continent, completely dry or self-care of catheter
              1 = accidents, less than one a day, help with device
              0 = any worse grade of incontinence

DRESSING   2 = dresses independently
              1 = some help with dressing
              0 = dependent or more help with dressing

TRANSFER   3 = independent
              2 = needs minor help
              1 = needs major help
              0 = unable

TOILET USE   2 = independent
              1 = needs help
              0 = dependent

WALKING   3 = independent
              2 = walks with aid
              1 = wheelchair independent
              0 = unable

OUTCOME
The level of independence/dependence will have been assessed in order to manage bladder and bowel elimination independently, with help, or totally dependent.

Table 12.4 (continued)

Standard 3
Treatment for urinary incontinence will commence following assessment and investigations.

STRUCTURE
Following the interdisciplinary assessment and investigations, the type of urinary incontinence will be diagnosed and recorded so that the correct treatment can be commenced.

PROCESS
1) Pelvic floor exercises will be taught to females and post-prostatectomy males where cognition and understanding remain.
2) Physiotherapists may consider interferential treatment.
3) Antibiotic therapy will be prescribed by the medical staff for proven urinary tract infection.
4) Anticholinergic therapy may be prescribed for detrusor instability by the medical staff where there is no significant residual urine (i.e. under 100ml).
5) Nursing staff will commence a bladder retraining programme for the patient where appropriate.
6) Timed voiding patterns will be maintained by the interdisciplinary staff.
7) Appropriate clothing and aids will be organised by the occupational therapists.
8) Intermittent catheterisation may be suitable for the person with an acontractile bladder.
9) Long-term catheterisation may be the treatment of choice.

OUTCOME
Each individual patient will have the correct method of treatment for the type of urinary incontinence which has been diagnosed.

(Dolman, 1993)

Discharge from Hospital

When an incontinent person is to be discharged from hospital, successful transition to coping at home depends on careful planning and liaison between hospital and community services. Written information to supplement verbal instructions, such as how to obtain help, manage equipment or obtain supplies, is advisable. Most units will have a discharge planning policy, and liaison with the community services is often carried out by the liaison visitors to the elderly. This will entail asking the district nurse to assess for and order supplies before the patient is discharged, so that there is no delay in supplies being available once the patient is home. Discharge planning should be commenced in plenty of time, although patients are all too frequently sent home without sufficient incontinence supplies for more than a day or two, and the carers experience much anxiety. Policies should be written to avoid such anxieties for the carers.

The Department of Health has emphasised the importance of ensuring that before patients are discharged from hospital, proper arrangements are made for their return home and for any community care which may be necessary. The Parliamentary Select Committee emphasised the need:

1) to provide families with the necessary information and reassurance about the care of the patient after discharge,
2) to check on day of departure that the patient was fit to leave hospital,
3) to inform the patient's general practitioner/community nursing services/social services of the patient's potential needs in time for them to be met,
4) to secure therapy assessment prior to discharge, and to ensure that facilities in the home are appropriate to the needs of the patient concerned.

If these criteria are followed, incontinent patients returning home should receive an unbroken chain of individualised care.

Staff Attitudes

Staff working in community units must have a positive attitude towards promoting continence and not merely accept incontinence as inevitable. Education for all grades of staff must be readily available on the causes and effects of incontinence. Most continence advisers organise educational sessions for community staff on a regular basis and also educate through nursing and midwifery colleges, ENB courses (post-registration) and universities. Today, there is no excuse for remaining ignorant about incontinence, and staff attitudes are changing to a much more positive approach.

RESIDENTIAL AND LONG-STAY CARE

Scott et al., (1990) found that incontinence in different types of care settings is by no means uniform (Table 12.5).

Table 12.5   Urinary Incontinence in Different Care Settings

SETTING	% INCONTINENT
Community	9%
Private Residential	18%
Local Authority	16%
Private nursing	32%
Psychogeriatric	57%
Geriatric medicine	59%
Continuing care	75%

(Scott et al., 1990)

Many of the conditions which lead to admission into care are associated with incontinence (Buchan, 1991). Incontinence is itself a major reason for admission to long-term care.

The factors contributing to incontinence in old age have been covered in Chapter 11 and the methods for promoting continence in the community, already discussed in this chapter, also apply to care in residential settings. Carers are often unqualified and may not understand why an elderly person is more susceptible to incontinence. Education for these carers is essential. Carers' attitudes become more and more important as dependence increases.

In residential homes, an individual's identity may all too easily be submerged in the institutionalisation of the surroundings, and in consequence loss of part or all of the person's motivation, self-respect and interest may occur, leading to institutional apathy with staff indifference (Irvine, 1991).

REFERENCES AND FURTHER READING

Buchan, R., 1991. A nursing trial of absorbent disposable incontinence pads. *Care of the Elderly*, 3, 2: 81–4.

Dolman, M. 1993. *Multidisciplinary Approach to Continence in the Elderly: Standards.* East Berkshire Community NHS Trust, Maidenhead.

Irvine, L., 1991. Paving the way to self-control: Maintaining continence in elderly people. *Professional Nurse*, November: 94–7.

King, M. R., 1979. A study on incontinence in a psychiatric hospital. *Nursing Times*, 75: 1133–5.

King, M. R., 1980. Treatment of incontinence. *Nursing Times*, 76: 1006–10.

Lepine, A., et al., 1979. The incidence and management of incontinence in a home for the elderly. *Health and Social Services Journal*, 89: E9–12.

Mahoney, F. I., Barthel, D. W., 1965. *Maryland State Medical Journal*, February. Rehabilitation Section: 61–5.

Scott, D. J., et al., 1990; Functional capacity and mental status of elderly people in long-term care in West Glasgow. *Health Bulletin*, 48: 17–24.

Thompson, J., 1990. Managing continence systematically. *Nursing Times* 86, 46: 60–2.

Chapter 13

Aids to Continence for People with Physical Disabilities

Helen White, RGN, RHV

Director, Continence Project, Prom-o-Con, Manchester

Many people with physical disabilities have a neurogenic bladder or bowel problem which impairs their continence. Chapter 8 discusses the different types of neuropathic bladder and their management, Chapter 10 discusses bowel problems. It is important to be aware that many people with disabilities will have urgency, others have difficulty emptying, or may need to use assisted techniques such as intermittent catheterisation or manual bowel evacuation.

However, many of these people are rendered incontinent not by a bladder or bowel problem, but by a poorly adapted environment. Even those with completely normal functions may become incontinent if their physical difficulties are severe enough. This chapter considers methods by which people with a physical disability may be helped to be independently continent. The aids to toileting mentioned in this chapter, together with many more, are listed in the Disabled Living Foundation *Hamilton Index* (1995) Part 3, section 14, and hand-held urinals can be found in the Continence Foundation *Directory of Continence Products* (1995). These directories give details of suppliers, approximate price and dimensions of items available in the UK.

Assessment for appropriate aids is often multidisciplinary and may be led by an occupational therapist, physiotherapist or nurse, as local circumstances and skills dictate. Most health authorities and social services departments supply some of these items, although the range may be limited in some areas. Disabled Living Centres generally offer an assessment service and have a range of items to view or even to try.

CONTINENCE IN PUBLIC PLACES

Many public buildings and amenities are poorly equipped for the needs of disabled people, especially regarding the provision of suitable lavatories (Cunningham and Norton, 1993). Although toilets adapted for people with disabilities are becoming more common, especially in new buildings, there are still many situations in which it is impossible for someone with limited mobility to reach a lavatory. Many obstacles are obvious, such as a flight of steps, a door too narrow to admit a walking aid or wheelchair, or an inwardly opening door in a cubicle too small to allow the door to be closed with a wheelchair inside. Other obstacles are more subtle, such as poor signposting or ambiguous labels on doors which disadvantage those with visual impairment. Where there are no specially adapted facilities, wheelchair access is seldom possible, and an escort of the opposite sex cannot accompany and help. Encouragingly, the new high-speed trains and certain airlines are introducing more accessible lavatories, but there is no certainty that these will be available when travelling. Facilities on most trains and planes remain difficult to use, even for people with minor levels of impairment.

All too often the person with a disability is excluded from activities because the lavatory facilities are inadequate. Journeys or holidays are difficult unless facilities are already known to the individual. Shopping must always be done in centres with an accessible lavatory. Visits to the cinema, theatre, or other places of entertainment must always be preceded by enquiries. Going to a pub for a drink is often impossible. Some people even have to give up a job which they are perfectly capable of doing because the nearest lavatory is two floors down. Even where there are specially designed facilities, access to them is not always guaranteed. Some are poorly designed, without reference to available guidelines, and may just have a grab-rail as a token gesture. Sometimes a tried and trusted convenience is suddenly closed because of vandalism, lack of staff, or as part of expenditure cut-backs. Time and time again the activities of people with physical disabilities are determined not by personal preference but by public provision for their needs.

This situation is improving, and public awareness increasing. Most new public buildings now have reasonable facilities. Even those not covered by legislation, such as private hotels, often have specially adapted rooms. Some districts have entered a scheme of keeping toilets for people with disabilities locked to avoid vandalism (National Key Scheme, administered by the Royal Association for Disability and Rehabilitation (RADAR), who will issue a key to individuals for a small fee). RADAR also publish a guide to accessible public lavatories, giving details of locations (RADAR, 1995). The Centre for

Accessible Environments publish a 'Good Loo Guide' which gives design guidelines.

LAVATORY DESIGN FOR PEOPLE WITH DISABILITIES

Public Conveniences

The Department of the Environment, in their Building Regulations (1992), gives guidance on lavatory design for people with disabilities. Funding is available through the Department of Employment to adapt existing premises for people working, or about to work, in premises where the toilet facilities are inadequate.

Figures 13.1 and 13.2 (overleaf) show a cubicle layout to accommodate wheelchair and ambulant people. The door should open outwards or slide, unless the room is large, because an inward-opening door takes up too much space. Handles, locks and rails should be large enough to grasp easily, simple to use with minimal strength, and low enough to reach easily from a wheelchair. A disposal bin large enough for used incontinence products should be provided.

A cubicle of at least 1.5m x 2m should allow transfer from a wheelchair either from in front or from the side. Some people can stand and turn with the chair in front of the lavatory; others prefer to remove one arm from the wheelchair and transfer sideways. A few use a chair with a zipped back so that they can transfer backwards. This is particularly appropriate for double amputees.

The British Standards Institution has revised BS 6465 (1995) which covers the provision of sanitary facilities in public buildings. This recommends at least one unisex facility in a range of public amenities.

Travers et al., (1992) have found toilet facilities in one large teaching hospital to be woefully inadequate. The worst toilets were found on a ward for elderly people, none of which was suitable for use by people with disabilities. Bedside commodes had to be used instead. It seems unlikely that this hospital is unique.

Private Lavatories

The lavatory in the person's own home can be tailored to individual needs. There may of course be limitations because of the needs of other members of the household. In certain cases a Disabled Facilities Grant from the local authority may be available to build a completely new bathroom where the existing facilities are inaccessible. A stairlift to transport the person from downstairs to upstairs may be a more appropriate alternative to a new downstairs bathroom. The usual

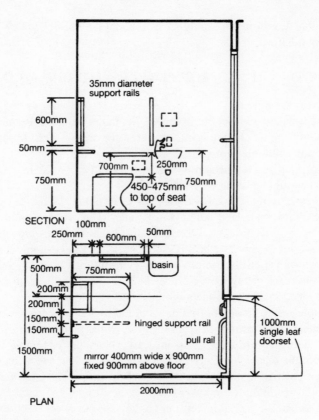

Figure 13.1   *Wheelchair cubicle.*

practice is for an occupational therapist to identify the individual's needs and the local authority to assess the client's financial contribution, according to his ability to pay. In practice, if the client is unable to make this contribution, alternative sources of finance may be available. This can take time, and temporary measures, such as a chemical commode, may be considered.

Note: Figures 13.1 and 13.2 are taken from *Approved Document M – Access and Facilities for Disabled People.* HMSO, London. Used by permission.

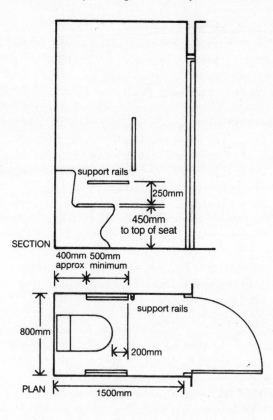

SECTION

support rails

250mm

450mm
to top of seat

400mm 500mm
approx minimum

PLAN

support rails

800mm

200mm

1500mm

Figure 13.2   *Cubicle for ambulant disabled people.*

Accessories for the Lavatory

The range of equipment available is vast (Equipment for Disabled People, 1995). In many regions the Disabled Living Centre carries a permanent display. Social Services may provide equipment free of charge, or on permanent loan, or may merely recommend what is most appropriate. It is important to distinguish between the needs of the person using the lavatory in achieving independence, and the needs of a carer, who may be frail or assisting a highly dependent person. In some cases it may be necessary to have equipment tailor-made. REMAP, a voluntary organisation of engineers and occupational therapists, can design or modify equipment to suit the needs of an individual.

Grab Rails, Seats and Support Frames

A wide variety is available. These can add greatly to the stability and confidence of someone unsteady on his feet, and give leverage for rising from a wheelchair or the lavatory. Some are free-standing. Flanges at the feet of a frame give added stability. For long-term use it is generally preferable to have rails fixed either to the floor or to the walls. Horizontal, vertical or diagonal variations are available, depending on the individual's needs. Horizontal rails assist a 'pushing up' movement, whilst vertical rails assist a 'pulling up' movement. The Disabled Living Foundation *Hamilton Index* Part 3, section 14 gives details ('Personal Toilet', updated annually).

The lavatory seat should be at a height that is easy to get on and off. People with stiff or painful joints may find it difficult to use a modern low-level lavatory. A footstool may be needed to give the correct sitting position on a high seat. This is especially important to promote effective bowel evacuation. People transferring sideways from a wheelchair to the lavatory must have each seat at the same height as the other. Detachable raised lavatory seats can be used to increase the height from between 50-150mm. It is important to use a model with an inner lip fitting directly into the bowl, not perched on top of the ordinary seat, as these are the most stable. Some raised seats have a cut-out front to facilitate wiping. Adjustable clips will ensure stability. Others slope forward or sideways to accommodate a rigid leg or calliper. The seat should be easily removable for cleaning, as well as for when the lavatory is used by others.

Spring-loaded or electrically operated elevating lavatory seats can be obtained if rising from the sitting position is a particular problem, although they should be used with care for a frail person, who might be catapulted forward.

Lower Limb Amputation

This is an increasingly common problem which gives rise to special needs. The rehabilitation team will teach the most appropriate method of transfer prior to discharge from hospital. This may be a stand or a sideways transfer, depending on the ability to weight-bear on the other leg. High amputation can cause problems of balance when sitting on the lavatory, or the stump may slip into the pan. This can be overcome by providing a wider support seat with a narrow aperture, while still allowing access for personal cleansing. A zipped back wheelchair is useful for backwards transfer for people with a double amputation.

Pressure Care
Pressure-relief oval toilet seats or commode rings provide greater body support for people who may take a particularly long time to empty the bladder or bowel (Figure 13.3). This is important where there is loss of sensation, sacral lesions or severe weight loss. Wooden seats tend to be more comfortable than plastic, and a bench seat will allow sliding for easy transfer.

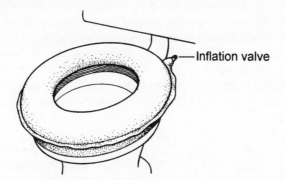

Inflation valve

Figure 13.3   *Oval pressure relief cushion.*

Cleansing
Toilet paper should be situated within easy reach, without the user having to stretch. For those with the use of only one hand, the paper must be situated on the side they can use. A roll of paper is very difficult to tear off with one hand, and people may be tempted to try dangerous manoeuvres such as holding the roll still with the forehead. Folded paper in a pull-out dispenser is much easier for the one-handed.

People who have a problem with wiping because of limited reach may find toilet tongs or a bottom wiper useful. These hold the toilet paper and extend the reach considerably. Alternatively, a portable bidet (Ganmill) which fits on top of the lavatory pan can be used. This will usually require the presence of a helper, as the bidet has to be filled with warm water, positioned on the pan, and emptied after use via a plug into the lavatory. Where finances and space permit, a permanent bidet with foot controls (e.g. Clos-o-Mat) may be useful. The Loo Top (Westholme), compatible with most lavatory bowls, can be programmed to an individual's needs and will clean and dry from underneath.

A person with limited dexterity may also need an adapted handle to enable easy toilet flushing.

ALTERNATIVES TO THE LAVATORY

It is often necessary to find an instant solution to an inaccessible lavatory. Commodes and handheld urinals provide an immediate answer, whilst chemical toilets and commodes can be quicker and cheaper alternatives to providing a new lavatory or adapting an existing one. Before recommending these alternatives, it is important to make sure that the user and the family will find this acceptable, as some people dislike the idea of a commode in living areas, or even in the bedroom, especially if there are other people around (Naylor and Mulley, 1993). It can also cause embarrassment to those who are dependent upon carers to empty the receptacle. It may be necessary to convince both client and carer of the potential benefits, especially if mobility is slow or painful, or if nocturia is very frequent.

Commodes

There are many different commodes available, from a simple stool to very sophisticated designs. They can be classified as static, chemical and mobile.

Some commodes are wooden rather than metal and can be disguised as an easy-chair. Generally, a commode will be between 475mm and 550mm high, although many are adjustable. Optional features include removable arms (for sideways transfer from a wheelchair or bed), wheels and footrests. Some are foldable so that they can easily be taken away on holiday. Some can be wheeled over a lavatory and so used as a sanitary chair with the pan removed. Others can be fixed to the side of the bed for stability in night use. Special commodes with splayed legs for added stability are available for people who are very obese.

A commode must be fitted with a compatible container which fits the aperture closely, to avoid soiling of the commode or floor. Usually, it is most convenient to be able to remove the pan from the back. The Institute of Consumer Ergonomics, Loughborough, has also recommended that commodes have a cover which is light and hinged at the back; padded arms, which are level and extend forward as far as the front of the seat; a seat and arms made from non-absorbent material; and a container which is easy to remove, carry and replace.

Chemical Toilets

Chemical toilets, designed for use in camping or caravanning, may be used instead of a commode, for instance in situations where the user is unable to empty a commode and has no regular helper. The chemicals ensure that even if it is not emptied for several days, urine and faeces do not cause a smell or infection risk. Chemical commodes do not normally accommodate a raised seat, but purpose-built frames with adjustable arms and legs and optional castors are available.

Illustrations and details of the types of commode are given in *Equipment for Disabled People*, 1995. General points to consider when selecting a commode are given in Table 13.1.

Table 13.1   General Points to Consider when Selecting a Commode

ASSESSING THE USER'S NEEDS

- *Height and weight.* Especially important if the user is grossly overweight.
- *Mobility and dexterity.* To enable independence for sitting and personal cleansing if possible.
- *Posture position and degree of neuromuscular control.* Safety straps or a harness may be necessary.
- *Dependence/independence.* It is advisable to check who is going to empty the commode, as this can prove difficult for people with poor dexterity or frail carers.
- *Storage.* Hospital and residential settings may prefer stacking commodes, whilst a solid wooden or upholstered style may blend more acceptably with furniture in the home.
- *Cost.* This can vary from a few to hundreds of pounds. Some people are willing and able to purchase the commode of their choice. Local authorities may offer a restricted range, or have a long waiting list.
- *Preference.* Decisions should always be made with the client, not for him.

COMMODE FEATURES

- *Stability.* The model must be suitable for the weight of the user. This is important for people who are obese or who have balance problems.
- *Height and comfort of the seat, back and arm rests.* Removable arms are available for sideways transfer. Models with adjustable height are recommended for multiple use.
- *Seat aperture, length and compatible container.* This will avoid soiling the commode or floor. Oval seats and containers are available.
- *Seat.* A cut-away seat may be necessary for people who need to wipe sitting down or who use manual bowel evacuation.
- *Container.* This should be easy to remove, carry and replace.
- *Mobile commodes or sanichairs.* These should have brakes fitted to castors for maximum safety. Check that the height will fit over the toilet seat. A glide-about is a commode on wheels which will slide over a lavatory and rotates on its own axis (and can be obtained with movable arms). It is useful if cubicle space is limited.

When either a commode or chemical toilet has to be used in a living room it may be possible to partition off a corner of the room with a ceiling-to-floor curtain, so that some privacy and separation is maintained. Before this equipment is issued or privately purchased, instructions on the use, cleaning and maintenance should be understood by the user or carer, as it is important that it is kept in safe working order.

Hand-Held Urinals

Hand-held urinals are useful for people with severe mobility restrictions, particularly when visiting places with inaccessible lavatories, travelling, or in bed. They can also help carers when lifting is a problem.

It is advisable to practice at home in private before trusting to the use of a urinal in a public place. Where grip or eyesight are a problem, a chair- or bed-pad will protect against possible spillage. Sometimes a travel rug over the knees will conceal what is happening. Other considerations include:

- Material of the urinal: lightweight plastic or papier maché are useful for people with frail wrists.
- Handles to hold the urinal: again where grip is a problem. Rubber round the handle will add extra grip. An extended handle may help if wrist movement is restricted.
- Spill-proof design: this is particularly important for people with restricted eyesight or shaky hands.
- Easy to use and clean.

Male Hand-Held Urinals

The standard male 'bottle' or urinal is familiar to most nurses (Figure 13.4(a)). It is available in metal, plastic or disposable papier maché, the latter two being lighter for those with a weak grip. Bottles usually have a capacity of 500ml or 1 litre. Some have a snap-close lid to avoid the danger of spilling after use. A bedside or chairside holder

Figure 13.4(a)   *Male bottle.*

is useful to prevent a full bottle being accidentally kicked or knocked over. A flatter version may be more stable to use and less easy to spill if placed between the legs in bed (Figure 13.4(b)). A non-spill adapter will fit most standard bottles (Figure 13.4(c)). The rubber sleeve fits snugly into the neck of the bottle with the air vent upwards. The valve allows urine to pass in but not to return. This is particularly useful for someone with a poor grip or shaky hands who tends to spill or drop the bottle, or someone who falls asleep with a used bottle in bed and then rolls over and knocks it over.

The Reddy Bottle (Figure 13.4(d), overleaf) is a completely disposable plastic urinal which folds flat and is therefore very easy to carry. It is useful for journeys and for those who suddenly get 'caught short' in public. The non-return valve and wire ties enable it to be carried after use until a suitable place is found for disposal. However, as it can only be used once (the non-return valve ensures that it must be cut to be emptied), it is too expensive for routine use, but good for special situations or locations.

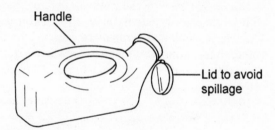

Handle

Lid to avoid spillage

Figure 13.4(b)   *Bottle with flat bottom for stability.*

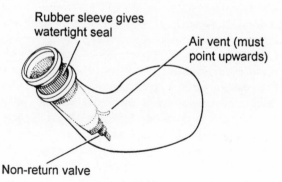

Rubber sleeve gives watertight seal

Air vent (must point upwards)

Non-return valve

Figure 13.4(c)   *Non-spill adaptor in the neck of a male bottle.*

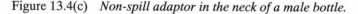

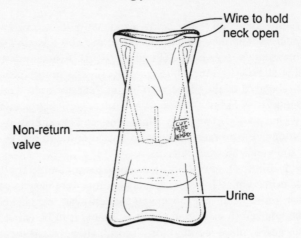

Figure 13.4(d)   *Disposable plastic urinal.*

The female swan-necked urinal (Figure 13.4(e)) is useful for men with a retracted penis who have difficulty in using a standard bottle. The whole penis and scrotum can usually fit inside the neck of the bottle, so that urine is caught at whatever angle it emerges.

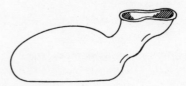

Figure 13.4(e)   *Swan-necked urinal.*

Female Hand-Held Urinals

Women who cannot get to a lavatory or commode, or who find sitting on one painful, have a variety of alternative urinals available. A standard hospital model bedpan can be used, although they tend to be rather large and cumbersome and are difficult to get onto without assistance. Many people with disabilities are too unstable to sit upright unaided on a bedpan, and they are very uncomfortable to use lying down. Smaller hand-held urinals tend to be easier to use independently, provided that the individual has reasonable manual dexterity.

Some women construct their own urinals from items such as household funnels, tubing and hot-water bottles. A narrow tall jug is useful if there is difficulty in abducting the thighs. The pan-type female urinal (Figure 13.5(a), William Freeman & Co.) is a shallow plastic dish with a rounded lip for comfort and to prevent spillage. It is emptied via the rubber cap on the handle. It can be used in bed or on a chair. Women who cannot raise their buttocks to position it can often roll onto it sideways, as it is shallow. Someone who is bedbound can empty it into a bucket by the bed and re-use it without assistance. Alternatively, a self-adhesive penile sheath can be attached to the handle and connected to a large capacity drainage bag, which can be discreetly supported underneath or beside the chair or bed (Figure 13.5(b)).

The slipper bed-pan (Figure 13.5(c)) is similar in use to the pan

Rubber stopper

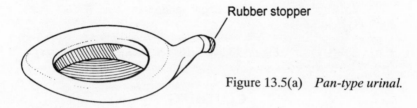

Figure 13.5(a)   *Pan-type urinal.*

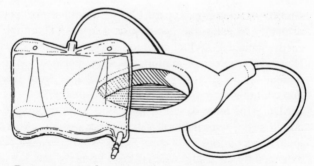

Figure 13.5(b)   *Pan-type urinal connected to a drainage bag.*

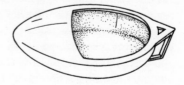

Figure 13.5(c)   *Slipper-type urinal.*

urinal, only larger. The St Peter's Boat (Figure 13.5(d)) is a pear-shaped dish with a handle which can be used either on the edge of a bed or chair, with the knees apart, or standing up. The Bridge urinal (Beambridge Medical) is popular (Figure 13.5(e)). A woman in a wheelchair may find a hand-held urinal easier to use with a specially adapted cushion with a removable U-shaped cut-out in front which leaves a gap for the urinal.

Figure 13.5(d)   *St Peter's Boat.*

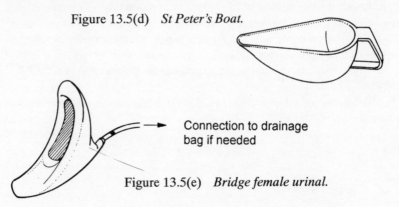

Connection to drainage
bag if needed

Figure 13.5(e)   *Bridge female urinal.*

CLOTHING

Choice of clothing is particularly important for people who have difficulty in using the lavatory or a urinal (Thornton, 1990). Loose, easily-managed styles and fastenings can be quicker to adjust. However, choice of clothing is very personal. It is important to remember that in asking someone to change from their normal style, you could be asking for a change in self-image.

Men with poor dexterity may find a fly-opening extended to the crotch seam, with dabs of Velcro for fastening, easier and quicker to undo than buttons or a zip (Figure 13.6). Pyjama bottoms with an extended fly are useful when using a urinal in bed. Loose-fitting boxer-style shorts can be easier to use than bikini briefs or Y-fronts. Shirts with long tails can dangle into the toilet bowl. Specially-adapted braces may be easier to manage, as trousers can be lowered without having to remove clothing or the braces.

Many women, especially older women, wear several layers of clothing (e.g. skirt, petticoat, corset, vest and pants). It can take considerable time and agility to get them out of the way, and accidental wetting or soiling is common. Tight skirts can be difficult to pull up in

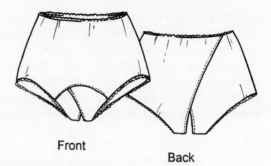

Front

Back

Figure 13.6   *Open-crotch pants.*

a hurry and trousers are not easy to remove quickly. It is better to
encourage the use of fewer layers and a choice of shorter vests and
lined skirts and dresses. Petticoats are best avoided.

A teddy (camiknickers, Figure 13.7) or ordinary knickers with
gusset extended and fastened with a dab of Velcro (Figure 13.8) can

Figure 13.7   *Camiknickers.*

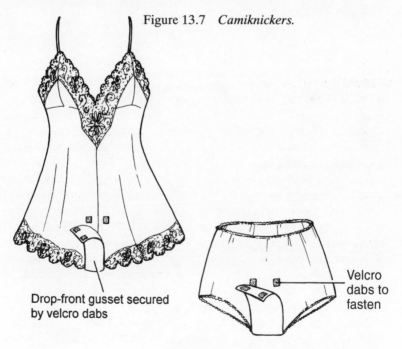

Drop-front gusset secured
by velcro dabs

Velcro
dabs to
fasten

Figure 13.8   *Pants with extended gusset.*

313

make fastening more convenient. Full-skirted or wrap-around skirts and dresses are easier to lift out of the way and can be tucked into a waist band or belt when balance is poor, or when transferring from a wheelchair to the toilet (Figure 13.9). Many women wheelchair-users prefer to wear trousers. An opening in the side seams allows the rear of the trousers to be dropped before transferring to the lavatory. Knee length or open-backed night-dresses with a generous overlap are easier at night.

Women who use a hand-held urinal may find that split-crotch pants and tights, or loose French knickers (Figure 13.10), can be pulled out of the way when using the urinal without having to take them down. Drop-front incontinence pants can also be useful (see Chapter 15).

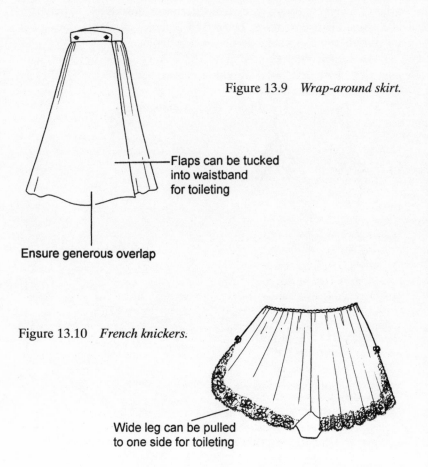

Figure 13.9   *Wrap-around skirt.*

Flaps can be tucked
into waistband
for toileting

Ensure generous overlap

Figure 13.10   *French knickers.*

Wide leg can be pulled
to one side for toileting

CONCLUSION

Many people with physical disabilities can be helped to be continent either by adapting lavatories to their needs or by providing acceptable alternatives. Increased public awareness has led to the needs of disabled people being more often considered, but there is still a long way to go before facilities are universal. Detailed individual assessment will indicate the most suitable solution for each individual. In this assessment the nurse, occupational therapist and physiotherapist should ideally work together with the disabled person and his or her family to arrive at an answer.

In some areas a Disabled Living Centre is run by the health authority or the social services department, or by a voluntary organisation. The disabled person and family, accompanied by a therapist, can receive expert assessment and help, and often try different aids before a decision is made to order an item.

REFERENCES AND FURTHER READING

British Standards Institution, 1993. BS 6465. BSI, London.

Centre for Accessible Environments, 1988. *Good Loo Guide*. CAE, London.

Continence Foundation, 1995. *Directory of Continence Products*. The Continence Foundation, London.

Cunningham, S., Norton, C., 1993. Public inconveniences: some suggestions for improvement. The Continence Foundation, London.

Department of the Environment and the Welsh Office, 1992. *Approved Document M – Access and Facilities for Disabled People*. HMSO, London.

Disabled Living Foundation, 1995. *Hamilton Index. Personal Toilet*. Part 3, section 14. DLF, London.

Disabled Living Foundation, 1988. *Clothing for Continence – Men; Clothing for Continence – Women*. DLF, London.

Equipment for Disabled People, 1995. *Personal Care*, 7th edn. Mary Marlborough Lodge, Nuffield Orthopaedic Centre, Oxford OX3 7LD.

Naylor, J. R., Mulley, G. P., 1993. Commodes: inconvenient conveniences. *British Medical Journal*, 307: 1258–60.

Royal Association for Disability and Rehabilitation, 1995. *National Key Scheme Guide*. RADAR, London.

Thornton, N., 1990. *Fashion for Disabled People*. Batsford, London.

Travers, A. F., Burns, E., Penn, N. D., Mitchell, S. C., Mulley, G. P., 1992. A survey of hospital toilet facilities. *British Medical Journal*, 304: 878–9.

The following Patient Organisations provide information sheets for members:
Alzheimer's Disease Society
Association for Spina Bifida and Hydrocephalus
Multiple Sclerosis Society
Sexual and Personal Relationships of Disabled People (SPOD)
Spinal Injuries Association
Stroke Association

Addresses of these organisations and others mentioned in the text can be found in Appendix 2.

Chapter 14

Acquiring Continence – Supporting People with Learning Disabilities

David Sines, PhD, BSc, RMN, RNMH, RNT, PGCTHE, FRCN

Co-ordinator of Nursing/Professor of Community Health Nursing, Ulster University

People with learning disabilities (or mental handicap) essentially have difficulties with learning. The majority of people, irrespective of their degree of disability, have the potential to attain some degree of continence. Incontinence usually represents a failure to learn the skills necessary for continence.

The concept of learning disability has been defined by the perceptions that society has held towards this client group. In the past twenty years the drive has been towards 'normalisation' (Wolfensberger, 1972). This approach dismisses earlier attitudes that people with learning disabilities should be treated as being disabled first and people second. The normalisation debate focuses upon a value system that recognises the need for all people to be regarded as equal members of society, with equal rights and responsibilities.

Underlining this approach is the need to avoid segregating people from the mainstream of ordinary society. Opportunities must be extended to ensure that purposeful integration occurs (Towell, 1991). This philosophy also presumes that people with learning disabilities will be free to experience the responsibilities, frustrations, failures and rejections shared by others.

This debate is primarily a human rights issue and suggests that long-stay specialist hospitals are no longer the place to care for and support people with learning disabilities. Because of this, learning disability is now set to challenge the skills and practices of many nurses working in the community, as an increasing number of people seek support from both specialist community mental handicap nurses and others working in primary health care teams.

WHAT DO WE MEAN BY 'LEARNING DISABILITY'?

It is all too easy to regard people as falling homogeneously into neat categories or 'labels'. This is particularly true of people with learning disability, who are in fact often very different from each other, with different learning abilities, needs and expectations. Essentially they all share one thing in common – their disability is almost always caused by organic or genetic changes very early on in life. The degree to which the symptoms of learning disability may impair normal functioning will depend much on the extent to which learning opportunities can be provided throughout life. Learning is a lifelong occupation, and when stimulating opportunities and experiences are presented to people with learning disabilities, accompanied by associated rewards, then new skills may be acquired which may increase their range of competence and potential for integration in the community.

Learning disability defies any more specific definition but it is sometimes helpful to regard it as a non-clinical condition, the symptoms of which may be ameliorated by the provision of positive learning experiences.

The extent to which individuals possess certain self-help skills, such as continence, or the degree to which they conform to 'normal' patterns of behaviour, will often determine the extent to which they are accepted in society. Categorisation still appears to be a pre-requisite for professionals as part of their assessment process, and this in turn enables them to make decisions about clients and their rights. Most of these decisions are based on assessments of achievements (functional assessments), but all too often the recipient is a passive contributor to the process and will almost certainly be dependent on carers and others to provide the learning opportunities needed to acquire skills such as continence. This situation is far from ideal, and it should be the aim of all nurses to empower their clients as active partners in determining their needs.

CURRENT PATTERNS OF SERVICE DELIVERY

Since its inception in 1948, the National Health Service (NHS) has provided extensive services for people with learning disabilities, albeit mainly in large hospitals for the first twenty-five years of its existence.

During the past twenty years local authority social services departments have been increasingly involved in the provision of residential, day and domiciliary services for people with learning disabilities, and have become equal partners in the provision of statutory services with the NHS. Although services are not uniform across the country, in the best cases this partnership has resulted in the provision of a comprehensive range of services, which now emphasises the importance of community care as a positive choice, without residential provision being the exclusive option. Hence, dependence on long-stay residential care is being rapidly reduced, and is being replaced by a range of options based on local need, flexible enough to meet the demands of local people in their neighbourhoods.

The NHS and Community Care Act (DoH, 1990) requires that planning agreements should be reached between health and social service departments which clearly identify which services will be provided by each agency, and which identify the processes to be adopted in assessing the needs of individuals in need of care. As a crude rule of thumb, it has been suggested that care for people with learning disabilities should be assessed on the basis of whether their needs fit in to two distinct categories – health and/or social care.

It is intended that resources will be concentrated in local communities through the provision of skilled, peripatetic support from a range of professionals including doctors, mental handicap nurses, clinical psychologists, physiotherapists, speech therapists and occupational therapists. These specialists usually work as members of specialist community learning disability teams, and in turn complement the work of local primary health care teams which will continue to provide the first point of contact for people with learning disabilities and their families. Such teams are made up of general practitioners, district nurses and health visitors who work in collaboration with social workers from the local social work office.

Health authorities will continue to be responsible for the provision of extensive preventive, screening and treatment services to pre-school and school age children. General practitioners are becoming increasingly vigilant in the provision of immunisation and screening programmes for young children with handicaps, as their involvement in the local community is further developed and encouraged, following the implementation of GP fund-holding.

The National Health Service will also continue to provide services directly or through other agencies such as the independent or voluntary sector, to meet health care needs of people with learning disabilities and their families. Changes are taking place within local authorities, and although health authorities may choose to place contracts within their own organisation, they should be closely monitored, reviewed and inspected by both the local authority and the health authority.

CARE MANAGEMENT

Contracts will be negotiated for each person with a learning disability, using a system known as *care management*. The principles of care management require that the needs, wishes and ambitions of individuals and their families are identified and acknowledged by skilled practitioners. The task of the care manager will be to match these needs and ambitions against a range of available resources in the community. The relevant skills of practitioners will be accessed to support people and their families. Many of these 'contracts' may be placed with community nurses.

The principles of care management will require nurses and social workers to identify their skills and competencies, and to match these to the specific needs of individual service users and their families. Such needs may require the introduction of specialist programmes to enable clients to acquire continence. In accordance with the monitoring role required of care managers, the degree of success that nurses and others demonstrate in assisting people to acquire these skills may be used to evaluate the effectiveness of nursing care delivered during the course of the contract period.

Consequently, opportunities for practice may require that the learning disability nurse assumes full responsibility for aspects of care and quality of life for the people for whom they work. The way in which this care is delivered is based upon a number of specific competencies which have been identified in response to needs of people with learning disabilities and their families over many years of practice. The nursing profession requires that all nurses preparing for such practice undertake three years training, including generic health care principles and a specialist training of eighteen months in learning disability care and practice.

It is during this training that the core competencies are identified and explored by student nurses, who upon qualification are registered as independent practitioners in learning disability nursing care (ENB, 1988, Syllabus for Mental Handicap Nurse Practitioners).

Learning disability nurse practitioners receive in excess of 80% of their training in community and domiciliary-based settings outside of hospital. During this time they are encouraged to foster close links with the primary health care team, with the local authority social services department, and with the voluntary and independent sectors. Sharing learning experiences with informal carers, social workers and others provides excellent opportunity for collaboration, enabling the learning disability nurse to develop a clear framework for a partnership with the local authorities. It also fosters coordination at local level between their skills and those of social workers.

The community learning disability nurse is therefore well placed, by specialist training and experience, to work with people with learning disabilities across a range of agencies, wherever they live. They have acquired considerable expertise in the use of behavioural skills, and may use a broad range of competencies to assist people with learning disabilities to acquire new skills such as continence.

CONTINENCE AND LEARNING DISABILITY

For the majority of people with learning disability, the acquisition of continence will require the introduction of learning programmes based upon the principles of behaviour modification. However, some people also suffer from additional difficulties such as coexistent physical disabilities, and others may have a neurogenic bladder problem as well. In such cases it is essential to investigate bladder function prior to initiating a training programme, as the training is not likely to be effective if there is a severe underlying bladder dysfunction. Likewise, if individuals have associated physical disabilities that restrict the acquisition of independence and self-help, any programme will have to be adapted or modified accordingly. The particular problems facing people with a neuropathic bladder and physical disabilities are discussed in Chapters 8 and 13 respectively.

Incontinence can be one of the most socially restricting aspects of learning disability, and it may become a major issue when determining a person's access to support services in adult life. If the person lives at home within the family (as many do), incontinence often presents one of the major challenges. Parents should be encouraged not to simply accept incontinence as an inevitable part of their child's disability from an early age, and not to wait until he reaches adulthood before attempting any training. The physical burden of laundry, spoilt furniture and clothing, especially for the older child and adult, may be overwhelming (Sines, 1985). Considerable extra financial costs are common, as a Disabled Living Foundation survey highlighted in 1978 (the conclusions of which are still applicable today, Bradshaw, 1978). This includes the additional costs associated with laundry, replacing clothing and bedding worn out by excessive washing, electricity, buying pads and equipment, new carpets and furniture.

The social aspects of incontinence may predominate for some people and may be associated with stigma. For example, the odour and embarrassment which may accompany long-term incontinence are also applicable to this client group and their families, and may encourage the family to become socially isolated. As the young person grows, persistent incontinence becomes an increasing burden and may result in request for admission to specialist residential provision for temporary or permanent care away from home.

In recognition of this problem, the community learning disability nurse may work in close liaison with specialist social workers and health visitors to offer a range of practical assistance. The model adopted by most workers is one of partnership with family carers. By sharing in the design of personal programmes of care, it is often possible to relieve some of the burdens associated with incontinence. Care packages involve: the provision of specialist advice and behavioural training; financial support (often from the Department of Social Security); practical support in the form of home-based sitting services; and an individually determined supply of disposable pads and appliances to alleviate the consequences of incontinence, where local budgets permit.

If the person with a learning disability requires a home away from the family, incontinence may be the deciding factor in placement. Many community-based services are now equipped to provide responsive support to people with a range of continence needs, although others are more selective, choosing to admit only those people who are able to care for most needs independently. Current government policy accepts that incontinence must not be used as a reason for excluding someone from health or social care provision. However, acquisition of continence is still regarded as a major aim of individually-designed programmes of care for people with learning disabilities. By gaining continence the majority will be enabled to avail themselves of an informed range of choice, whenever the decision to seek an alternative home becomes necessary.

Some people (22,000 in 1995) still remain resident in long-stay specialist hospitals for people with learning disabilities, and in excess of 50% have been shown to have some difficulty with continence

(Craft et al., 1985). However, as the more able people are discharged from hospital to live in the community, the number of staff available to work with those that remain increases proportionally in many instances. Additional staff numbers, and a more proactive approach to assisting people to acquire self-help skills, has led to many people acquiring some form of continence before they leave the hospital to live in the community. Learning disability nurses provide therapeutic interventions with their clients with the aim of maximising each person's potential, to improve the quality of life both within hospital and in preparation for a move to the community. The majority of health and local authorities are now engaged in extensive programmes to make provision for community living for people with learning disabilities who were previously resident in hospital.

Wherever people with learning disabilities live, incontinence is now regarded as being a manageable problem for the majority. Thankfully, the problems associated with low baseline skills in the acquisition of continence can be relieved, and in many cases compensated for, by the introduction of comprehensive toilet training programmes. In the majority of places, community learning disability teams now operate to support clients in their own homes and community facilities. Community learning disability nurses work as independent therapists, but have the support of clinical psychologists and others whenever additional advice is required. However, nurses often feel frustrated in their work in the community and must depend upon the skills and commitment of families and other carers in non-NHS facilities to implement the programmes of care consistently. Similarly, they may have to depend on others to prescribe and provide incontinence aids in support of their behavioural programmes, and this requires careful coordination and collaborative inter-professional teamwork.

THE IMPORTANCE OF EARLY INTERVENTION

As with most skills, teaching people with learning disabilities to be continent is more likely to be successful the earlier it can be started. The ideal time to start training is probably before the second birthday (or earlier if the family and child feel ready), i.e. the same age at which most children are toilet-trained. Some training can commence as early as 12–15 months, for example introducing the child to sitting on the potty. This will usually be part of a larger programme aimed at achieving maximum independence in skills of daily living. Home-

Table 14.1 Model for Shaping Toilet Behaviour

FINAL TARGET BEHAVIOUR	Patient goes to the toilet independently	Patient removes his clothing independently	Patient sits down on the toilet independently	Patient eliminates only in the toilet and is otherwise continent
INTERMEDIATE TARGET BEHAVIOUR	Patient asks to go to the toilet	Patient removes or actively attempts to remove some of his clothing	Patient is helped to sit down on the toilet and sits unrestrained	Patient eliminates in the toilet regularly and has only infrequent episodes of incontinence
	Patient indicates his need to eliminate	Patient actively assists when clothing is removed by nurse	Patient is placed on the toilet and sits unrestrained	Patient has established some regularity and uses toilet more frequently than is incontinent
BASE TARGET	Patient is taken to toilet by nurse	Patient cooperates passively when clothing is removed by nurse	Patient is placed on toilet and is restrained to sit	Patient uses toilet when placed on it but is incontinent at all other times

Tierney, 1973, reproduced by courtesy of the Editor, *Nursing Times* based training programmes will often commence at this time and will be introduced by the community learning disability nurse or specialist health visitor. One such programme is Portage (Revill and Blunden, 1978) which provides goal plans and home teaching schedules for the promotion of continence for young children with learning disabilities.

However, if training has not been started early, this by no means indicates that the chance has been lost, and very high success rates can be achieved with older children, adolescents and adults who have either missed out or failed with training earlier in life.

Toilet-training people with learning disabilities is not a simple or easy procedure. It should never be started lightly, without consideration of the full implications. All those connected with the individual's care must be enthusiastic and willing to cooperate and work hard together as a team. Ideally, the programme should be supervised by a professional trained in working with this client group (nurse, psychologist, or other), usually with additional experience in using behaviour modification and operant conditioning techniques. The Registered Nurse for the Mentally Handicapped (RNMH) receives extensive instruction in such techniques during training, and the popularity of additional courses is increasing.

Without such support, whether in residential care or in the community, any toilet-training programme will be more difficult to implement and will stand less chance of success. It is probably wise for those inexperienced in these methods not to attempt a programme without support and supervision, because the additional work and effort involved can rapidly lead to frustration and disillusionment with failures.

TRAINING METHODS

The ideal aim of toilet-training is independent toileting and continence. This may not be realistic for all individuals. Certainly, there are so many elements involved that it is usually best to break down the skills required into a series of intermediate target steps or behaviours, which can be worked on separately or in combination. One method of dividing the steps, devised by Tierney (1973), is shown in Table 14.1 (facing). The ultimate goal is to achieve the top final target behaviour in all four columns. Progress is indicated by ascending any of the columns from the base target behaviour, via intermediate targets, towards the final target. An end point may have to be accepted short of the top in one or more of the goals, depending upon a realistic assessment of the individual's physical and mental potentials.

Most programmes are based on the theories of behaviour modification. The underlying principle is that behaviours which result in pleasant consequences are thereby 'reinforced', and will tend to continue and become an established element of the individual's behaviour repertoire. Behaviours which result in neutral or adverse consequences are not reinforced and tend to be discontinued or 'extinguished'. By close observation and careful planning, a programme is worked out to shape the desired behaviour gradually, by the use of appropriate rewarding until a carefully defined target behaviour is attained.

Many different training methods to enhance continence have been used with people with a learning disability, and most achieve a reasonable degree of success. The programme must be acceptable to and understood by those who will carry it out, whether family or staff. The main differences between approaches are in the timing of toileting and the use of reinforcers, and in residential settings, whether people are trained individually or in groups. Probably the most successful method is individualised intensive training using regular time-interval toileting and mild correction for incontinence (Smith, 1987). Whichever method is chosen, the most crucial factor in success will be a consistent approach to training, i.e. having everyone who is involved with the individual approaching the training in an identical manner throughout the training period.

Intensive individual training involves a great commitment on the part of the trainer and may be very time-consuming during the initial stages. A method outlined and found successful by Smith and Bainbridge (1991) is shown in Table 14.2. This method used regular toileting, timed by the clock rather than to coincide with any pre-charted likely times for incontinence. This regular-interval training has usually been found to be simpler to carry out than toileting based on the individual's own natural bladder functioning, and as effective as individual programmes. Long-term follow-up of people who achieved independent toileting with an intensive individual programme has shown that continence is significantly better for this group than matched people who received group training. Ten years after the initial training, people who had received an individual regular toileting programme retained an 88% improvement on their pre-training continence (as compared to 52% for those who had group training). It was estimated that, although the initial training was very

Table 14.2   Bladder Training Procedure

- Seat the trainee in view of the toilet for the duration of the training day.
- Increase fluid intake (approximately 200ml every half hour).
- Every half hour, prompt the trainee to the toilet using the minimum possible prompt.
- Get the trainee to sit until urine is passed or for a maximum of ten minutes. If no urine is passed, the trainee simply comes off the toilet and waits until the next prompt.
- Reward with praise and other appropriate rewards as soon as he/she *begins* to pass urine on the toilet.
- 'Fade' out prompts to toilet, fading out physical prompts first, then verbal prompts next, leaving gestural prompts which are then faded down to eye pointing. At, or around this point, self-initiated toileting should begin to occur.
- When self-initiated toileting is reliably established, move the trainee gradually back from the toilet towards the normal living area ('backward chaining').

Dry Pants Procedure
- Every fifteen minutes, on the quarter hour, guide the trainee's hand to feel his or her pants, and ask if his or her pants are dry.
- Praise him or her lavishly and reward for 'having dry pants'.

From Smith and Bainbridge, 1991.

costly in nursing time, this was recouped in time saved well within one year. Over 10 years it was estimated that 5200 hours of nursing time were saved per client (Hyams et al., 1992).

The use of punishment in training is a controversial issue. Certainly many earlier studies, especially in the USA, used punishment or 'over-correction' to eliminate undesired behaviours. Today this is usually seen as unethical, especially the use of physical punishment. It has also been found to be largely unnecessary, and indeed may be counterproductive if it produces a high level of anxiety, since learning is impeded. However, a reprimand, or 'time out' from reward or attention for a specified time interval, are a commonly-used response to avoidable mistakes. This is probably helpful if given consistently and promptly. Some training methods also require the individual to participate in rectifying the consequences of incontinence (i.e. changing the bed or clothes), and this has in some instances been found to hasten learning (Barker, 1979).

BASELINE OBSERVATION

All toilet-training programmes should start with a baseline observation period. This involves regular checks at predetermined intervals to ascertain whether the individual is wet or dry, and careful recording of results. Close observation should be made of episodes of incontinence as well as the preceding and consequent behaviours of both the person and care giver.

Families or staff can develop styles of coping with and reacting to incontinence that could actually be eliciting the behaviour. The most common mistake is to give a lot of attention and create a lot of activity when incontinence occurs, and to almost ignore the person when dry or self-toileting. It is easy to see how this situation can arise. Incontinence is experienced as a nuisance, because if not dealt with promptly it can soil the environment and lead to odour. It is a natural reaction to hurry the incontinent person to the bathroom to clean up. While washing and changing the individual, most people will give him at least some attention and contact, both physical and verbal. Even if the content of the verbal exchange is a rebuke it constitutes attention, and some people with a learning disability tend to respond to any form of attention as if to a reward. The incontinence is actually being rewarded. Conversely, dryness is seldom rewarded so consistently. When observing this behaviour pattern in carers it is important not to apportion blame to parents or staff, who are probably very caring, but to tactfully point out that this kindness may be counterproductive, and suggest how the attention might be reversed to reward continence rather than incontinence.

Observation of the client will indicate whether any warning is given of imminent micturition. Many will have no verbal skills, so this will usually be non-verbal, such as general agitation, getting up, or repetitive actions. Does the individual seem to be able to discriminate when he is wet? This might again be by agitation or wandering or by pulling at clothing or crying. Is he ever toileted, and if so, is the toilet used appropriately? How many other para-toilet skills does he already have? Being able to walk, put on and remove clothing, sit upright unaided, wash hands, communicate simple needs verbally or non-verbally, and follow simple commands are all useful although not essential. Sometimes specially adapted clothing can improve the potential for self-care.

During this baseline period it is also important to establish what constitutes a reward for each individual. To an even greater extent than with other people, this group are not capable of conceptualising a distant, albeit worthwhile, reward once the goal has been achieved. Something must be found which acts as a reinforcement to behaviour and which can be delivered immediately, simply, reliably and frequently. This may be verbal – saying 'well done', or giving a cheer. More often, non-verbal rewards may be better understood and appreciated. This might be anything from a smile or pulling a funny face, to clapping, a pat, a hug or a kiss. The reward may be a drink or a sweet or other food. Care should be taken with edible rewards as the calories involved can lead to a weight problem and increase tooth decay. Likewise, fluid intake may already be excessive (which will exacerbate incontinence), because it has been found by carers that drinks act as pacifiers. This will not be harmful during training, since the greater the fluid intake, the more training opportunities will occur, but excessive frequency once trained will be undesirable. Also, if drinks are used as a reward during training, they should be strictly reserved for the relevant purpose and not given at indiscriminate times as well. Sometimes the reward can be linked to the toilet itself, e.g. using a musical toilet alarm or setting up an apparatus which will produce a noise when urine is passed onto it.

It can never be merely assumed that something will act as a reward unless it has been proved that the individual will respond to it in some way. If the reward selected is actually disliked, or seen as neutral, it will not reinforce the desired behaviour. A noise might be found frightening for example, or a selected food disliked. Often a small reward such as a sweet which can be easily kept in the trainer's pocket and delivered immediately is the best choice. The effectiveness of rewards should be reviewed regularly, as the desire for a given reward may reach satiation point, so that it becomes ineffective. If this occurs, new rewards should be introduced.

To be selected as suitable for toilet-training, the individual should be able to hold urine for at least one hour on some occasions and respond to simple rewards, and there should be someone, either a relative or a professional, prepared to carry out the programme.

THE TRAINING PROGRAMME

Most training programmes will take several weeks, and in some cases several months, to be effective. It is essential to keep accurate records throughout, so that progress can be monitored and any necessary adjustments made (Woods and Guest, 1980). Records will also provide feedback to help keep up the motivation of all involved. This is probably the most crucial factor in success, together with the programme being rigidly and consistently adhered to and not abandoned too soon. The community learning disability team has a very important supportive role in the home, and although not always actually able to carry out the training, should be freely available for advice and encouragement to help maintain motivation.

Once any target behaviour is achieved, prompts should gradually be withdrawn, i.e. from actually escorting the client to the lavatory, to verbal and then gestural prompts, so that the behaviour becomes increasingly spontaneous and independent. This process is called 'fading'. Rewards should also change from being continuous (a reward for every correct achievement) to intermittent, with gradually decreasing frequency of reward (termed 'changes in reinforcement schedule').

Eventually the comfort and independence afforded by continence become reward enough in themselves to maintain the behaviour for some individuals. Others will need intermittent reinforcement and reminders to maintain continence after the programme itself is over. Some will never achieve total continence and will always need some help and reminders.

The introduction of toilet training in an institutional setting where it has never been used before often involves a considerable change in attitudes, and particularly re-thinking of professional roles. This cannot be imposed from above or outside, as the staff must actively want to participate. At first it is often seen as a lot of extra work, and pessimism about the outcome is common. It is usually best to introduce the idea by means of staff training sessions such as study days and seminars, and start toilet-training in those areas where staff express an interest or request a programme. Likewise, it is a good idea to select patients for training whom the staff feel are appropriate and have a chance of attaining continence, certainly in the first instance. Pointing out the potential long-term benefits of reducing the proportion of time spent in toilet-related activities, and a more satisfying workload, may help gain enthusiasm for the project. All residential and day care staff, including ancillary and domestic personnel, must understand the training, so that consistent responses are shown by all members of the care team.

A significant number of people with learning disabilities exhibit other behavioural challenges in addition to incontinence. It has often been found that these improve during a toilet-training programme. General levels of self-help skills and independence are also often increased as an additional benefit. This is probably a result of the increased attention and stimulation offered within the learning environment afforded by toilet-training.

Sometimes using a pants alarm (see Figure 5.3, page 116) or toilet bowl alarm will help greatly during the training. These enable carers to know immediately when urine has been voided, whether continently or incontinently, and to take the appropriate action promptly. The more closely the consequence is paired with the act, the stronger will be the conditioning effect. Care should be taken, however, that the individual does not respond paradoxically to alarms – that is, a few might enjoy hearing the pants alarm and wet intentionally to create the noise or, alternatively, might be frightened by the toilet alarm and withhold urine when on the toilet.

Nocturnal enuresis can be corrected by similar but obviously less intensive behaviour modification programmes. Dry beds should be rewarded and regular toileting encouraged at predetermined intervals. Participation in changing wet beds aids learning. An enuresis alarm can be effective if *well supervised* (Chapter 5) and used as part of a broader behavioural programme.

FAECAL INCONTINENCE

A minority of people with learning disabilities may also have difficulty in managing faecal continence. In some instances this may be attributed to neurological deficits or to emotional difficulties which may present as encopresis. In the latter instance children and adults may soil following the acquisition of continence. Community learning disability nurses may be particularly useful in introducing behaviour programmes to assist with this problem.

For emotional problems, the community learning disability nurse may work in close association with social workers, consultant psychiatrists and clinical psychologists as co-therapists, and may enable the individual and the family to explore and understand some of the underlying stressors that may contribute to causing this difficulty.

Sometimes clearing of the bowel by administering a series of enemas is necessary before a behavioural or bowel training programme can be successfully implemented.

NURSING FOR COMPETENCE

The majority of people with learning disabilities will acquire continence, but for those persons who may not be able to attain the goal of independent social competence other measures will be necessary. A minority of people may be unresponsive to toilet training, and for those persons every effort must be made to contain the situation with respect and dignity. The use of individually selected appliances and pads will be one way of alleviating some of the distress associated with long-term incontinence.

However, the behavioural approach does appear to offer a solution for many people. This method of intervention has been described in this chapter but cannot operate in isolation from the existence of positive staff attitudes, the aim of which will be to enable all members of the organisation to commit themselves to enhancing the quality of life and care for their clients.

The behavioural approach is dynamic and facilitates the involvement of staff members in the identification and implementation of a skill or competence enhancement programme. The following principles underpin this model:

● The objectives of all programmes will be 'driven' by the needs of service users and by standards and criteria set by the organisation (vis-à-vis service agreements and care plans).

● Service responses will be measurable and include criteria relating to the outcomes of care.

● Performance against agreed criteria is monitored regularly, and corrective action is taken as appropriate.

This chapter presents an outline framework for the provision of a quality service for clients with learning disabilities who may have difficulties with the acquisition of continence. The aim will be to provide high quality services to people and their families, and to provide a stimulating and competent workplace within which a highly trained and professional workforce may respond to the needs of their clients. John O'Brien (1982) has described a range of service accomplishments for people requiring longer term support from health and social care agencies. In his paper 'A Guide to Personal Futures Planning' he suggests that five key accomplishments are necessary if high quality care is to be offered and received:

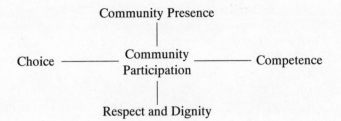

This model has received universal acclaim in both the United States and Canada and it has also been adopted in many services for people with learning disabilities in the United Kingdom. The model suggests that human relationships, skill acquisition (competence), respect and dignity, and integration and participation in the community are key features and aims of modern day services for this client group.

The combination of the behavioural approach and the five service accomplishments described above provides opportunities for people with learning disabilities to attain their maximum level of independence in all areas of function, which of course includes the acquisition of continence skills.

REFERENCES AND FURTHER READING

Azrin, N. H., Foxx, R. M., 1971. A rapid method of toilet-training the institutionalised retarded. *Journal of Applied Behaviour Analysis*, 4: 289–99.

Barker, P., 1979. Nocturnal enuresis: an experimental study involving two behavioural approaches. *International Journal of Nursing Studies*, 16: 319–27.

Bradshaw, J., 1978. *Incontinence, a Burden for Families with Handicapped Children*. Disabled Living Foundation, London.

Craft, M., Bicknell, J., Hollins, S., 1985. *Mental Handicap: A Multi-Disciplinary Approach to Care*. Balliere-Tindall, London.

Davies, B., 1988. *Case Management: Why We Must Develop Policy, Argument and a Research Agenda*. Personal Social Services Research Unit, Discussion paper 559, University of Kent.

Department of Health, 1989. *Caring for People – Community Care in the Next Decade and Beyond*. Cm 849. HMSO, London.

English National Board for Nursing, Midwifery and Health Visiting, 1988. *Project 2000 – Syllabus for Mental Handicap Nurse Practitioners*. ENB, London.

Hampshire Social Services and Winchester Health Authority, 1989. *Andover Project of Case Management for People with a Mental Handicap – A Briefing Paper*, Winchester.

H. M. Government, 1990. *The NHS and Community Care Act*. HMSO, London.

Hyams, G., McCoull, K., Smith, P.S., Tyrer, S.P., 1992. Behavioural continence training in mental handicap: a 10-year follow-up study. *Journal of Intellectual Disability Research*, 36: 551–8.

O'Brien, J., 1982. *A Guide to Personal Futures Planning*. Responsive Systems Associates, Georgia.

Revill, S., Blunden, R., 1978. *A Manual for Implementing Portage Home Training for Developmentally Handicapped Pre-School Children*. NFER, Oxford.

Sines, D. T., Bicknell, J, 1985. *Caring for Mentally Handicapped People in the Community*. Harper & Row, London.

Sines, D., 1983. Incontinence: helping people with mental handicap. *Nursing Times*, 79, 33: 52–5.

Smith, L. J., Bainbridge, G, 1991. An intensive toilet training programme for a boy with a profound mental handicap living in the community. *Mental Handicap*, 19: 146–50.

Smith, P. S., 1979. A comparison of different methods of toilet-training the mentally handicapped. *Behaviour Research Therapy*, 17, 1: 33–43.

Smith, P. S., Smith, L. J., 1987. *Continence and Incontinence: Psychological Approaches to Development and Treatment*. Croom Helm, London.

Tierney, A. J., 1980. Toilet-training the mentally handicapped. *Nursing*, 1, 18: 795–7.

Tierney, A. J., 1973. Toilet-training. *Nursing Times*, 69: 1740–5.

Towell, D., Beardshaw, V., 1991. *Enabling Community Integration*. King's Fund College, London.

Wolfensberger, W., 1972. *The Principle of Normalisation in Human Services*. National Institute on Mental Retardation, Toronto.

Woods, P. A., Guest, E.M., 1980. Toilet training the severely retarded: the importance of evaluation. *Nursing Times* occasional papers, 76, 18: 53–6.

Chapter 15

The Use of Continence Products

Ian J. Pomfret, RGN, NDN Cert, PWT
Continence Adviser, Chorley & South Ribble
NHS Trust

A huge range of products is produced to help incontinent people. These aids aim to preserve the individual's dignity and self-respect by making it possible to conceal and manage incontinence. By containing urine or faeces, the product should enable the person to achieve 'social continence'. In the past the provision of aids has too often been seen as the be-all and end-all of incontinence management. The nurse has assessed the incontinent patient with the selection of the most suitable pad or appliance paramount in mind. This outdated practice has to a great extent been superseded by a more positive, problem-solving approach. However, even with the best available nursing and medical care, not all incontinent people can be completely cured. There is always likely to remain a sizable minority whose problem persists despite all efforts. There will also be those who are too ill for therapy, or who make an informed decision not to undergo recommended treatment. Some may be improved considerably but still wish to use a product to allow confidence in public, and many will need a temporary supply while awaiting or undergoing treatment.

SELECTION OF INCONTINENCE PRODUCTS

People require and expect many different things from a continence product. The ideal aid should fulfil the following criteria. It should:

1) Be fail-safe, i.e. contain the excreta completely and prevent any leakage through to clothing or the environment at any time and under any circumstances.
2) Be comfortable to wear and protect vulnerable skin from soreness, chafing or pressure sores.
3) Be easy for the incontinent person to use and manage independently. Where this is not feasible due to physical or mental disability, it should be easy for the carer to use.

335

4) Disguise or contain any odour.
5) Be easily concealed under clothing, neither bulky nor noisy, and so be inconspicuous in use.
6) Be easy either to dispose of, or wash and clean, as appropriate.
7) Be reasonably priced and easily available.

Some people will also have their own particular requirements, such as being reasonably attractive so as to fit their personal body image, or easy to pack and transport for travellers. Some like disposable items, others prefer to wash and re-use products. This list could be extended almost indefinitely. Each incontinent person's priorities will be unique to him as an individual.

There continues to be considerable confusion over the proliferation of incontinence aids. The Continence Foundation (1995) produces a Directory of Continence Products, a comprehensive catalogue of products available in the UK. Sections are updated on an annual basis. Over 3,000 different products are listed, together with over 130 different manufacturing companies and distributors. The catalogue does not aim to give detailed recommendations on selection, or to be a 'best buy' guide. It gives simple, practical advice on the use of generic types of products. Some manufacturers also produce booklets and leaflets giving advice on product selection and use, relevant to both professionals and the general public.

Historically, many items produced for use by incontinent people have been poorly designed, with little thought put into the real needs of the user. Often pads have been conceived merely as larger versions of babies' nappies, without realising that the needs of an ambulant adult are likely to be very different. Many appliances were very heavy and cumbersome, with multiple straps, belts, and connections which were difficult to use and provided many potential weak spots for equipment failure. Today, considerably more thought is going into product design, and modern science and technology are employed for the benefit of the user. Many companies have realised that there is a potentially vast market for incontinence products, particularly if those who at present hide their problem can be persuaded to come forward and seek help (see prevalence of incontinence figures, Chapter 1).

Increased public awareness about incontinence and increased advertising of incontinence products is leading to more discriminating users. Many retail pharmacists now stock incontinence products openly on their shelves.

Substantial investment by companies in recent years has resulted in new product developments. For example, super-absorbent polymers are now commonly incorporated in disposable incontinence pads. Many types of reusable aids are available; and urine collection aids have become more simple to fit and use. This process is on-going and with continuing investment, research and development, we will see better, more effective products becoming available.

Growing recognition of the problem by health and social service care providers were reflected by industry in their work with C.E.S.T. (the Centre for Exploitation of Science and Technology), which convened a consortium of companies producing products for the British market, established links with the Government and higher education, and produced a comprehensive report on advanced medical textiles in 1991.

This in turn led to the formation of a manufacturers' group, S.P.A.C.C. (Suppliers and Producers Association for Continence Care), founded in 1993. This Association is now (1995) incorporated within the Absorbent Hygiene Product Manufacturers Association (A.H.P.M.A.), promoting research and the development of products for continence care.

Despite some efforts in this and other countries, there continues to be little high quality research into the function of continence products (Cottenden, 1992). With the notable exceptions of the Department of Health funded projects in Bristol (Urological Disposables Evaluation Centre) and London (absorbent products, based at St Pancras Hospital), work has been poorly coordinated.

There remains a need for measurable quality standards for all incontinence products. To date, only urinary catheters (BS 1695) and urine collection bags (BS 7126) benefit from British standards.

Recent work on the inclusion of super-absorbents into incontinence pads, and studies of both body-worn and bed/chair protection and reusable aids, are helping professionals to advise suppliers, carers and patients on the optimum product for their needs. However, much work on objective performance criteria and clinical applications remains to be done.

In some respects, there is still a reluctance to try new aids. Both users and professionals continue to have low expectations of performance. It is expected and accepted that products will be uncomfortable, smelly and leak from time to time. Nobody enjoys having to wear a continence product, but if one is needed it should not be necessary to expect a poor performance.

SUPPLY OF PRODUCTS

The supply of incontinence aids is not always straightforward or easy.

Prescription

Fewest problems are encountered in the community with collection devices such as catheters, bags and male appliances, as most are available on prescription currently by the general practitioner and soon by designated community health nurses with nurse prescribing. The Drug Tariff (Part IXB) lists incontinence items available on prescription and gives basic guidance on the usual expected life of the product. However, some advice given conflicts with manufacturers' recommendations for their products and would benefit from review and clarification.

Most general practitioners have no specific training and still find selection from the many items difficult, especially if there is no fitting service available. The GP sometimes writes a prescription for a generic type of product and leaves the selection of a specific item to the retail pharmacist, who may be equally lacking in knowledge or training. Some pharmacists deal with only one wholesaler, who may not stock the exact item requested and will provide a substitute. Others have difficulty in obtaining small quantities, and will only order and stock certain sizes or types.

The provision of an appliance on prescription, without a fitting service or follow-up supervision of its use, cannot be ideal for the patient. Dispensing Appliance Centres (DACs) have emerged to provide a fitting and dispensing service for a range of prescription items, including incontinence aids (Platts, 1990). However, there is no quality control on the service provided by appliance contractors – some merely deliver, with no fitting.

In many areas, continence advisers, either alone or via a multidisciplinary continence link group, are seeking to improve this aspect of patient care. Study days, seminars and meetings are held with medical practitioners and wholesale and retail pharmacists to discuss and share knowledge on product selection and use. Equally importantly, professionals are beginning to recognise the essential need to include the users of products in these discussions, as the user has invaluable, first-hand knowledge on the effectiveness (or otherwise) of individual aids.

Non-Prescription Items

The health authority (in Scotland, the health board) takes responsibility for the supply of absorbent aids to the patient in the community, usually via the district nursing service, although sometimes jointly with the social services department, and occasionally via the social services department alone. In Scotland, bedpads (but not body-worn pads) may be obtained with a general practitioner's prescription, provided that they meet specifications laid down by the Department of Health (1972).

In general, regulations about what should be made available to the patient are permissive rather than directive. Contracts for the supply of absorbent products have often been awarded regionally, and each Unit or Trust is encouraged to purchase within the contract. With little evidence except price to go on when awarding contracts, it was not uncommon for the contract to be awarded to the contender whose price was the lowest, regardless of quality.

This situation is slowly changing with the formation and development of regional or divisional commodity advisory groups for continence products. In some regions this has led to the publication of 'Best Buy Guides' for products, combining clinical information on the selection and use of individual items, with ordering and commercial information on packaging, pricing and so on. These give a wider freedom of choice to the purchaser and enable comparison of similar products on basic performance criteria, in addition to cost.

However, individual health authorities and Trusts continue to vary greatly in what they are prepared to provide for incontinent people. Most have certain 'stock' items that are easily available. Some hold a reasonable selection of absorbent aids from which it should be possible to meet most needs; others provide a bare minimum. Some authorities will only buy from within the regional contract or divisional agreement; others are prepared to negotiate separately if they feel their clients' needs cannot be met from within the contract. The difference between authorities, even those immediately adjacent geographically, can be quite startling, and there is a great inequality of provision of absorbent aids across the country. Most authorities do have a 'special order' system whereby an item that is not kept in stock may be obtained by a special requisition. Usually this is authorised by a senior nurse manager. In practice this system functions badly in many instances, and in some areas it is impossible to obtain items to suit individual requirements.

Many community nurses are becoming more aware of the vast range of aids which are available through attending educational events where manufacturers exhibit their products. It is often financial constraints that limit product choice, either in regard to quantity, quality – and more often both – rather than a lack of knowledge by the nurse.

Supply problems in hospital likewise depend on local circumstances. Some hospitals insist on buying in bulk, and so will only order a single item for all needs. Others will allow ward managers and senior nurses to be more flexible and order a range of items.

In view of the fact that a good reliable product can make such a difference to the life and well-being of an incontinent person, those areas where supply is problematic warrant investigation and an appropriate remedy. A person with continence problems has to live with and depend on their product, often on a daily basis. Naturally there are many competing needs for money in the National Health Service, but it should not be beyond the realms of feasibility to devise a system by which a selection of thoroughly tried and tested aids is available free of charge to anyone who has need of them.

There is a huge variability of arrangements for providing incontinent people with products between different European countries (Norton, 1992). Possibly the UK could learn from Sweden in this respect. There, all community nurses have a catalogue of 'approved' and tested aids which they can prescribe for their patients. These prescriptions are processed centrally and then sent to a distribution centre, for direct delivery to the patient. It is likely that a similar system could operate in the UK. However, it is unlikely that retail chemists could cope with this as they lack both storage space and delivery facilities, so the health service needs to look at its own supplies system. Not only could the quality of the incontinent person's life be improved, but in the long term such a system could also be cost-effective, enabling patients to stay in the community and live independent lives rather than possibly needing institutional care.

In practice, many incontinent people currently buy their own continence products. For those who can afford to do so, or have minimal leakage, this matters little. However, some people who can ill afford it are forced to purchase their own aids, either because they will not seek professional help, or because National Health Service provision is inadequate in quality or quantity. It is not uncommon to meet an incontinent elderly woman who is 'rationed' to a fixed number of pads per week, but who really needs twice as many and has to make up the balance from her own pocket. Usually this means buying sanitary towels or baby diapers from a chemist, which can be very expensive, especially to someone on a pension or low income. Some will buy by mail order from newspaper advertisements. A few seek personal help from commercial appliance-fitters or showrooms.

Some people prefer to buy products privately, but for the majority it represents a financial burden, coupled with the fact that they often receive no advice or help on selection or suitability; and if obtained by mail order, no fitting or guarantee of performance. There is also a tendency for those who can disguise their incontinence to delay indefinitely the point at which they pluck up the courage to seek professional help.

The need to provide information on services and resources for people with incontinence problems has been identified by health care professionals and manufacturers of products. This could be achieved by publishing clear, concise information as to where help may be obtained, either on packaging material for products or by inclusion of advisory leaflets within the package itself. The Continence Foundation runs a national database of products.

ASSESSMENT

The key to the success or failure of product use will usually lie in an accurate initial assessment of the individual patient's needs. There is no single aid that will suit everyone. The nurse must make an assessment, with the range and uses of the available aids in mind, so that a decision can be made with the patient (and carers, if relevant) as to the item or items most suited to the individual's needs. It should never be forgotten that a patient's needs may change with time, so the assessment of suitability must be a continuing process, and the supply systems must be flexible enough to accommodate changes. Nurses must challenge policies such as 'All incontinent people get one box of pads per fortnight' as being unlikely to meet the needs of any but a few individuals.

When making an assessment for the provision of aids, the following points will be of particular significance:

The Incontinence Itself
Including type (urinary or faecal); amount (how much is lost in total volume?); pattern (is this a single flood, occasional large amounts, frequent small amounts, or a continuous dribble?); precipitants of incontinence (e.g. is it stress, urge, or passive incontinence?); timing

(night only, only when out, only after diuretics, only when suffering bronchitis). Also of note are other urinary symptoms, such as frequency and urgency.

Mobility
The bedbound, chairbound and ambulant patient have different needs. The sportsman or woman will have different requirements from someone who leads a more sedentary life.

Manual Dexterity and Eyesight
If dexterity is poor, some products cannot be managed easily or independently. For example, particular disabilities may determine the particular type of outlet tap that can be used. Impaired vision may preclude the use of certain products or mean that extra teaching is needed.

Local Anatomy
Features of the genital skin condition or anatomy may indicate or preclude certain items. Of particular note are a retracted penis, hernias or scrotal swellings, skin sensitivities or lesions, obesity, and any particular deformities.

Mental Function
A confused or demented person will seldom be able to manage a complex aid unless help is available. Some will not even be able to put on a pad correctly, if at all. If the patient denies any problem of incontinence it will usually be fruitless giving them a product, as it will not be used.

Personal Hygiene
People vary greatly in their levels of hygiene. The fastidious may use a product differently or require a different aid from someone with poor hygiene. Washable and reusable aids are often inappropriate for those unlikely to wash them properly.

Personal Preference and Perception of Need
Some people take a like or dislike to certain products. For example, some men dislike the idea of pads. The look and feel of a product may influence choice, and some people will refuse to try something just because of the way it looks or because they do not like the idea of it. These personal preferences should be respected wherever possible; it

is, after all, the patient who has to wear and rely on the product. Incontinence can be very damaging to an individual's body-image and self-confidence. An incontinence product should not add to such problems.

Official Services
The availability of help from the district nurse, care assistant, laundry or disposal services may influence management.

Availability
An easily and reliably available aid may be preferable to a more suitable but unreliably or intermittently available one, where there are supply problems. However, this situation should not be allowed to continue indefinitely, and the nurse should make every effort to get the most suitable aid reliably supplied.

Domestic Facilities
People with poor facilities for washing and drying may find using washable products difficult. Disposal may be problematic.

Regular Help
For those with impaired mental or physical abilities, some aids will only be usable if someone else is regularly available to help.

Financial Considerations.
The NHS has to be cost-conscious, and cost must be a factor if several items are genuinely equally suitable. Additional equipment which might be necessary in order to use certain aids, such as a washing machine, might also be precluded because of cost.

It cannot be emphasised too often that products will seldom be the first or only management for incontinence. Nobody's incontinence should be presumed to be intractable until it has been fully investigated. The majority are curable.

The remainder of this chapter outlines broad types of aids. Currently available examples and addresses of suppliers/manufacturers are given in the Continence Foundation *Directory of Continence Products* (1995).

Users need to become more involved in the choice of products for their own use. People have a huge variety of reactions to the same product, and choice is very individual. No single product will suit all needs. When supplying any product it is essential to teach the patient and carers how to use it correctly, including application, removal, cleansing or disposal. The nurse should also check periodically that the aid is being used appropriately (written instructions may be useful for the forgetful). A suitable aid will be ineffective if it is used wrongly, and it is surprising how many patients will use even the simplest aid inappropriately – for example, applying a pad with the plastic backing next to the skin. Regular re-evaluation of the use of the aid should ensure both that the patient's needs have not changed and that a newer, more suitable aid is not now available.

PADS AND PANTS

The use of an absorbent pad worn or incorporated inside a retaining garment is the most common way of managing incontinence. For women, there is no satisfactory external collection appliance and pads are the only way of collecting leakage. Many men, especially those with a retracted penis or poor manual dexterity, also use pads, although some feel that pads are 'feminine' and prefer to use an appliance if at all possible for urinary leakage.

A considerable amount of technology lies behind the design of a good incontinence pad, and much thought has been put into the manufacture of the better products. However, there are also many low-quality products in existence, often using cheap materials. Unfortunately it is extremely difficult to spot inferior products until they are in use, when their performance is usually poor. It is very important to ask the manufacturer what a pad is made from and to try it in practice, or refer to relevant research, before making large purchasing decisions. At present, there is still no central quality control of pads in the UK, although the International Standards Organisation is in the process of developing standards for absorbent products.

The most readily available and most commonly used pad is a sanitary towel. If a brand with a plastic backing is used, it will cope successfully with minimal leakage. The advantages of using a sanitary towel are that it is small and unobtrusive under clothing, reasonably comfortable, easily available, and easy to dispose of in a public convenience. They are 'normal' for women to wear, so may not make the user feel conspicuous as 'incontinent'. The disadvantages are that, for greater than minimal leakage, several of them may have to be worn at a time; if a brand without plastic backing is used, urine tends to leak straight through onto clothing; the cost can be considerable; and many elderly women feel embarrassed buying them. For those with slight or occasional incontinence who can afford sanitary towels, they are the best solution. For anything heavier, a specially designed incontinence pad is usually more satisfactory.

The use of pads and pants may present problems with washing the pants. If so, the light mesh pants are usually easiest to wash, although they do not stand up well to hospital laundries. Disposal of pads can also be problematic if incontinence is heavy.

Three broad categories of garments may be distinguished: pads with waterproof backing worn inside a retaining garment; an absorbent pad worn inside waterproof pants; and all-in-one garments ('diaper' system). Each is available in both disposable and washable versions.

Pads with Waterproof Backing

These pads are usually composed of three layers – a non-woven surface, absorbent wood-pulp or tissue-paper, and a waterproof backing. Claims made that the non-woven cover is a 'one-way membrane' to keep the skin dry have never been proven and are possibly a myth. The backing should either be completely covered or micro-embossed to minimise skin contact with the plastic. Many different sizes, shapes and thicknesses are available, and generally those which use the best quality materials will perform best.

Pads were traditionally oblong and uniform throughout their length. There is now a move towards shaping pads for comfort between the legs and distributing materials unevenly, according to absorption demands. Some pads have ridges or channels designed to encourage dispersion and holding of urine.

Attempts have been made to prevent the persistent problem of leakage from the sides of pads by overlapping the backing around the edges, by including super-absorbent materials, designed to absorb and 'hold' the urine within the pad, by incorporating layers of pulp with differing degrees of compression to aid the passage and holding of fluid in the pad and by elasticating the edges and including splash-guards.

Despite all these measures, no pad has yet been manufactured which will remain free from leakage under all circumstances. Indeed, evidence suggests that up to one third of all pads leak before being changed – a surely unacceptable failure rate.

For Light Incontinence (50–100ml per void)
Small, discreet pads are available in a variety of makes and designs
both with and without super-absorbents (Figure 15.1).

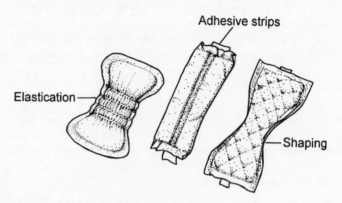

Figure 15.1 *Pads for light incontinence.*

For Moderate to Heavy Incontinence (100ml+ per void)
People voiding larger amounts of urine per void require larger pads, in
order to contain the loss until the absorption process is completed and
to provide sufficient material, pulp (and super-absorbents, where used),
to hold the urine until the pad can be changed. It is nearly always
immobile dependent people who lose volumes greater than 150ml at a
time.

Pads for moderate to heavy incontinence may be rectangular or
body-shaped (Figure 15.2). Rectangular pads are, in general, cheaper
than shaped pads. The largest growth area appears to be in shaped
pads, which are perceived to offer greater comfort and security by
carers and users. They are available in a wide range of sizes and
absorbencies.

Disposable plastic-backed pads are suitable for urinary or faecal
incontinence. Washable pads with waterproof backing are suitable for
urinary loss only. It has been found that the larger washable pads tend
to leak a lot and may give rise to laundry problems. They do, however,
stay intact, whereas the pulp in some disposables may clump when
wet, and are compact to carry when travelling (Philp et al., 1993).

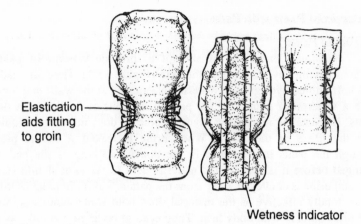

Elastication
aids fitting
to groin

Wetness indicator

Figure 15.2   *Pads for heavy incontinence. May be rectangular or shaped.*

Pants

Pads with waterproof backing are usually worn inside simple, inexpensive stretch pants, designed only to hold the pad in place (Figure 15.3). Some have an open mesh, others are more closely knitted. Ordinary underwear may not provide the necessary support to prevent leakage, particularly in cases of heavy loss, and may lead to the false assumption that the pad is inadequate. People who wish to wear their normal underwear should be encouraged to wear it on top of a pair of stretch pants.

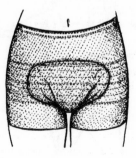

Figure 15.3   *Stretch pants hold absorbent plastic-backed pad securely in place.*

Pants with Waterproof Gusset

Some fabric pants have a waterproof gusset or crotch (Figure 15.6). Newer versions attempt to resemble normal attractive underwear.

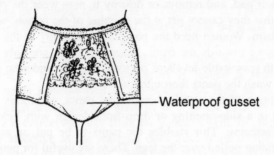

Waterproof gusset

Figure 15.6 *Pants with waterproof gusset.*

Washable Pants with an Integral Pad

Fabric pants may have an integral absorbent gusset with a waterproof lining (Figure 15.7). These have been found to be good for people with light incontinence in the community, despite problems with leakage (Hanley, 1992). Their appearance of being similar to ordinary pants is liked, and people who have difficulty in positioning a separate pad may find that they enhance independence. For some people they are a great success. They are also used in addition to a disposable pad for additional security by some users (Philp et al., 1992, 1993). They are also useful for people with infrequent or intermittent incontinence, to be in place 'just in case'.

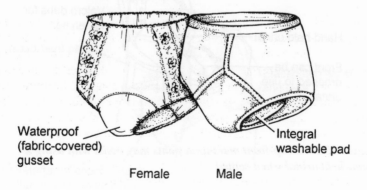

Waterproof
(fabric-covered)
gusset

Integral
washable pad

Female   Male

Figure 15.7 *Washable pants with absorbent gusset.*

Plastic Pants

Plastic pants were for many years the only form of incontinence pants available. Many designs are simply large versions of babies' plastic pants made from polyvinylchloride (PVC) with elasticated legs and waist. Some have straps to retain the pad in position. Drop-front and side-opening varieties fastened with tapes or poppers are also available.

Some people feel that plastic pants are very safe and would trust nothing else. They are also reasonably cheap. They do have many disadvantages in that they tend to be uncomfortable, hot and sticky, and rustle a lot. With repeated washing the 'plasticiser' which makes the PVC soft leaks out and the plastic soon becomes hard and brittle, with cracks developing. Plastic pants can be the cause of considerable skin damage and cause excessive perspiration.

They are also so closely associated with babies and nappies that many adults find wearing them degrading. Their use cannot be recommended except in special circumstances (such as for the young patient with very healthy skin for a limited period of time); most patients who are using them can easily be weaned off them when they discover that the alternatives are just as safe and much more comfortable.

Attempts have been made to improve plastic pants. Some are made from heavy-duty plastic in order to prolong their life. This generally results in the pants being very stiff and even more noisy and uncomfortable. Others are lined with material to prevent direct skin contact with the plastic, which may reduce discomfort to some extent.

The development and manufacture of ever-widening ranges of alternatives has led to the decline in use of plastic pants.

Pads

Pads which go inside pants with waterproofing usually have no waterproof backing themselves, and are therefore relatively cheap. Many different sizes and thicknesses are available, and selection should be tailored to the patient's needs. Rolls of absorbent material which can be cut to any length have the advantage of flexibility for varying needs, but some patients cannot manage to cut a roll easily. Some rolls are of very poor quality and the absorbent material falls apart in use. Additionally, excessive padding may be used inappropriately and occasionally misuse may occur, e.g. as absorbent material for wound dressings. This has resulted in a decrease in the use of this type of incontinence product in many areas.

Marsupial pants have specially designed pads which fit into the pouch. These may be single or double, depending upon the absorbency required.

Washable insert pads are also available.

Diaper Systems (All-In-Ones)

Diaper systems are all-in-one disposable garments with a plastic wrap around and integral pad (Figure 15.8). They are based on much the same concept as babies' disposable nappies and are used for the management of heavy incontinence, especially with elderly people in long-term care. This relatively expensive method is acceptable in some situations, especially if versions with elasticated legs, self-adhesive patches, and a non-woven material lining the plastic are used. However, many people react unfavourably to the association with babies, and they do tend to rustle and be rather hot.

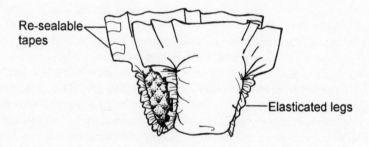

Figure 15.8   *All-in-one diaper.*

Recent developments in all-in-ones include re-sealable adhesive tapes which allow the garment to be removed and replaced if required (for example, for toileting purposes), the inclusion of super-absorbents, and wetness indicators to alert carers when the garment needs changing.

They are becoming more popular in the UK in long-term care. Some evaluations have been conducted but as yet no standard exists for their manufacture or performance. The main role for all-in-one diapers is in coping with heavy or double incontinence in an immobile person, and where the user must be left for long periods between changes, e.g. overnight when living at home.

Reusable versions of the all-in-one are available, but performance tends to be poor with the heavy incontinence for which they are intended. They are bulky and tend to take a long time to dry. Although a few people do like them, and they may provide a solution to certain idiosyncratic problems, it has been concluded that there is no scope for issuing them as a routine stock item (Philp et al., 1992, 1993).

MALE APPLIANCES

The male anatomy offers greater potential for the successful use of appliances than does that of the female. The penis can be inserted into a collection device or have an appliance attached to it, thus avoiding the distribution of urine over the entire perineum. Men with faecal incontinence or a retracted penis usually have to use absorbent pads rather than an appliance.

There are three distinct types of male appliances: dribble pouches, penile sheaths, and body-worn appliances.

Dribble Pouches
Dribble pouches, as the name suggests, are suitable for men with a very slight or dribbling incontinence. It only takes a few millilitres of urine to leak through clothing and form a wet patch, so even very occasional dribblers may like to wear a pouch for security.

Pouches may be made of waterproof backing with absorbent pulp inside. These tend to be bulky and difficult to disguise under trousers. More successful are pouches with waterproof backing lined with a super-absorbent material and pulp (Figure 15.9). These can be worn inside mesh pants or the patient's own close-fitting pants.

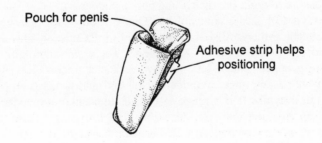

Pouch for penis

Adhesive strip helps positioning

Figure 15.9   *Male drip collector.*

Washable dribble pouches may be worn on a waist-belt, jock-strap style. The pouch may be filled with wadding and changed as necessary (Figure 15.10). Dribble pouches are not available on prescription.

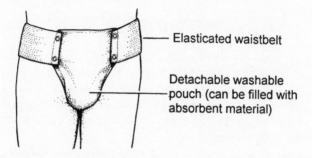

Elasticated waistbelt

Detachable washable pouch (can be filled with absorbent material)

Figure 15.10 *Male dribble pouch.*

Penile Sheaths

A penile sheath is a soft, flexible, latex sleeve which fits over the penis and attaches to a urine collection bag. It may also be referred to as a condom urinal, an incontinence sheath, or an external male catheter. Sheaths are designed to collect urine voided incontinently from the penis and store it in the bag until it can be conveniently emptied. A sheath is suitable for men suffering moderate to severe urinary incontinence, and may also be used for men with urgency or frequency in circumstances where it would be difficult to make repeated visits to the lavatory. It may be worn continuously or intermittently, for example just at night or when going out.

Two types of sheath are available. One is a very soft, thin, one-size latex sheath gathered distally into a rigid outlet tube. It may have a foam ring to cushion the tip of the penis. These twist and kink easily and are generally much less successful than a thicker, less flexible sheath with a reinforced moulded distal end and outlet tube (Figure 15.11). It is available in a range of sizes from paediatric to extra large. It may or may not have an 'anti-kink' bubble type moulding outlet. Different sheath systems suit different men. It is worth trying different systems to find the best for each individual. The selection of a bag is as important as the sheath itself.

Penile sheaths are not suitable for men with a very small or retracted penis, as attachment is impossible. Some men have a skin sensitivity to

Figure 15.11   *Penile sheaths.*

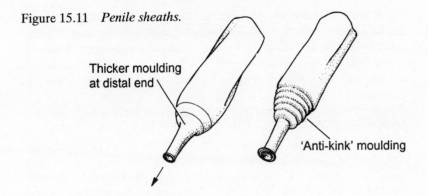

Thicker moulding
at distal end

'Anti-kink' moulding

Connect to drainage bag

the latex and therefore cannot use sheaths. Non-latex sheaths are a new
development to overcome this. If the patient is to apply and manage his
own sheath, a reasonable degree of manual dexterity, good eyesight,
and a fair mental capacity are needed. Demented or confused patients
may repeatedly pull a sheath off and will almost certainly be unable to
cope alone.

Adhesives
Some people use no method of attachment with a sheath, relying on
having the correct size to hold it in place. Generally only non-ambulant
patients can manage this, and most ambulant men need some method
of holding the sheath in place. The simplest, but probably least
effective, method is a strip of tape or adhesive foam wrapped around
the outside of the sheath. Because no adhesive attaches to the skin, the
sheath easily slips off. If inflexible tape is used, this may constrict the
penis if the man gets an erection. Somewhat more effective is a
foam-and-elastic re-usable band fastened with Velcro, but again there
is no direct skin adhesion (Figure 15.12).

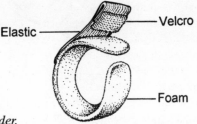

Elastic

Velcro

Foam

Figure 15.12   *Sheath holder.*

The most effective way of securing a sheath is by direct adhesion to the skin of the penis. This should never be done with ordinary surgical tape, as this is not designed for the sensitive penile skin. Repeated application can cause skin problems, the incidence of skin sensitivities is high, and there is seldom enough elasticity in the tape to allow for erections.

Four methods of skin adhesion are designed for use with sheaths. Double-sided adhesive foam strips tend not to have good elasticity and not to return well to their former length if stretched. Some tend to absorb urine and then to lose their adhesive qualities. Hydrocolloid strips are adhesive on both sides, and can be applied around the penile circumference and the sheath then rolled up and over and pressed down to stick. The better makes have elasticity and 'memory' (i.e. return to their former length after stretching), to accommodate changes in penile size.

Medical adhesives probably give the most secure fixation of all. They may be spray-on or in a tube of glue. The adhesive is applied around the circumference of the penis, allowed to dry for a few moments, and the sheath is then rolled over it and pressed down. However, the spray version tends to be difficult to direct accurately. A brush-on version is easier to target accurately. Many men find the adhesive rather too adherent, and repeated removal may cause sore skin.

This is also true of the self-adhesive types of sheaths which have become available, with and without applicators (Figure 15.13). For those who have a reaction to adhesive or to latex, the use of skin protective wipes, of the type used by ostomy patients, may be of benefit. Less allergenic materials may offer wider choice in the future.

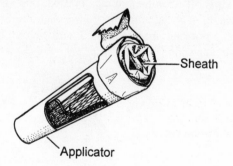

Figure 15.13   *Self-adhesive sheath in applicator prior to positioning.*

Other developments include sheaths with an inflatable cuff to hold it in place. For men with a retracted penis who are unable to wear penile sheaths, a retractile penile pouch, similar to an ostomy appliance, has been designed and manufactured (Pomfret, 1990).

Selecting and Using a Sheath
The selection of sheath and adhesive will depend on the patient's preferences and any known skin sensitivities. The sheath should always be large enough to fit easily over the penis and to allow for changes in penile size. A sheath which is too tight can be very dangerous, even causing necrosis of the penis. Some companies supply a measure to assist in the selection of the best size. Prior to applying the sheath, the genital area should be washed and thoroughly dried. It is best to avoid using any creams or powders if adhesive is to be used. Long pubic hairs around the base of the penis should be trimmed short. If adhesive is used, this should be applied about half-way along the shaft of the penis (Figure 15.14), the sheath unrolled about 3cm and then, making sure the foreskin is not retracted, unrolled over the penis. It is important to leave a gap between the tip of the penis and the outlet tube to allow a small reservoir for sudden gushes of urine and to avoid pressure on the penis. If, however, this gap is too large the sheath may tend to twist, so that drainage is impossible. This is a particular problem with very thin sheaths.

If the sheath has a reinforced ring around the base of the penis, the

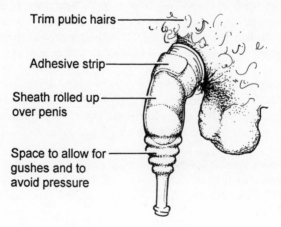

Trim pubic hairs
Adhesive strip
Sheath rolled up over penis
Space to allow for gushes and to avoid pressure

Figure 15.14 *Positioning adhesive on penis.*

ring may be cut to prevent pressure problems. The outlet tube is then connected to a suitable drainage bag. All bags used with indwelling catheters are suitable for use with sheaths, and their selection will depend on assessment of the patient's needs and wishes (see Chapter 9). Wide-bore drainage tubes may facilitate efficient drainage.

When first applied as a new method of management, a penile sheath should be observed and checked regularly to look for any signs of constriction, skin sensitivities, or pressure. The sheath should be changed daily at first and the skin carefully inspected. Once the sheaths have proved satisfactory, each sheath can safely be left in place for one to three days between changes, depending on circumstances, the manufacturer's instructions and the user's wishes. To remove a sheath applied with adhesive, simply roll both off together. The medical adhesives often have their own remover to take off any glue left behind. Simple soap and water will remove most others. If adhesive is used, the sheath has to be disposed of and a new one used. If the sheath has not been stuck it may be washed, dried and re-used. If the patient voids normally at times, it is usually best to disconnect the sheath from the bag for micturition, rather than remove it completely each time.

Most penile sheaths, adhesives and drainage bags are available on prescription in the community.

Body-Worn Appliances
There is a proliferation of male appliances and many variations are available. All of these devices are expensive, and skilled fitting by an expert is essential. Many of the older models were very cumbersome, with multiple straps and connections, and were made of heavy rubber. The more modern versions are lighter and simpler, but there remains scope for improvement, especially in comfort and ease of use.

Drip-type urinals are designed for men with light to moderate incontinence. They comprise an internal sheath and an external cone to collect urine, with waist and groin straps (Figure 15.15). An additional collection bag may be attached to give a greater capacity.

Pubic-pressure urinals have a semi-rigid pubic-pressure flange which is held closely to the pubis by waist and groin straps. This pressure may correct retraction and allow the penis to protrude into the urinal (Figure 15.16).

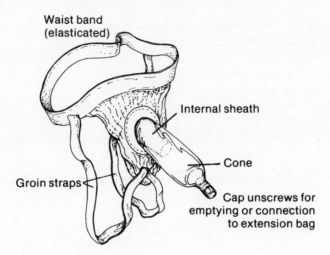

Figure 15.15   *Drip-type urinal.*

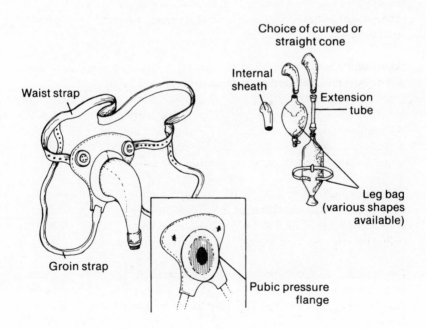

Figure 15.16   *Pubic pressure urinal.*

359

Diaphragm urinals have a flexible diaphragm, held by straps through which the penis passes into the urinal (Figure 15.17).

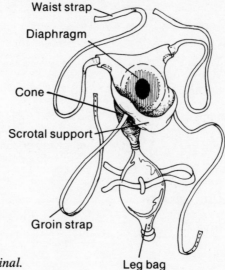

Waist strap

Diaphragm

Cone

Scrotal support

Groin strap

Leg bag

Figure 15.17
Diaphragm urinal.

Penis and scrotal urinals contain the whole genitalia and can be used with a severely retracted penis (Figure 15.18).

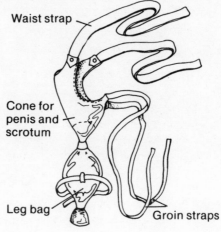

Waist strap

Cone for penis and scrotum

Leg bag

Groin straps

Figure 15.18
Penis and scrotal urinal.

Male appliances come with many variable features. Some have an internal sheath to hold the penis and prevent backflow. Some have a scrotal support. Some are all rubber, others have material or elastic straps and plastic drainage bags. Bag capacity can range from 100ml to 750ml. Some bags are free-hanging, others have leg-straps. Bags may be thigh-worn or used on the calf with an extension tube. Some are one size only and must be cut to fit the individual; others come in graduations of one-eighth of an inch of penile circumference (measured next to the body with penis in a flaccid state). Outlet taps, connections and straps may all vary and be easier for some patients than others.

The patient must have a reasonable level of personal hygiene and be willing to wash and clean the appliance regularly. Each patient will need two urinals, one in use and one being washed and dried. A mild antiseptic solution for cleaning may help to reduce any odour.

Many of the companies who make these devices have a specialised fitting service, and a nurse who is new to this field will usually do best to ask for their help or advice. Special items can often be made up individually if the patient has a particular problem. Most of these appliances are available on prescription.

COLLECTION DEVICES FOR WOMEN

A variety of devices have been designed for use by women with urinary incontinence problems. These have included adhesive and appliance types of aids but none have proven to be very effective to date, and none are available on prescription in the UK.

BED PROTECTION

When a heavily incontinent person is in bed, some method of protecting the bed and skin will be needed unless an appliance is being used. Good quality body-worn pads should generally prevent wetting or soiling of the bed. If worn at night, bed protection may be unnecessary.

Mattress Covers
Various grades of waterproof mattress cover are available to fit single or double beds. For long-term use the heavier-grade plastics are best. Elasticated edges make putting the cover on and keeping it in place easier. Many mattress covers are hot, uncomfortable and noisy. Covers

should be wiped clean when changing bed linen, to prevent odour occurring. Newer 'breathable' fabrics, although more expensive, tend to be much more comfortable.

Drawsheets

If urine loss is not too heavy, a drawsheet may be preferred to a full mattress cover. Restless patients may find a drawsheet is easily displaced. A drawsheet may be a simple plastic sheet to be used under a linen washable drawsheet, or a completely disposable sheet with an absorbent surface and waterproof backing. These disposable sheets can be very useful for someone at home with washing difficulties.

Disposable Underpads

Disposable underpads or bedpads are possibly one of the least effective and most misused of all the items that nurses use. The National Health Service consumes vast quantities (estimated use was 80 million pads in 1990) and yet very little research has been done to study their effectiveness (Thornburn et al., 1992). The most commonly used pads are made from five layers of low-quality tissue-paper or wadding with a plastic backing. This type does not meet official standards for absorbency (DHSS, 1972) and will not cope with anything but the smallest leak. Any sizable leak results in the patient lying in a puddle, and very often the undersheet gets wet as well. The pad protects neither the patient nor the bed. Claims that one-way covers protect the skin are unfounded.

Thicker, better-quality underpads are available. Although more expensive, they are much more likely to protect the bed and possibly the patient.

Where underpads are used they should be laid across the bed with the sealed edges at top and bottom, so that if urine is going to leak out it will do so away from the patient, rather than towards his head and feet. The commonly-seen nursing practice of using several underpads on top of each other is both expensive and senseless. 'Packing' a patient at night – i.e. wrapping him in five or six underpads – is costly and does little for the patient or bed. It is much more effective to use one good-quality pad than several cheap ones, and also usually cheaper in the long run. Underpads should really only be used for faecal incontinence or slight urinary leakage in bed, or as a back-up in case a body-worn pad tends to leak in bed. They have been found to be unacceptable for use as sole protection for people with moderate to severe leakage (Thornburn et al., 1992).

Care should be taken when selecting the type of disposable under-pad to be used. Ryan-Woolley (1987) advised the use of sterilised fluff pulp products in areas such as theatres and maternity units and in any situation where a wound exists.

The Department of Health (1984) has stated that the choice between using sterile and non-sterile products is a matter for professional judgement. Virgin fluff pulp bedpads should be used in clinical areas where there is a higher risk of infection. Recycled paper bedpads are designed for bed protection only for incontinent patients, and should never be used near open wounds or pressure sores.

Reusable Bed Pads

There has been a large growth in the range of absorbent, reusable bed pads available in the UK. There is a wide range of sizes, with or without tuck-in flaps to suit a variety of needs.

A choice of upper fabric layer is available, i.e. the one next to the skin. Brushed polyester does not absorb urine itself, allowing it to pass into the core of the pad to be dispersed and absorbed, leaving the skin relatively dry. Cotton, although it absorbs urine itself and becomes wet, is said to be cooler in use when not wet and reduce the risk of pressure sores.

The central absorbent or soaker layer, which is composed of viscose, polyester or rayon acts as a wick, absorbing urine loss.

In those products with a third, waterproof layer, this is made from a number of water-resistant or impermeable materials. Some are non-slip and so stay in place more easily. A backing usually makes the product harder to dry.

A washable sheet is especially popular in residential homes and in the community, where washing facilities allow. If there is no helper on hand to change the incontinent person, and where he or she cannot manage alone, it can allow an undisturbed and comfortable night's sleep. However, their use will not be cost-effective unless staff or carers are taught that routine changing is no longer necessary. Some people do not find it acceptable to wear no nightclothes below the waist. Good washing and drying facilities are essential.

THE FUTURE FOR INCONTINENCE PRODUCTS

On-going research and development, together with vigorous commercial activity, has made many items now obsolete. Health care professionals are more aware of developments and are coming together with manufacturers to develop better products for our patients. The trend towards involving patients directly in the development of products is welcome. These initiatives and the momentum of change must continue to be encouraged and be supported by all involved in continence care.

REFERENCES AND FURTHER READING

Association for Continence Advice, 1993. *Directory of Continence and Toileting Aids*. ACA, London

Centre for Exploitation of Science and Technology, 1991. *Advanced Medical Textiles*, Dr J. Savin, CEST, London.

Continence Foundation, 1995. *Directory of Continence Products*. Continence Foundation, London.

Cottenden, A., 1992. Aids and appliances for incontinence. In: Roe, B. H. (ed). *Clinical Nursing Practice*, Prentice Hall, Hemel Hempstead.

Department of Health and Social Security, 1972. Specification for disposable underpads. TSS/D/300000. DoH, London.

Department of Health, 1984. *Non-sterile Packaged Surgical Supplies*. Safety information bulletin No. 19(84)64. DoH, London.

Hanley, J., 1992. Choosing garments to aid incontinence. *Nursing Times*, 88, 27: 50–1.

HEI, 1986. *Incontinence Garments, Results of a DHSS Study*. Health Equipment Information, Department of Health, London.

Malone-Lee, J., McCreery, M., Exton-Smith, A. N., 1983. A community study of the performance of incontinence garments. Department of Health and Social Security, Aids Assessment Programme, London.

Norton C., 1992. Continence provision. *Nursing Times*, 88, 44: 76–8.

Philp, J., Cottenden, A., Ledger, D., 1993. A testing time. *Nursing Times*, 89, 4: 59–62.

Philp, J., Cottenden, A., Ledger, D., 1992. The reuser's guide. *Nursing Times*, 88, 44: 66–72.

Platts, L., 1990. Dispensing advice. *Nursing Standard*, 5, 8: 14–15 (Suppl.).

Pomfret, I., 1990. All shapes and sizes. *Journal of District Nursing*, 8, 12: 9–10.

Ryan-Woolley, B., 1987. *Aids for the Management of Incontinence*. Kings Fund Project Paper, 65. Kings Fund, London.

Thornburn, P., Cottenden, A., Ledger, D., 1992. Undercover trials. *Nursing Times* 88, 13: 72–8.

Chapter 16

Continence Services

Jill Beadle, DMS, RM, RN, NDNC, RT

*Operational Manager, Services for Physically Disabled
People, Southampton Community Health NHS Trust*

CONTINENCE IS EVERYBODY'S BUSINESS

The Utopian view that the majority of incontinent people have the
potential to regain continence, if accurately diagnosed and correctly
treated, is not so unrealistic. It is estimated that of the 3 million incontinent people in the United Kingdom, 70 per cent will show a good
response to treatment, the necessary therapy often being simple in
nature (DoH, 1991). The remaining 30 per cent may not have complete
urinary and/or faecal control, but their incontinence can be managed in
an appropriate way. So why do so many people remain without help?

The myths, fallacies and the taboo upon talking about micturition
and defaecation are major problems which result from a general
lack of knowledge about bladder and bowel function. Changing
attitudes towards elimination is a key responsibility of all health care
professionals, in order to ensure that incontinence is not accepted
as either an irreversible or an inevitable condition. Education can
be instrumental in changing attitudes, starting from toilet training
onwards. The emphasis should be on healthy bladder and bowel
function in the context of total body functions. It is inappropriate to
concentrate solely on the bladder and bowel, since so many other
physiological, psychological and environmental influences contribute
to maintaining continence.

Almost every day most health care professionals, including
nurses, midwives, health visitors, doctors, occupational therapists and
physiotherapists, regularly encounter incontinent people. Incontinence
may not be the reason for the initial professional contact, but it is each
health care professional's responsibility to elicit health-care problems
from the patient and to initiate a response that will help to resolve those
problems.

What better opportunity to promote continence than during a home
visit by a district nurse or health visitor? Home visits present an ideal

opportunity to detect early symptoms of a problem and an ideal time to teach the principles of good bladder and bowel care. This can often be repeated, rather than the one-off opportunity of a clinic appointment. Who is more likely to detect incontinence than a practice nurse during cervical screening or a family planning consultation, a physiotherapist during an exercise class or an occupational therapist during an assessment for aids to mobility? There is no better time to start bladder rehabilitation than during hospital admission for an acute disease or injury which has caused incontinence. Yet the fact remains that many opportunities to prevent, detect, treat or manage incontinence are missed because many health care professionals lack the knowledge, awareness or motivation to assess and effectively tackle the problem.

Education for health care professionals on the promotion of continence and management of incontinence should be a continuous process, commencing in basic training and continued in post-basic education courses. Many post-basic courses now include continence as a topic and the opportunities always exist for updating by study days, seminars and exhibitions. For trained nurses who wish to explore the subject in greater depth, the English/Welsh National Board Course 978: 'An Introduction to the Promotion of Continence and Management of Incontinence' offers the opportunity to gain detailed knowledge.

Each professional contact affords the opportunity to educate and promote continence with the patient, family and carers, with potential for beneficial results in health gain and improvement in quality of life, and possibly in preventing problems. It is therefore important that all professionals are knowledgeable. Knowledge should encompass what local services have to offer, and to whom, and how to gain access to them through an identified referral process.

THE MAIN ACTIVITIES OF A CONTINENCE SERVICE

The development of continence services throughout the United Kingdom has been extremely diverse, and there is considerable variation in the role and functioning of continence advisers. Growth has been haphazard with no central coordination or guidance. The variety in posts and services offered is influenced by the employer's commitment to the service. Now that more than a decade has passed since the employment of the first continence adviser, far more information and knowledge is available to enable people to set up continence services that will meet the health needs of the local population in a constructive and proactive way.

The Department of Health carried out a review of continence services in England in 1991 and, in a lengthy report, has made recommendations on the key elements of a continence service (Table 16.1).

Table 16.1 Key Elements of a Continence Service

The Department of Health (1991) has identified six key elements for an effective service:
- active, enthusiastic consultant and general manager involvement;
- continence advisers with management and teaching skills and who carry a small patient caseload to keep their clinical skills up to scratch;
- the effective use of a computer to store, monitor and review patient information;
- a sympathetic and knowledgeable person answering the telephone;
- the public being well aware of the service through active publicity work;
- a separate budget.

(DoH, 1991).

It was envisaged that a small team of specialist nurses should work within a supporting network of other professionals. A comprehensive continence service will involve the skills and input of a wide range of agencies (Table 16.2, overleaf). Incontinence is essentially a problem for the multidisciplinary team, and one of the challenges in organising a service is the coordination of these elements (see Chapter 4 for a discussion of different professions' roles). Table 16.3 (page 369) lists the professionals who should be involved in multidisciplinary planning (Norton, 1995).

Table 16.4 (page 369) gives more detailed guidelines on the components of a continence service (Royal College of Physicians, 1995).

Table 16.2 Continence Services Network – A Model

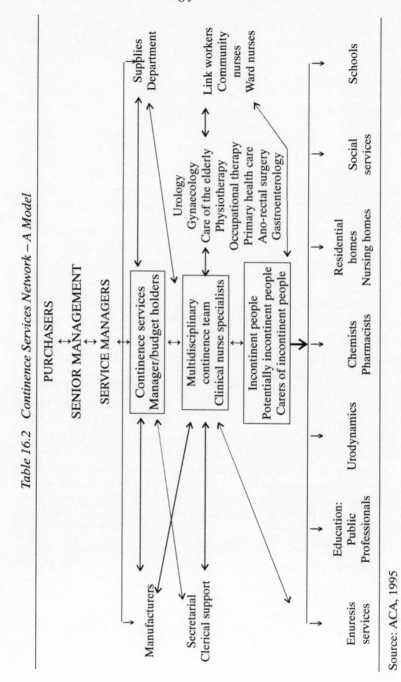

Source: ACA, 1995

Table 16.3 Multidisciplinary Planning

MEDICAL	NON-MEDICAL
Urologist	Continence adviser
Gynaecologist/Urogynaecologist	Nurses, midwives and health visitors
Physician	Physiotherapist
Geriatrician	Occupational therapist
Neurologist	Dietitian
General practitioner	Clinical psychologist
Consultant in rehabilitation	Social worker & Social services staff
Psychiatrist/Child & adolescent	Community learning disability team
psychiatrist	Supplies staff
Paediatrician	Manager
Coloproctologist	Appliance practitioner
Gastroenterologist	Stoma care nurse
	Voluntary bodies/Community health
	council
	Users/carers

Source: Norton, 1995

Table 16.4 Components of a Continence Service

The ideal continence service should embrace the following:

- A defined method of entry for patients referred by general practitioners, nurses, hospital staff and patients themselves.
- Access to appropriate diagnostic facilities, including urodynamic and anorectal investigations.
- Access to medical and surgical consultants with a special interest in incontinence.
- Integration of continence services for children with other paediatric services.
- Attention to the wishes of patients and carers.
- Access to nurses and physiotherapists with special training in treatment modalities for incontinence.
- A role for one or more specialist continence advisers in the education of the public and professionals in continence maintenance.
- A policy concerning the purchasing and supply of containment materials and equipment in the community, in residential and nursing homes and in hospitals.
- Well-defined audit and quality assurance systems.

The structure required to achieve these aims might include:

- A designated manager.
- An expert advisory panel.
- A budget to provide staff, their training and support services, and containment materials and equipment.

Source: RCP, 1995.

369

This chapter focuses on the nursing element, and in particular the role of the continence adviser. There are three main areas of functioning that can be identified for a continence service: health education; promotion of continence; and management of incontinence.

Health Education

Health Education campaigns often focus on 'attractive', high interest subjects, for example the heart, healthy diet and dental care. Little has been done on maintaining and promoting continence. And yet the maintenance of continence is a health matter which directly affects the quality of life of many people. The cost of incontinence to the National Health Service has been estimated at £56 million per year for pads and appliances (CEST, 1990), but just 'mopping up' will neither sufficiently contain the problem nor contribute to a reduction in the incidence of incontinence.

The current reforms of the National Health Service place an emphasis on assessing and promoting health gain of a local population in an efficient and effective way, and particularly highlight cost-effectiveness. In relation to continence, this can be achieved through health education activities that encompass all age groups, in two major areas. Firstly, in getting the population to 'Think Bladder and Bowel' to ensure, over the long term, that these vital organs of the body are not abused or compromised through lack of knowledge. Secondly, in educating incontinent people and their carers to seek help and not to accept it as an inevitable, unresolvable problem. The Department of Health and the Continence Foundation held the first ever major public awareness initiative on incontinence in 1994, resulting in a substantial public response, which has been maintained via a continued media interest in the subject.

In order to undertake a health education campaign, it is essential that continence advisers work closely with local health education departments and ensure the development of well-focused campaigns, which are progressively directed at specific sections of the population. Liaison achieved with the health education department will enable continence campaigns to be coordinated with other health education initiatives and activities within the district or unit, so that maximum effects can be gained. The potential for preventive work remains almost entirely unexplored.

Promoting Continence

For those people who are incontinent, the promotion of continence should be the main objective of any intervention. Often one of the greatest barriers to this is a negative attitude, and intervention should focus on motivating the patient, providing the right support mechanisms, and ensuring that he or she is followed up by the appropriate health care professionals.

Holistic patient care facilitates full integration of bladder and bowel management with other care that the patient receives. Few, if any, of the suggestions for nursing intervention made in this book are beyond the capability of *any* trained nurse who has the appropriate knowledge. Pelvic floor exercises, bladder retraining, behavioural techniques, modification of the environment and appropriate use of products are all within the scope of the nurse. Nor is making an assessment of the problem very difficult, given adequate time and an understanding of what information is needed. A clear common continence assessment strategy, with a well designed continence assessment form, will enable all nurses to carry out individualised continence care.

There should be a clearly defined referral process for incontinent people (RCP, 1995). This should be communicated widely to all health care professionals. The general practitioner is the first point of contact for most incontinent people. The GP will often refer to a nurse for a detailed individual continence assessment. Following assessment, the nurse may be in a position to promote continence or may consider referral to a doctor, continence adviser or other professional necessary for further investigation and treatment. Whichever method of assessment and treatment is followed, it is important that the management and resolution of the continence problem is the objective.

Management of Incontinence

The provision of free absorbent products is a concessionary service from health authorities, which explains the considerable geographic variance. Each health authority can determine the level of provision in the light of local needs and circumstances. Inevitably there are budgetary constraints, which lead to local policies being developed identifying criteria for provision. Several models currently exist. One of the most common is that of provision through a home delivery service, whereby, following an assessment of need by the district nurse, free products are delivered to a client's home on a regular basis. The NHS is not permitted to charge for this service.

The provision of continence products to people for the appropriate management of incontinence should only be initiated following a nursing assessment to ensure correct selection and fitting. A trial period with a few selected products will help to ensure that the correct one has been selected and that it does contain the incontinence being experienced by the client. A strategy for regular reassessment will ensure the correct provision on an ongoing basis. More detail is provided on this in Chapter 15.

THE ROLE OF THE SPECIALIST CONTINENCE ADVISER

In 1981, there were seventeen full-time continence nurse specialists employed in the UK. By 1990 there were over 300 continence advisers, with at least one in 86% of all health authorities, the majority being nurses (a few are physiotherapists) (Norton, 1990). In 1995 this figure had risen to over 400 (Continence Foundation, 1995). If continence is the responsibility of every health care professional and all should be able to deal with it, what role is there for the specialist 'continence adviser'? Not for day-to-day management, perhaps, nor for the assessment and treatment of every incontinent person, but as a catalyst for improved care and coordination of services, as a clinical support for nurses who have incontinent patients, and as an educator and researcher.

The continence adviser has developed as a clinical nurse specialist. There are many roles to accommodate, a number of support mechanisms to develop and employ, and key functional areas to maintain to ensure the efficiency and effectiveness of service provision in meeting the continence needs of the local population.

In providing education, advice and support, the specialist continence adviser will, initially, be guided by the terms of employment. This will be influenced by the employing authority, which may be a Trust or a joint-funded position with Social Services. Developing the role and coordination of service activities will require careful time management and extensive managerial and communication skills, to ensure the achievement of demonstrable results.

The role of the continence adviser remains largely unevaluated. Early work (Ramsbottom, 1982; Badger, 1983) was inconclusive as to the effectiveness and identified many methodological difficulties in such research. More recently, the Social Policy Research Unit (York University) has conducted a descriptive study commissioned by the Department of Health (Rhodes and Parker, 1993).

Most advisers in post fulfil all or most of the role outlined below. Continence advisers themselves rate management and teaching as more important than clinical functions (RCN, 1992). A detailed interpretation of the job needs to be adapted to local circumstances, and not be defined so rigidly as to restrict the development of the individual post-holder's interests and activities. However, any job description should contain elements of the following: teaching, management, resource and information person, caseload, budget management, liaison with companies and supplies staff, and research.

Teaching
Teaching should be the primary role of the continence adviser. Teaching should not be confined to *incontinence*, as maintaining and improving continence is equally – if not more – important, to ensure that continence is maintained throughout life. Health education models for healthy bladder and bowel function are easy to develop, and should form the foundation of any teaching carried out by the continence adviser.

As most incontinence management is within the scope of all nurses, with a little additional instruction, teaching other nurses is obviously one of the best uses of the adviser's time. This should be achieved by teaching both learners and qualified nurses and in keeping trained staff updated by regular in-service training. Formal lectures, seminars, workshops, exhibitions and more informal meetings can all be used for education, as well as clinic visits and working with the adviser for a short period. Indeed, one of the best teaching opportunities is in the one-to-one situation of the joint assessment of a patient. The adviser can teach assessment skills which the referring nurse could then use in assessing the next incontinent patient.

Teaching should not be confined to nurses. All professional groups can benefit from the continence adviser's knowledge and expertise. Medical students, qualified doctors, physiotherapists, occupational therapists, social workers, pharmacists and unqualified staff, such as care assistants and home care assistants, can improve their practice with increased knowledge about continence.

The patient and relatives or carers will also benefit from teaching. This will usually be on an individual basis, but talks may also be given to groups, for example the local branch of the Womens' Institute, the Multiple Sclerosis Society or other groups of people with disabilities, or pre-retirement courses and relatives' support groups. Advice on services, products and management methods is often sought from the adviser by a diverse range of groups, and many teaching opportunities present themselves once the service becomes known. There is a lot of evidence that information and knowledge enhances patient outcomes (see Norton, 1983).

Where the adviser wishes to, the teaching role can be extended to writing articles for the nursing and paramedical press, in order to educate a wider audience. Each adviser will need to develop a plan for educational activities to ensure that all staff and others who could benefit are offered regular educational opportunities. All teaching activities should be evaluated, both for their impact upon knowledge and for subsequent changes in clinical practice.

Management

The continence adviser will need many different skills as the manager of an effective service. All managers in today's NHS need to be able to prepare a coherent business plan with realistic objectives defined. The objectives must be amenable to clinical and budgetary audit (i.e. their achievement or otherwise must be measurable). The service will also need an active quality assurance programme, ideally with consumer involvement in both planning and evaluating the service. As part of a Unit or Trust, the continence adviser may become involved in bidding for contracts and making a case to purchasers (both health and social services) for continuing with, and preferably expanding, the service.

It should be part of the continence adviser's role to become involved in drawing up local policies and standards for continence care. There will also be a need to devise a strategy for publicising the service, not only to other professionals, but also to the general public. In 1992, less than one third of services were advertised directly to potential clients (Rooker, 1992). For a taboo subject, with such a low presentation rate, this is surely unacceptable.

Resources and Information

The continence adviser should act as a local resource and information person. The adviser should keep up to date with all the current literature, research and trends in the field, and be available for consultation, whether by telephone or in person, on all aspects of continence and incontinence. Building up a small reference library can be beneficial to anyone undertaking a project on incontinence.

A resource display of incontinence products, as a permanent exhibition, can be an invaluable resource both to professionals and the general public. It is important that it is kept up to date, and this can be

achieved through successful negotiation and liaison with manufacturers. The site of the exhibition is important in allowing access and, if
sufficient space is available, the potential exists for its development as
an assessment centre with a continence clinic attached.

Assessment and Management of Patients
The continence adviser will usually see individual patients to assess
and manage incontinence. Referrals may be taken from a wide
spectrum of other professionals. In some situations a self-referral
telephone line or clinic may also operate. When the referral is from a
nurse, the adviser should be used for advice only, and not be expected
to take over the management. The ideal situation would be a joint
assessment with the referring nurse, collaboration over the formulation
of a care plan, advice and support during implementation, and help in
evaluating its impact. The adviser should not, indeed cannot, expect or
encourage referral of *every* incontinent patient, because of the numbers
involved. The referring nurse should be taught how to carry out a basic
assessment and be encouraged to try the obvious remedies first, only
referring problematic cases for advice in future. The referring nurse
must retain responsibility for the patient's care, using the adviser as an
outside pair of eyes to view the problem from a fresh angle, and as a
nurse with additional specialised expertise who may know of treatment
or management methods which have not yet been tried for the
particular patient.

Some patients are referred from other professionals and may not
already have a nurse involved in their care. Provided that they are not
in need of nursing care, but only require incontinence advice, the
continence adviser may accept such people on to a personal caseload,
depending upon local operational policies. Self-referrals may be treated
likewise. It is important for the adviser to retain a small caseload in
order to maintain clinical competence and to have practical experience
of all methods recommended to others.

As well as advising nurses on the management of individual
patients, the continence adviser should be available to offer suggestions on general points of patient care, such as ward routines and
policies. Clinical nurses should be able to consult the adviser on the
best current concepts of patient management and the promotion of
continence. In fulfilling this role, the adviser has to tread very
carefully. Arriving uninvited and criticising current nursing practice
will not lead to an easy acceptance of the specialist's advice. It is best
to implement changes gradually, introducing new ideas one at a time.

There should not be an expectation of changing attitudes overnight, nor should unrealistic expectations be raised.

Where urodynamic investigation facilities are available locally, the continence adviser may become involved in actually working in the clinic. This can provide invaluable clinical insights. If this is not practicable, a mechanism for very close liaison must be devised.

Budgetary Management

The Department of Health (1991) recommends that budgetary management should be the responsibility of the continence adviser. However, considerable diversity exists from one district to another, with only some continence advisers managing a budget. If responsibility for a budget is within the remit of a continence adviser, knowledge of and training in financial management will be critical to success.

Commonly a continence budget has several divisions, the largest being for the purchase of absorbent incontinence products, and it is this aspect of the budget that requires considerable skill to manage. Problems arise predominantly because of the indirect responsibility that a continence adviser has over the nursing staff who order incontinence products. This is found both in the community and in controlling the use of products in the hospital situation.

Within the total continence service, money is needed both for health education and the promotion of continence as well as the long-term management of incontinence. The budget should, ideally, be divided to accommodate all three aspects. Failure to plan for and achieve this will result in all of the available money being spent on products. There are two main effects of this. Firstly, the time taken to monitor and control the expenditure on products interrupts time management; and secondly, frustration is incurred through not being able to achieve all the goals of the service.

Budgetary responsibility requires the establishment of information systems in order to be able to provide regular reports to key personnel on expenditure patterns (Thompson, 1990). Computerised information systems are available, either as stand alone software or as part of a supply and delivery package from some manufacturers. An information system is not only vital for keeping all users of the service informed, but also for forecasting expenditure and in formulating annual financial reports. Trends of service activity can be monitored, and negotiation for additional resources, where needed, can be made on the basis of accurate information.

Monitoring Market Trends on Products

Incontinence products are being developed continuously, and it is important for the continence adviser to monitor the quality and cost of all items. Evaluation of products should always be done using sound research methodology and, if appropriate, with the approval of the local ethical committee. The continence adviser needs to know and understand different methodological approaches to product evaluation, so that reports can be read critically and interpreted and applied appropriately. Too often a 'trial' is said to have been carried out when really only a small number of people have been asked to use a product without any identified evaluative process.

A good trial should produce recommendations for the selection of products. To be credible and influence change to the benefit of incontinent patients, whilst being cost effective, a trial must be well designed, involve sufficient subjects to be statistically significant, and the results analysed using relevant methodology. Qualitative research has its uses, but must always be recognised as such. There is a need for more evaluations to be on a collaborative, multicentre basis to achieve the numbers to make results meaningful.

With so many companies involved in making or marketing incontinence aids, the continence adviser must maintain good links with industry. This can be of mutual benefit. The nurse can tell the manufacturer of any faults in products, and suggest improvements. Industry can then obtain sensitive feedback on product performance and ideas for future developments. Progressive companies are willing to invest in educational programmes and the production of information booklets and teaching aids, taking the view that the greater the awareness among professionals about incontinence, the greater the potential market for the better quality products.

Liaison with Supplies Departments

Good liaison with supplies officers and the product distribution service is vital. When selecting items for stock or for contracts, the adviser can form a link between users and purchasers and may need to organise product appraisal or even formal clinical trials. This liaison may be formalised in a supplies working group which would include the continence adviser, infection control nurse, supplies officer, and representation from interested parties such as nurse managers and administrators. This work aims to ensure coordination within and between areas, for example community and hospital, such that the users (patients and nurses) receive both the quality and quantity of products they need. Waste can be minimised by decreasing over-ordering or inappropriate orders, and implementing more effective stock control. When new items are introduced, the adviser will often help with training all staff involved in how to use them. This can be essential to the success or failure of new products.

As well as involvement in local groups, the continence adviser may be involved in regional adjudication meetings. Regional contracts awarded to manufacturers should be influenced by continence advisers and supplies officers, who can identify the needs and preferences of the local population. Communication and cooperation amongst districts on the award of regional contracts will contribute to economies of scale in purchasing.

Often nurses and patients feel they do not have a channel of communication with those who buy products, and that they have no control over the products which they receive. The adviser can open communication channels, and help to ensure that the patient is getting what is needed to maintain continence or to contain incontinence.

Link Nurses

The continence adviser often works alone with the mammoth task of counteracting incontinence. One solution is to develop a network of link or resource nurses. These are nurses or, in some cases, other professionals, with a special interest in continence, from a wide variety of clinical areas and specialities. Commonly, these nurses form a 'continence interest group' and meet regularly with the continence adviser for education and discussion of research. The group forms a vital channel of communication, as the link nurses can disseminate information to their colleagues, enabling a large number of people to be updated in a comparatively short space of time (Hall et al., 1988).

Most link nurses should undertake the ENB 978 course in order to be in a stronger position to advise colleagues on continence. This subsequently leaves the continence adviser more time to fulfil other roles.

Link nurses can develop their own continence clinics, with the support of the continence adviser as a peripatetic teacher. Clinics can be set up and the support of the continence adviser progressively withdrawn as each link nurse gains confidence and competence. Continence clinics provide increased opportunities to attract people in for help in different settings – for example, an occupational health department (Steele and Pomfret, 1992). Clinics can be supported by a consultant or general practitioner; they can be by appointment or 'drop-in' (Macaulay and Henry, 1990). With any continence clinic it is important to monitor and evaluate effectiveness through demonstrable health gain or improvement in quality of life, in order to be able to bid successfully for money to support additional clinics.

Research

Continence advice is becoming a recognised and respected area of specialised nursing practice. Yet while some practice is research-based, and some research has been carried out over the past decade, there remains an urgent need for more. It is essential for continence advisers to have research skills.

Small-scale descriptive studies can document the current situation and practice. It is as important with small as with major research projects to identify the research protocol, publish results and implement change in practice at a local level based on those results. With major research projects an appropriate level of funding, resources and support will be essential to ensure the successful coordination of research activities with the other daily activities of the continence adviser. Too often 'research' is tacked on to the end of a job specification, almost as an afterthought, without any provision for resourcing or supervising it.

Nursing should be a research-based profession, and it is no longer acceptable to base practice on techniques that 'have always been used'. The growth of knowledge on the promotion of continence and the management of incontinence enhances the clinical practice of continence advisers and all health care professionals. It is up to the key professionals to ensure that this knowledge is used for the benefit of incontinent people.

Communication Systems and Channels

As a result of having mainly indirect responsibility for and involvement in care, it is essential that continence advisers act as communication coordinators to ensure that people are kept informed of what is happening within the continence service. This can be achieved through a regular news-sheet, time spent at meetings or formal education sessions, and the appropriate use of link nurses and information technology. Information can be made available to everyone through the integration of information systems amongst different specialities.

Consultation is critical to successful results when implementing change. Excellent communication skills and the involvement of professionals in working parties and meetings will help to avoid antipathy towards the continence adviser and help others to feel that they 'own' the change, rather than that it has been forced upon them. For example, standards of clinical care should be developed with, rather than imposed upon, clinical practitioners. Resistance to change may be associated with a fear of fragmentation of care. If effective management of change is linked with efficient information and communication channels, it will facilitate high standards of care and the integration of service activity, with the resultant 'seamless care' that everyone is striving to achieve.

Seamless care requires an effective interface between specialist nurses, other nursing and medical specialities, social services, voluntary agencies and carers, family and patients. It facilitates continence being seen as an integral part of total care, not an isolated, specialist nursing activity. The continence adviser can help to bring about this integration by coordinating assessment and reassessment strategies, facilitating the integration of information systems, sharing data and applying the findings to clinical practice.

SUPPORT FOR THE CONTINENCE ADVISER

The post of continence adviser can be a lonely one, especially when first appointed. Adequate managerial and peer group support can make a great difference. Management support will usually come from a line manager, and peer support is found by meeting others in similar posts locally and sharing information and expertise.

The Association for Continence Advice was founded in 1981 with the aim of opening up communication channels between interested professionals. Membership is multidisciplinary and not confined to continence advisers. The Association holds a national conference each year, has a quarterly newsletter and a network of Regional groups which meet regularly. The Royal College of Nursing also has a continence care forum for nurses with an interest in continence.

It is essential that the continence adviser is permitted both the time and a budget to obtain both adequate peer support and ongoing professional education (ACA, 1992). It is impossible to function as an effective educator and resource person unless there is a regular top-up of personal knowledge and enthusiasm.

Achieving the optimum possible care for incontinent people is dependent upon gaining a multidisciplinary approach to the promotion of continence and management of incontinence, supported by wide communication channels, and gaining and building on material and manpower resources. For the incontinent person, achieving accurate diagnosis and treatment is critical if continence is to be gained or the appropriate management of incontinence implemented. The continence adviser must work with all nurses, other professionals and the incontinent person and her or his relatives, to increase awareness, knowledge and the facilities for tackling and alleviating this most distressing condition.

REFERENCES AND FURTHER READING

ACA, 1993 and 1995. *Guidelines for Continence Care*. Association for Continence Care, London.

ACA, 1992. *Action on the Agenda*. Association for Continence Advice, London.

Badger, F. J., Drummond, M. F., Isaacs, B. 1983. Some issues in the clinical, social, and economic evaluation of new nursing services. *Journal of Advanced Nursing*, 8: 487–94.

Baker, K., Foster, P., 1989. Objective continence: assessment is the key. *Journal of District Nursing*, 7, 11: 12–14.

Brink, C., Wells, T., Diokno, A., 1983. A continence clinic for the aged. *Journal of Gerontological Nursing*, 9, 12: 651–5.

Brown, J., Thomas, E., White, H., McCallum, A., 1991. An incontinence helpline service. *Nursing Standard*, 5, 38: 25–7.

Carter, P., Winder, A., Budd, M., Shepherd, A., Feneley, R., 1992. Organising a continence advisery service. *Health Trends*, 24, 1: 27–9.

CEST, 1990. Advanced Medical Textiles. Centre for Exploitation of Science and Technology, London.

Continence Foundation, 1995. *Index of Continence Services*, Continence Foundation, London.

DoH, 1991. *An Agenda for Action on Continence Services*. Department of Health, London.

Hall, C., 1990. Advising on continence. *Nursing Times Community Outlook*, July: 38 & 43.

Hall, C., Castleden, C. M., Grove, G. J., 1988. Fifty-six continence advisers, one peripatetic teacher. *British Medical Journal*, 297, 6655: 1181–2.

Hamilton, B. H., Badger, F. J., Drummond, M. J., Isaacs, B., 1985. The work of the Nurse Adviser on incontinence. *Geriatric Nurse* (New York), 6, 2: 199–202.

HM Government, 1990. The NHS and Community Care Act. Westminster.

Incontinence Action Group, 1983. Action on incontinence: report of a working party. King's Fund Centre project paper 43. Kings Fund, London.

KPMG Peat Marwick McLintock, 1990. Marketing for health care providers. *Developments in Health Care*, No. 4.

KPMG Peat Marwick McLintock, 1989. Your services – planning, acting and monitoring. *Developments in Health Care*, No. 2.

McGrother, C. W., Castleden, C. M., Duffin, H., Clarke, M., 1986. Provision of services for incontinent elderly people at home. *Journal of Epidemiology and Community Health*, 40, 2: 134–42.

Macaulay, M., Henry, G., 1990. Drop in and do well. *Nursing Times*, 86, 46: 65–6.

Norton, C., 1995. Commissioning comprehensive continence services: guidelines for purchasers. The Continence Foundation, London.

Norton, C., 1990. A success story. *Nursing Times*, 86, 33: 72.

Norton, C., 1984. Challenging speciality. *Nursing Mirror*, 159, 19: xiv–xvii.

Norton, C., 1983. Training for urinary continence. In: Wilson-Barnett, J. *Patient Teaching*. Churchill Livingstone, Edinburgh & London.

Patterson, H., 1990. Education wanted (training for continence advisers). *Nursing Times*, 86, 46: 71.

Ramsbottom, F., 1982. Advising the nurse. *Nursing Times*, 78, 5: 24–8.

Rhodes, P., Parker, G., 1993. *The Role of the Continence Adviser in England and Wales*. Social Policy Research Unit, University of York.

Rooker, J., 1992. *Community Continence Services*. The Labour Party, London.

Royal College of Nursing Continence Care Forum, 1992. *The Role of the Continence Adviser*. RCN, London.

Royal College of Physicians, 1995. *Incontinence: Causes, Management and Provision of Services*. RCP, London.

Shepherd, A. M., Blannin, J. P., Feneley, R.C.L., 1982. Changing attitudes in the management of urinary incontinence – the need for specialist nursing. *British Medical Journal*, 284: 645–6.

Smith, N. K. G., 1988. Continence advisery services in England. *Health Trends*, 20, 1: 22–3.

Snaith, A. H., 1985. Planning and managing a health service in the United Kingdom. In: Holland, W. W. (ed). *The Oxford Textbook of Public Health*, Volume 3. Open University Press.

Steele, W., Pomfret, I., 1992. Promoting continence at work. *Community Outlook*, January: 15–16.

Swaffield, J., 1986. Avoiding incontinence – health education and preventive care for women. *Nursing* 3, 10: 6–7.

Thompson, J., 1990. Managing continence systematically. *Nursing Times*, 86, 46: 60–2.

Watson, R., 1989. Good nursing practice: the only basis for effectiveness. *Senior Nurse*, 9, 5: 28–9.

White, H., 1982. Setting up an advisery service. *Journal of Community Nursing*, September: 4–6.

Young, P. 1986. Setting up an advisory service. *Nursing Times*, 82, 48: 68–71.

See also Appendix 3: Reports Relevant to Continence Care.

Appendix 1

Continence Organisations in the UK

The Continence Foundation is a charity which acts as a national resource centre for information, education and research on urinary and faecal incontinence. A range of publications for professionals and the public is available, as is a database of services and products. The Continence Foundation's Information Helpline, staffed by nurse continence advisers, welcomes calls from the public or professionals.

The Continence Foundation, 2 Doughty Street, London WC1N 2PH. Tel: 0171–404 6875. Incontinence Information Helpline (Monday–Friday 9am–6pm): 0191–213 0050.

The Association for Continence Advice (ACA), a multidisciplinary professional body for anyone with a special interest in continence. The ACA has a quarterly newsletter, an annual conference, and a national network of Regional groups which meet regularly for peer support and educational activities. The ACA have published guidelines for continence services which recommend strongly that continence care has to be multidisciplinary, involving all members of the team.

Association for Continence Advice, 2 Doughty Street, London WC1N 2PH. Tel: 0171–404 6821.

The Enuresis Resource and Information Centre (ERIC) offer a comprehensive service to children and teenagers with day or night wetting. Advice is given by phone or post; a range of publications is available; a database of services and research can be consulted; and alarms and bed protection can be obtained by mail order. ERIC have recently published minimum standards for enuresis services which will be of great use to anyone who sees children with bedwetting.

Enuresis Resource and Information Centre, 65 St. Michael's Hill, Bristol BS2 8DZ. Tel: 0117–926 4920.

InconTact (National Action on Incontinence) is the consumer self-help group for people with continence problems and their families. A quarterly newsletter is published.

InconTact, 2 Doughty Street, London WC1N 2PH.

International Continence Society (UK). The UK branch of the ICS holds an annual meeting as a forum for clinical and basic science researchers to exchange views.

ICS (UK), c/o Graham Hosker, Hon. Sec., Department of Urological Gynaecology, St. Mary's Hospital, Whitworth Park, Manchester M13 0JH. Tel: 0161–276 6332.

Royal College of Nursing Continence Care Forum is a group for RCN members with a special interest in continence. An annual conference is held in the autumn and a range of reports have been published.

c/o Royal College of Nursing, 20 Cavendish Square, London W1M 0AB. Tel: 0171–409 3333.

Irish Continence Interest Group. An all-Ireland multidisciplinary group.

c/o Maire Doyle, Continence Adviser, 66 Andersonstown Park, Belfast BT11 8FG, Northern Ireland. Tel: 01232 611679.

Appendix 2

Useful Addresses and Organisations
(See Appendix 1 for Continence Organisations)

Age Concern (England), Astral House, 1268 London Road, London SW16 4EJ. Tel: 0181–679 8000.

All Mod Cons, c/o The Continence Foundation, 2 Doughty Street, London WC1N 2PH. Tel: 0171–404 6875. (A campaign for better public conveniences.)

Alzheimer's Disease Society, Gordon House, 10 Greencoat Place, London SW1P 1PH. Tel: 0171–306 0606.

Association for Spina Bifida and Hydrocephalus (ASBAH), ASBAH House, 42 Park Road, Peterborough PE1 2UQ. Tel: 01733 555988.

Association of Chartered Physiotherapists in Women's Health (formerly ACPOG – Association of Chartered Physiotherapists in Obstetrics and Gynaecology), c/o The Chartered Society of Physiotherapists, 14 Bedford Row, London WC1R 4ED. Tel: 0171–242 1941.

British Colostomy Association, 15 Station Road, Reading RG1 1LG. Tel: 01734 391537.

British Digestive Foundation, 3 St Andrew's Place, Regent's Park, London NW1 4LB. Tel: 0171–486 0341.

Carers' National Association, 20–25 Glasshouse Yard, London EC1A 4JS. Tel: 0171–490 8818.

Centre for Accessible Environments, 35 Great Smith Street, London SW1P 3BJ. Tel: 0171–222 7980.

Counsel and Care for the Elderly, Twyman House, 16 Bonny Street, London NW1 9PG. Tel: 0171–485 1550.

Department of Health, Medical Devices Agency, 14 Russell Square, London WCI. Tel: 0171–972 8080 (adverse incidents); 0171–972 8181 (product evaluation).

Department of Social Security, Benefits Information Helpline: 0800–666555. Disability benefits: 0800–882200.

Disabled Living Centres Council, 286 Camden Road, London N7 0BJ. Tel: 0171–700 1707.

Disabled Living Foundation (DLF), 380-384 Harrow Road, London W9 2HU. Tel: 0171–289 6111.

English National Board for Nursing, Midwifery and Health Visiting, Victory House, 170 Tottenham Court Road, London W1P 0HA. Tel: 0171–388 3131.

Family Fund, P.O. Box 50, York YO1 1UY.

Health Education Authority, Hamilton House, Mabledon Place, London WC1A 9TY. Tel: 0171–383 3833.

Help the Aged, 16–18 St. James' Walk, London EC1R 0BE. Tel: 0171–253 0253.

Ileostomy Association, Amblehurst House, Black Scotch Lane, Mansfield NG18 4PF. Tel: 01623–28099.

Interstitial Cystitis Support Group, c/o Council for Voluntary Service, Northampton & County, 13 Hazelwood Road, Northampton NN1 1LG.

Irritable Bowel Syndrome Network, c/o The Wells Park Health Project, 1A Wells Park Road, Sydenham, London SE26 6JE.

Kidney Foundation, 3 Archers Court, Stukley Road, Huntingdon, Cambs PE18 6XG.

Medical Devices Agency – see Department of Health (above).

Mencap, 123 Golden Lane, London EC1 3PP. Tel: 0171–454 0454.

Multiple Sclerosis Society, 25 Effie Road, Fulham, London SW6 1EE. Tel: 0171–736 6267.

National Association for Colitis and Crohn's Disease, 98a London Road, St. Albans, Herts AL1 1NX. Tel: 01727 844296.

National Childbirth Trust, Alexandra House, Oldham Terrace, London W3 6NH. Tel: 0181–992 8637.

National Pharmaceutical Association, Mallinson House, 40–42 St. Peter's Street, St. Albans, AL1 3NP. Tel: 01727 832161.

NASPCS – the organisation for parents of children who have a stoma or congenital incontinence, 51 Anderson Drive, Darvel, Ayrshire KA17 0DE.

Parkinson's Disease Society, 22 Upper Woburn Place, London WC1H 0RA. Tel: 0171–383 3554.

RADAR (Royal Association for Disability and Rehabilitation), 250 City Road, London EC1V 8AS. Tel: 0171–250 3222.

Relatives' Association, 5 Tavistock Place, London WC1H 9SS. Tel: 0171–916 6055.

REMAP. Technical Equipment for Disabled People, c/o John J. Wright, National Organiser, Hazeldene, Ightham, Kent TN15 9AD.

SCOPE (formerly Spastics Society), 12 Park Crescent, London W1N 4EQ. Tel: 0171–636 5020.

Spinal Injuries Association (SIA), Newpoint House, 76 St. James' Lane, London N10 3DF. Tel: 0171–444 2121.

SPOD (The organisation for sexual and personal relationships of disabled people), 286 Camden Road, London N7 OBJ. Tel: 0171–607 8851.

Stroke Association, CHSA House, Whitecross Street, London EC1Y 8JJ. Tel: 0171–490 7995.

Urinary Conduit Association, 36 York Road, Denton, Manchester.

Urostomy Association, Buckland, Beaumont Park, Danbury, Essex CM3 4DE. Tel: 01245 224294.

Appendix 3

Reports Relevant to Continence Care

Association for Continence Advice, 1993. Guidelines for continence care. ACA, London.

Association for Continence Advice, 1991. Guidelines on the role of the Continence Adviser. ACA, London.

Cunningham, S. and Norton, C., 1993. Public in-conveniences: some suggestions for improvements. The Continence Foundation, London.

Department of Health, 1991. Community Services Division (Sanderson, J.). An agenda for action on continence services. ML(91)1, Department of Health, London.

Department of Health, 1988. Health services development – the development of services for people with physical or sensory disabilities. HN(88)26. HN(FP)(88)25. LASSL(88)8. Department of Health, London.

Enuresis Resource and Information Centre (ERIC), 1993. Guidelines on minimum standards of practice in the treatment of enuresis. ERIC, Bristol.

Hopkins, A., Brocklehurst, J. and Dickinson, E., 1992. The Care Scheme (Continuous Assessment Review and Evaluation) clinical audit of long-term care of elderly people. The Royal College of Physicians, London.

Medical Research Council, 1993. Report of an MRC workshop to examine the research opportunities in urinary and faecal incontinence. MRC, London.

National Health Service Management Executive, 1993. Priorities and planning guidance 1994–95. EL(93)54. Department of Health, Leeds.

Norton, C., 1995. Commissioning comprehensive continence services: guidelines for purchasers. The Continence Foundation, London.

Parker, G. and Williams, J., 1991. Social Policy Research Unit, University of York. Secondary analysis of OPCS disability survey data on incontinence. Report One: Services, aids and equipment for incontinent adults and children in private households. DHSS 774.

Parker, G. and Williams, J., 1991. Social Policy Research Unit, University of York. Secondary analysis of OPCS disability survey data on incontinence. Report Two: Expenditure on incontinence for disabled adults and children in private households. DHSS 826.

Rhodes, P. and Parker, G., 1993. The role of Continence Advisers in England and Wales. Social Policy Research Unit, University of York.

Rooker, J., 1992. Community Continence Services. The Labour Party, London. (A Review of this Report was published in the British Medical Journal, February 1992. Volume 304, pp 464–5.)

Royal College of Nursing Continence Care Forum, 1994. Guidelines on male catheterisation – the role of the nurse. Royal College of Nursing, London.

Royal College of Nursing Continence Care Forum, 1992. Role of the Continence Adviser. Royal College of Nursing, London.

Royal College of Physicians of London, 1992. High-quality long-term care for elderly people – Guidelines and Audit Measures. A Report of the Royal College of Physicians and the British Geriatrics Society. Royal College of Physicians, London.

Royal College of Physicians, 1993. Multiple Sclerosis: A working party Report of the British Society of Rehabilitation Medicine. Royal College of Physicians, London.

Royal College of Physicians, 1995. Incontinence: *Causes, Management and Provision of Services.* RCP, London.

Appendix 4

Books on Incontinence

General

Absalom, M., Betts, C. (eds), 1992. *Endoscopic Urology for Nurses.* Royal London Hospital Trust, London.

Doughty, D. B., 1991. *Urinary and Fecal Incontinence: Nursing Management.* Mosby Year Book, St Louis.

Drife, J. O., Hilton, P., Stanton, S., 1990. *Micturition,* Springer-Verlag, Berlin.

Freeman, R. M., Malvern, J. (eds), 1989. *The Unstable Bladder.* Wright, London.

Gosling, J. A., Dixon, J. S. Humpherson, J. R. (eds), 1982. *Functional Anatomy of the Urinary Tract.* Churchill Livingstone, Edinburgh and London.

Jolleys, J. V., 1994. *Incontinence – Diagnosis and Management in General Practice.* Royal College of General Practitioners, London.

Lofting, D. (3rd edn). *A Guide to Continence Assessment and Bladder Retraining.* Dove Publishing, Warminster, Bath.

Mandelstam, D. (2nd edn), 1986. *Incontinence and its Management.* Croom Helm, London.

Moody, M., 1990. *Incontinence – Patient Problems and Nursing Care.* Heinemann Nursing, Oxford.

Roe, B.H., 1992. *Clinical Nursing Practice: the Promotion and Management of Continence.* Prentice Hall, London.

Smith, N., Clamp, M., 1991. *Continence Promotion in General Practice.* Oxford Medical Publications (Oxford University Press), Oxford.

Smith, P., Smith, L., 1987. *Continence and Incontinence: Psychological Approaches to Development and Treatment.* Croom Helm, London.

Steg, A. (ed), 1992. *Urinary Incontinence.* Société Internationale d'Urologie/Churchill Livingstone, Edinburgh. (Presentations from the 1991 SIU Conference, Seville.)

Women

Cardozo, C., Cutner, A., Wise, B., 1993. *Basic Urogynaecology.* Oxford University Press, Oxford.

Polden, M., Mantle, J., 1990. *Physiotherapy, Obstetrics and Gynaecology.* Butterworth-Heinemann, Oxford.

Stanton, S.L. (ed), 1977. *Female Urinary Incontinence.* Lloyd-Luke, London.

Stanton, S. L. (ed), 1978. *Clinics in Obstetrics and Gynaecology: Gynaecological Urology.* W. B. Saunders, London.

Stanton, S. L. (ed), 1984. *Clinical Gynecologic Urology.* C.V. Mosby Company, St Louis.

Stanton, S. L., Tanagho, E. A. (eds), 1980. *Surgery of Female Incontinence.* Springer Verlag, Berlin.

Children

Bellman, M., 1966. Studies in encopresis. *Acta Paediatrica Scandinavica* (Suppl.), 170, 7–132.

Blackwell, C., 1989. *A Guide to Encopresis.* Northumberland Health Authority. (Distributed by ERIC – see address below.)

Blackwell, C., 1989. *A Guide to Enuresis.* ERIC (Enuresis Resource and Information Centre), 65 St Michael's Hill, Bristol BS2 8DZ.

Bollard, J., Nettlebeck, T., 1989. *Bedwetting: A Treatment Manual for Professional Staff.* Chapman and Hall, London.

Buchanan, A., 1992. *Children Who Soil.* John Wiley and Sons, Chichester.

Butler, R. J., 1989. *Nocturnal Enuresis.* Butterworth Scientific, Guildford.

Butler, R. J., 1987. *Nocturnal Enuresis: Psychological Perspectives.* Wright/IOP Publishing Ltd, Bristol.

Clayden, G. S., Agnarsson U., 1991. *Constipation in Childhood.* Oxford University Press, Oxford.

Kolvin, I., MacKeith, R. C., Meadow, S. R., (eds), 1973. *Bladder Control and Enuresis.* William Heinemann Medical Books, London.

Lovibond, S. H., 1964. *Conditioning and Enuresis.* Pergamon Press, Oxford.

Morgan, R., 1984. *Behavioural Treatments with Children* (Chapter 4, bedwetting; Chapter 8, faecal soiling). William Heinemann Medical Books, London.

Bowels/Faecal Incontinence

Avery-Jones, F., Godding, E. W. (eds), 1972. *Management of Constipation*. Blackwell Scientific Publications, Oxford and London.

Cavarra, K., Prentice, A., Wellings, C., Gardiner, J., 1991. *Caring for the Person with Faecal Incontinence: a compassionate approach to the management of faecal incontinence for the state enrolled nurse*. Ausmed Publications, Australia.

Henry, M. M., Swash, M. (eds), 1992. *Coloproctology and the Pelvic Floor* (2nd edn). Butterworth Heinemann, London.

Kamm, M. A., Lennard-Jones, J. E. (eds), 1994. *Constipation*. Wrightson Biomedical Publishing, Petersfield, UK.

See also 'Children' (above).

Elderly

Brocklehurst, J. C. (ed), 1984. *Urology in the Elderly*. (Medicine in Old Age series). Churchill Livingstone, Edinburgh and London.

Fader, M., Norton, C., 1994. *Caring for Continence: a Care Assistant's Guide*. Hawker Publications, London.

O'Donnell, P., 1994. *Geriatric Urology*. Churchill Livingstone, Edinburgh.

Ouslander, J., 1986. *Clinics in Geriatric Medicine: Urinary Incontinence*. W. B. Saunders, Philadelphia.

Palmer, M. H., 1986. *Urinary Incontinence*. Slack Thorofare, New Jersey, USA.

Willington, F. L. (ed), 1976. *Incontinence in the Elderly*. Academic Press, London.

Investigation

Chapple, C. R., Christmas, T. J., 1990. *Urodynamics Made Easy*. Churchill Livingstone, Edinburgh and London.

Griffiths, D. J., 1980. *Urodynamics: The Mechanisms and Hydrodynamics of the Lower Urinary Tract*. Adam Hilger, Bristol.

Mundy, A. R., Stephenson, T. P., Wein, A. J. (eds), 1994 (2nd edn). *Urodynamics: Principles, Practice and Application*. Churchill Livingstone, Edinburgh and London.

Books For Patients

Burgio, K. L., Pearce, K. L., Lucco, A. J., 1990. *Staying Dry – A Practical Guide to Bladder Control*. John Hopkins University Press, Baltimore and London.

Butler, R., 1989. *ERIC's Wet-to-Dry Bedtime Book* (a self-help manual for children who wet the bed). Nottingham Rehab, Nottingham. (Distributed by ERIC, Bristol.)

Castleden, C. M., Duffin, H., 1991. *Staying Dry: Advice for Sufferers of Incontinence*. Quay Publishing, Lancaster.

Chiarelli, P., 1991. *Women's Waterworks: Curing Incontinence*. Gore and Osment, NSW, Australia.

Chiarelli, P., Markham, S., 1992. *Let's Get Things Moving: Overcoming Constipation*. Gore and Osment, NSW, Australia.

Dobson, P. *Bedwetting – A Guide for Parents*. ERIC (Enuresis Resource and Information Centre), Bristol.

Dobson, P. *Your Child's Alarm – A practical guide for parents to help their children overcome bedwetting*. ERIC (Enuresis Resource and Information Centre), Bristol.

Dobson, P. *You and Your Alarm* – A self-help guide for children to overcome bedwetting. (ERIC) Enuresis Resource and Information Centre, Bristol.

Feneley, R. C. L., Malone-Lee, J. G., Stanton, S. L., 1989. *Incontinence*. British Medical Association (family doctor booklet), London.

Gartley, C. B., 1988. *Managing Incontinence: a guide to living with loss of bladder control*. Souvenir Press. London.

Habets, B., 1993. *The Complete Incontinence Handbook*. Carnell, London.

Haslett, S., Jennings, M., 1992. *Hysterectomy and Vaginal Repair* (3rd edn). Beaconsfield Publishers, Beaconsfield.

Hunt, G., Whitaker, R., Oakeshott, P., 1993. *The User's Guide to Intermittent Catheterisation*. Family Doctor Publications, London.

Mandelstam, D., 1989. *Understanding Incontinence*. Chapman & Hall, London.

Mares, P. *In Control – Help with Incontinence*. Age Concern, London.

Meadow, R., 1980. *Help for Bedwetting: A Patient Handbook*. Churchill Livingstone, Edinburgh and London.

Medill, M. 1989. *Try for Dry*. Care Taker, Cheltenham. (The Mead House, Sherbourne, Glos GL54 3DR.)

Millard, R. J., 1993. *Overcome Incontinence*. Thorsons, London.

Montgomery, E., 1989. *Regaining Bladder Control* (2nd edn). Clinical Press, 26 Oakfield Road, Bristol BS8 2AT.

Morgan, R., 1988. *Help for the Bedwetting Child.* Methuen, London.

Nicol, R., 1989. *Coping Successfully with Your Irritable Bowel.* Sheldon Press, London.

Nicol, R., 1990. *The Irritable Bowel Diet Book.* Sheldon Press, London.

Nicol, R., 1991. *The Irritable Bowel Stress Book.* Sheldon Press, London.

Reynolds, R., 1993. *Coping Successfully with Prostate Problems.* Sheldon Press, London.

Reynolds, R., 1993. *Bladder Problems.* Thorsons, London.

Stokes, G., 1987. *Incontinence and Inappropriate Urinating* (Common Problems with the Elderly Confused series). Winslow Press, Bicester, Oxon.

The Kidney Foundation., 1994. *Cystitis.* (Available from The Kidney Foundation, 3 Archers Court, Stukeley Road, Huntingdon, Cambs. PE18 6XG.)

Welford, H., 1993. *Successful Potty Training.* Thorsons, London.

INDEX

abdominal massage 249
acontractile bladder 21, 22, 175, 295; *see also* underactive bladder
acupuncture 94
ageing (effect on continence) 9, 31, 258, 259, 261–71
alarms: enuresis 114–8, 331; pants 108–9, 115–6, 331; toilet bowl 329; vibrating 115
alcohol 26, 43, 45, 155, 211, 267
all-in-one pads: *see* diaper-style pads
alpha-blockers 84, 158, 161
amputation 301, 304
anal plug 254
ano-rectal manometry 234
anterior repair 144
antibiotics 84, 99, 109, 157, 235, 262, 295: catheter 208, 211, 216, 222; intermittent catheterisation 190; neurogenic bladder 177
anticholinergic drugs 26, 81, 82, 109, 177, 213, 243, 267, 295 (*see also* individual drug names)
antidiuretic hormone 84
anxiety 30, 46
artificial sphincter 87, 166–8, 180
assessment 33–75: behavioural 53, 274–7, 331, 328–9; children 106–7, 111–3; constipation 245; by continence adviser 375–7; day wetting 106–7; dementia 253; faecal incontinence 231–4, 251; home 287–8; learning disabilities 328–9; neurogenic 176; nocturnal enuresis 111–3; pelvic floor 133–4; products 341–4; prostate 155–6; residential care 291–2; stress incontinence 131; urinary incontinence 33–75
atrophic urethritis/vaginitis 24, 40, 42, 96, 203, 213, 264
attention-seeking 30, 271, 275
attitudes 8, 34, 45, 112, 259, 260–1, 268–9, 296–7, 365
autonomic dysreflexia 172, 191

balloon dilatation 159
bedpads 339, 361–363

bedwetting: *see* nocturnal enuresis
behavioural assessment 53: EMI 274–7; faecal incontinence 331; learning disability 328–9
behavioural challenges 330
behaviour modification 278–9, 324–31
benign prostatic hyperplasia (BPH): *see* prostate
bereavement 30, 271
bethanechol 81, 82, 84, 180
bidet 45, 103, 305
biofeedback 93–4, 109, 140, 143
biofilm 201, 208
bisacodyl 247
bladder: age changes 262–3; baby 12–14; congenital abnormalities 120; diverticula 74; normal 15–16
bladder-neck obstruction 162
bladder instability: *see* unstable detrusor
bladder training 49, 83, 87–94: catheter 219; children 108; post-prostatectomy 165
bladder washouts 208, 211, 216, 217–8, 237
bottom wiper 305
bowels 24–5, 43–4, 100, 226–57; *see also* faecal incontinence
budget management 376

caffeine 27, 37, 43, 91, 99
carbuncle 263
carcinoma 238: bladder 28, 42, 176; bowel 173, 235, 241, 242, 249; prostate 156, 160–1
carers 31, 46–7, 80, 259, 297: at home 285–6; products 343
catheter 81, 96, 194–225: balloon 199–200, 220–1; clamping 219–20; conformable 202, 217; elderly 263; fluids 212; Foley 194–221; neurogenic 172, 174, 180, 191; suprapubic 210, 221–2; terminal care 280; urethral stricture 161; urine specimen 211; -valve 207, 217
cauda equina 172, 239
cerebrovascular accident 18, 170, 171, 173, 238

– NOTES –

– NOTES –

– NOTES –

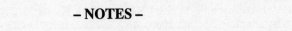

– NOTES –